Delivery of Speech-Language Pathology and Audiology Services

Delivery of Speech-Language Pathology and Audiology Services

Richard M. Flower, Ph.D.

Professor and Vice Chair
Department of Otolaryngology
University of California, San Francisco
San Francisco, California

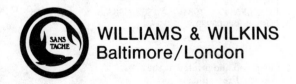

WILLIAMS & WILKINS
Baltimore/London

Editor: William Hensyl
Copy Editor: Deborah Tourtlotte
Design: Bert Smith
Illustration Planning: Lorraine Wrozsek
Production: Raymond E. Reter

Made in the United States of America

Library of Congress Cataloging in Publication Data

Flower, Richard M.
Delivery of speech-language pathology and audiology services.

Includes index.
1. Speech, Disorders of—Practice. 2. Language disorders—Practice. 3. Audiology—Practice. I. Title. [DNLM: 1. Speech pathology. 2. Speech pathology—Economics. 3. Audiology. 4. Audiology—Economics. 5. Delivery of health care—Organ. WM 475 F644d]
RC423.F584 1984 362.1′96855 83-6818
ISBN 0-683-03299-2

Composed and printed at the
Waverly Press, Inc.
Mt. Royal and Guilford Aves.
Baltimore, MD 21202, U.S.A.

To Wilda

Preface

This text was written for students preparing for careers in speech-language pathology and audiology, and for more experienced professionals who have discovered deficiencies in their own education. It discusses matters related to the organizational, interprofessional, economic, legal, and ethical aspects of delivering speech, language, and hearing services. Therefore, it aspires to introduce its readers to what are often aggregated as administrative topics—"administrative" as contrasted with "professional." But as our profession has emerged from a cozy, albeit obscure, cocoon into the mainstream of human services, successful speech-language pathologists and audiologists are increasingly confronting problems relating to these topics. We cannot, on the one hand, assert that we represent a fully independent and responsible profession and, on the other hand, restrict our purview to whatever occurs in immediate interactions with clients, dismissing all other aspects of service delivery as beyond—or beneath—our concern. The continuing prosperity, and perhaps even the ultimate survival, of our profession will depend to a significant degree upon the amount of responsibility each of us assumes for all aspects of the delivery of speech, language, and hearing services.

Two cautions will be reiterated throughout the text. First, although some major principles remain constant in the delivery of human services, essential details are ever-changing as laws and regulations are modified, as the requirements and policies established by professional associations are revised, and as the financial base for those services expands in eras of prosperity and contracts in eras of adversity. Consequently, all readers, and most especially the instructors who use this text, must supplement it with reviews of the current scene to ascertain whether important changes have occurred. Second, many facets of service delivery depend upon state and local regulations and practices, and those regulations and practices may differ at specific points from what is presented in this text. Often, differences are merely semantic, but occasionally they are substantive.

Above all, I hope the discussions that follow will assist readers to solve problems they encounter in delivering what are among the most essential of all human services—services that seek the amelioration of disorders of human communication.

Richard M. Flower
San Francisco, 1983

Acknowledgments

I once considered acknowledging, by name, all the people who contributed to my education about the delivery of speech-language pathology and audiology services: the professors who first introduced me to the field, faculty and staff members of the several institutions where I have been employed, colleagues on countless committees and boards of the American Speech-Language-Hearing Association, and sundry cohorts in other state and community activities. I have been singularly fortunate in my associations with many of the most creative and enterprising members of our profession and of related professions. Two factors led me to reconsider that notion. First, many of those people may not wish to have their names associated with this enterprise. Second, I do not aspire to being listed as name-drop champion in the next *Guinness Book of Records.*

There are some people, nevertheless, who must be acknowledged. Maurice H. Fouracre, then Chairman of the Division of Education of Exceptional Children at the State University of New York College for Teachers at Buffalo, introduced me to the mysteries of delivering human services in school settings. The late George J. Fortune, first Director of the Cleveland Hearing and Speech Center, with consummate patience, taught me about community services and community agencies. Francis A. Sooy, former Chairman of the Department of Otolaryngology and now Chancellor Emeritus of the University of California, San Francisco, and Roger Boles, the current Chairman of that Department, have offered unwavering support while I learned from the errors I have committed in directing a speech-language pathology and audiology program in a protean university medical center.

During the writing of this book, several people have remained immediately available to provide assistance. Katharine G. Butler can be credited with launching me on the project initially, and, in succeeding years, she pored over dim photocopies of the reams of grubby yellow paper that constituted preliminary drafts, making unfailingly helpful suggestions. A substantial segment of the superb professional staff of the national office of the American Speech-Language-Hearing Association willingly provided missing information and instructed me in areas of my ignorance. John L. Darby, Director of The Hearing Society of the San Francisco Bay Area, was, as always, a limitless repository of wisdom about the delivery of human services.

I have also been endowed with an editor-in-residence in the person of Ann Utter, administrative assistant to the program in speech-language pathology and audiology at the University of California, San Francisco. Finally, Tina Guerin spent the hours necessary to produce a clean manuscript out of those reams of grubby yellow paper.

R.M.F.

Contents

Preface vii
Acknowledgments ix

PART 1. THE ROLES OF SPEECH-LANGUAGE PATHOLOGISTS AND AUDIOLOGISTS IN THE DELIVERY OF HUMAN SERVICES

CHAPTER 1. Delivery of Speech-Language Pathology and Audiology Services: An Overview 1
CHAPTER 2. Speech-Language Pathology and Audiology in the Constellation of Human Services Professions 15
CHAPTER 3. Speech-Language Pathology and Audiology Services in Different Settings 47
CHAPTER 4. Referral Patterns and Procedures 77

PART 2. CLINICAL INFORMATION MANAGEMENT

CHAPTER 5. Clinical Reporting 102
CHAPTER 6. Systematic Record Keeping 128
CHAPTER 7. Storing and Retrieving Clinical Records 165
CHAPTER 8. Coding Systems for Clinical Information 174

PART 3. THE ECONOMICS OF DELIVERING SPEECH-LANGUAGE PATHOLOGY AND AUDIOLOGY SERVICES

CHAPTER 9. Computing the Costs of Speech-Language Pathology and Audiology Services 195
CHAPTER 10. Paying for Speech-Language Pathology and Audiology Services 222

PART 4. PROTECTING THE CONSUMERS OF SPEECH-LANGUAGE PATHOLOGY AND AUDIOLOGY SERVICES

CHAPTER 11. Legal and Ethical Considerations in Delivering Speech-Language Pathology and Audiology Services 252
CHAPTER 12. Assuring the Quality of Clinical Services 291

Index 329

PART 1

The Roles of Speech-Language Pathologists and Audiologists in the Delivery of Human Services

CHAPTER ONE

Delivery of Speech-Language Pathology and Audiology Services: An Overview

A popular social comment comedian of the 1960's told a story about the visit of a Lady Bountiful to an institution for delinquent adolescents. At one point, aghast, she asked the superintendent, "How can you expect to rehabilitate these young people in an institution surrounded by a high barbed-wire fence?" "Madam," replied the superintendent, "How are we to rehabilitate them if they aren't here?"

Although few of us in the "helping" professions resort to barbed wire, we all share the reality that we can only assist clients who are "here" to receive that assistance. We speech-language pathologists and audiologists have devoted most of our attention to developing approaches to the evaluation and amelioration of communicative disorders. Yet, the finest clinical services are of little use unless clients avail themselves of those services.

This book is mostly about matters related to getting, keeping, and efficiently managing clients, wherever we speech-language pathologists and audiologists provide our services: in rehabilitation facilities, in hospitals, in schools, in community centers, in private practice offices, and in the myriad other settings in which we work. This text will not be concerned with specific approaches to evaluation and intervention. It will focus on the "delivery" rather than on the services to be delivered, considering such topics as the place of our profession in the spectrum of human services professions, referral procedures (i.e., how clients come to and from members of those professions), storing and communicating clinical information, legal and ethical considerations in providing clinical services, and, most importantly, the economics of professional practice.

In titling this text, I referred unabashedly to the "delivery of clinical services." Many of our colleagues object to the use of "delivery" with respect to the services they provide. They contend that delivery refers to the missions of milkmen, the Postal Service, or the Fuller Brush Company, and insist that the term "delivery" is too dehumanized, too simplistic, even too crass, to apply to human services.

Yet, when members of our profession recognize that clinical services must indeed be delivered, they become infinitely more effective clinicians. We once behaved as though clients should seek us out like pilgrims journeying to gurus in Himalayan caves. We even implied that seeking out potential clients somehow represented unethical conduct. Furthermore, although we wanted to be paid as well as possible for our services, we preferred that several administrative layers be imposed between us and the original sources of the money: taxpayers, philanthropists, subscribers to insurance plans, or even, as a last resort, the clients themselves. In recent years, we have discovered that these attitudes have severely restricted the scope of our services. Many of the people who need our help do not join the pilgrimage to find us. Furthermore, we found many serious limitations in delivering our professional services only within the context of large institutions.

The notion that speech-language pathology and audiology services can and should be delivered represents a significant step forward. Delivery is a dynamic process. To deliver a commodity or service one must seek out consumers and ensure, insofar as possible, that they are offered and accept what they need.

The concept of delivery also entails the consideration of efficiency. After all, delivery is extraneous to the commodity or service. However necessary, it stands between the consumer and the product. The most economically efficient manufacturer faces bankruptcy if it is too expensive to get his product to the consumer. Similarly, human services fail when too many obstacles intervene between the provider and the consumer.

The services of the most skilled speech-language pathologists or audiologists are of little value without delivery systems that ensure their availability to the clients who need them. On the other hand, when the delivery systems become exorbitantly inefficient, the services soon become unavailable.

Some broad definitions may help to characterize the author's perspectives, prejudices, and points of view about the profession we represent, the services we deliver, and the essential characteristics of good service delivery systems. These definitions assume applicability in all of the settings where we deliver our services. While it is quite true that some significant setting-dependent differences exist in the delivery of speech, language, and hearing services, similarities generally outweigh differences. Many differences are essentially semantic, as, for example, the terms we use to refer to the consumers of our services. Since it seems most neutral, the term "clients" is used throughout this text, even though it differs from the language habits acquired in the setting where I work. Other terms will be used only in direct quotations or in contexts where that usage seems ridiculous (as in referring to a "physician's client" or a "client in the sixth grade"). It is hoped that this usage will create no semantic stumbling blocks and that readers can translate my terminology into the native language of the setting in which they are employed.

DEFINING OUR PROFESSION

Before defining the profession of speech-language pathology and audiology, or any other profession for that matter, one must first inquire whether it does, indeed, constitute a profession.

Attributes of a Profession

One of the most frequently quoted descriptions of the salient features that distinguish professions from other occupations was published by Cogan in 1955. He proposed five different criteria:

1. It must be founded upon an understanding of the theoretical structure of some department of learning or science.
2. It must involve some abilities—or competencies—that derive from that understanding.
3. It must have applicability to the vital practical affairs of man.
4. Its practice must be modified by knowledge of a generalized nature and by the accumulated wisdom and experience of mankind.
5. It must consider its first ethical imperative to be altruistic service to the client.

If these constitute the distinctive features, it should be possible to determine whether speech-language pathology and audiology qualifies as a profession by assessing this field against each of them.

IS SPEECH-LANGUAGE PATHOLOGY AND AUDIOLOGY FOUNDED UPON AN UNDERSTANDING OF THE THEORETICAL STRUCTURE OF SOME DEPARTMENT OF LEARNING OR SCIENCE?

Although our profession may suffer from inconsistencies in requirements for the various certificates, licenses, and credentials that define its practitioners, all of these requirements share one characteristic. They all require some preparation in the physical, biologic, social, and behavioral sciences from which our field derives.

The Position Paper on the Single Profession and its Credentialing, presented to the American Speech-Language-Hearing Association in 1982, defined the discipline basic to all professional endeavors in our field as "That branch of knowledge, both theoretical and applied, which focuses on human communication and its disorders," and observed further:

> The concept of a scholarly discipline underlying professional practice is not new. Curtis (1963) offered an affirmative answer to the question, "Is there a central nucleus of knowledge and thought concerning human communication that is significant to each of us, irrespective of our specialized interests?" and Peterson and Fairbanks (1963) wrote that "A service profession without a discipline, however, is not likely to achieve an attractive status.... Speech and hearing science may be considered a unified academic discipline, and is more generalized than is often recognized." Since the early days of the profession, however, the contents of that underlying discipline have both broadened and deepened. In addition to theoretical and applied knowledge about speech, language and hearing disorders and the traditional speech and hearing sciences, the discipline has come to include the full range of information about language structure and language use in comprehension and production, as well as the relevant knowledge in the cognitive, social, and physical domains that relates to the acquisition, use and dissolution of communicative systems.

There is considerable disagreement among practitioners of speech-language pathology and audiology as to what constitutes optimal preparation in the theoretical structures of the sciences that undergird the field. Nevertheless, there is virtually unanimous agreement that some knowledge of those theoretical structures is absolutely essential.

DOES SPEECH-LANGUAGE PATHOLOGY AND AUDIOLOGY INVOLVE ABILITIES AND COMPETENCIES THAT DERIVE FROM THAT UNDERSTANDING?

Some critics of the various standards for the practice of speech-language pathology and audiology propose that the standards are inadequate because virtually all are based on the completion of academic and practicum requirements rather than on the achievement of a specified set of competencies. Yet, even the most enthusiastic proponents of competency-based standards have failed to identify all of the competencies that are requisite to successful practice in this infinitely complex field.

No setter of standards, however, has ever proposed that we need be concerned only for what people know when they enter our field. We must also be concerned with what they can do and how well they can do it. Clearly, then, abilities and competencies are crucial elements in speech-language pathology and audiology.

DOES SPEECH-LANGUAGE PATHOLOGY AND AUDIOLOGY HAVE APPLICABILITY TO THE "VITAL PRACTICAL AFFAIRS OF MAN"?

At the core of the field of speech-language pathology and audiology is concern for human communication and its disorders. Surely, few processes equal communication in importance to the practical affairs of humankind.

ARE THE PRACTICES OF SPEECH-LANGUAGE PATHOLOGY AND AUDIOLOGY MODIFIED BY KNOWLEDGE OF A GENERALIZED NATURE AND BY THE ACCUMULATED WISDOM AND EXPERIENCE OF MANKIND?

Even a cursory analysis of the influences on speech-language pathology and audiology of generalized knowledge and accumulated wisdom and experience would require a sizeable volume. However, the following assertions should suffice here.

Our field has emerged from concerns for human rights that seek to achieve for all people the fullest possible participation in society. Therefore, speech-language pathology and audiology tend to prosper in eras when those concerns predominate and to wane in eras when other concerns claim higher priorities. Furthermore, the expressions of those concerns influence our field. When the expressions were paternalistic, the practices of speech-language pathology and audiology tended to be paternalistic. When the expressions emphasized each individual's right to self-determination, our practices focused on client participation in clinical processes.

Our practices reflect broader changes in prevalent views of human behavior. They are not solely influenced by studies of human communication but, rather, derive from theoretical formulations of broader aspects of human behavior. For example, one can chart prevalent views of phonologic disorders during the past 40 years from developmental, to behavioral, to generative, to cognitive. These views parallel trends evident in most fields whose practitioners study human behavior. Their influences did not merely represent changing fashions, however, since each exerted a cumulative effect on practices in the treatment of phonologic disorders.

Major achievements in technology are virtually always assessed for applicability to the methods of inquiry and the clinical practice of speech-language pathology and audiology. Many, such as the technologies of sound amplification and transmission and discrete acoustic analysis, artificial generation and modeling of speech signals, and the measurement of electrophysiologic responses, find a permanent place in the armamentarium of speech-language pathologists and audiologists. Others, such as technologies related to biochemical analyses and the use of electrodermal responses, still radiography, and thermography, although once considered promising, have been abandoned pending more convincing demonstrations of their utility.

Each of these assertions seems to illustrate that the practice of speech-language pathology and audiology has indeed been substantially modified by knowledge of a generalized nature and by the accumulated wisdom and experience of humankind.

DOES SPEECH-LANGUAGE PATHOLOGY AND AUDIOLOGY CONSIDER ITS FIRST ETHICAL IMPERATIVE TO BE ALTRUISTIC SERVICE TO THE CLIENT?

From its inception, the leaders in the field of speech-language pathology and audiology have begun each definition of the responsibilities of practitioners in this field with the declaration that the primary obligations center on the delivery of optimal services to clients. The first principle stated in the Code of Ethics of the American Speech-Language-Hearing Association is, "Individuals shall hold paramount the welfare of persons served professionally."

Defining Speech-Language Pathology and Audiology

At least according to Cogan's (1955) criteria, then, we should feel secure in referring to speech-language pathology and audiology as a profession. If we appraise our field against other criteria, however, we may temper that conclusion. Freund (1965) proposed three standards for measuring professions: (1) independence, (2) availability, and (3) learning. Independence is expressed through loyalty to clients, independence from government control, and authority over professional standards and discipline. Although speech-language pathology and audiology may generally rate well in terms of loyalty to clients and moderately well in self-regulation as to standards and discipline, the majority of its practitioners are substantially controlled by governmental jurisdiction.

Our profession would also win only a "fair" rating with respect to availability. Despite the expansion of clinical services in the past two decades, speech-language pathology and audiology services are not readily available in many locations nor to many members of our society.

Freund suggests two facets of the learning criterion: the degree to which a profession is capable of using available information and the degree to which that information is up to date. Unquestionably, many practitioners of our profession would be found wanting with respect to one or both of these criteria. On the other hand, the same conclusion could probably be applied to virtually every profession. Perhaps, then, this criterion and the other criteria, as well, may be more useful in the appraisal—or, even better, the self-appraisal—of individual professionals, rather than in the appraisal of an entire profession.

It is not enough merely to assert that we represent a profession. We must also define that profession. Like all professions, we are defined in many ways. The ASHA Position Paper on the Single Profession and Its Credentialing espoused the principle that speech-language pathology and audiology represents a single profession with designated areas of practice. The profession is defined by the concern for "the delivery of human services to individuals with speech-language-hearing disorders, aimed at the amelioration of communication difficulties stemming from such disorders." The designated areas of practice, specifically speech-language pathology and audiology, were defined as "specific ranges of clinical endeavor within the scope of the profession."

The Dictionary of Occupational Titles (1979), published by the United States Employment Services, is usually regarded as the most authoritative source for definitions of occupations represented in our nation's work force. It offers separate definitions for speech-language pathologists (referred to as speech pathologists) and audiologists.

SPEECH PATHOLOGIST

Specializes in diagnosis and treatment of speech and language problems, and engages in scientific study of human communication. Diagnoses and evaluates speech and language competencies of individuals, including assessment of speech and language skills as related to educational, medical, social and psychological factors. Plans, directs, or conducts habilitative and rehabilitative treatment programs to restore communicative efficiency of individuals with communication problems of organic and nonorganic etiology. Provides counseling and guidance to speech and language handicapped individuals. May act as consultant to educational, medical, and other professional groups. May teach scientific principles of human communication. May direct scientific projects investigating biosocial phenomena associated with voice, speech, and language. May conduct research to develop diagnostic and remedial techniques or design apparatus.

AUDIOLOGIST

Specializes in diagnostic evaluation of hearing, prevention, habilitative and rehabilitative services for auditory problems, and research related to hearing and attendant disorders. Determines range, nature, and degree of hearing function related to patients' auditory efficiency (communication needs), using electroacoustic instrumentation, such as pure-tone audiometers, and acoustic impedance equipment. Coordinates audiometric results with other diagnostic data, such as educational, medical, social and behavioral information. Differentiates between organic and nonorganic hearing disabilities through evaluation of a total response pattern and use of acoustic tests such as Stenger and electrodermal audiometry. Plans, directs, conducts, or participates in conservation, habilitative and rehabilitative programs including hearing aid selection and orientation, counseling, guidance, auditory training, speech reading, language habilitation, and speech conservation. May conduct research in physiology, pathology, biophysics, and psychophysics of auditory systems. May design and develop clinical and research procedures and apparatus. May act as consultant to educational, medical, and other professional groups. May teach art and science of audiology and direct scientific projects. May specialize in fields such as industrial audiology, geriatric audiology, pediatric audiology and research audiology.

Although these definitions are "official," they do not have the force of law, and in the final analysis legal definitions are probably the most important. In general, laws define professions according to their scopes of practice. This characterizes most state licensure laws. Although each law differs in its terminology, California's Speech Pathologists and Audiologists Licensure Act, found in Chapter 5.3 of Division 2 of the

Business and Professions Code, is essentially typical. It defines a speech pathologist as "a person who practices speech pathology" and then proceeds with this definition:

> "The practice of speech pathology" means the application of principles, methods, and procedures for measurement, testing, identification, prediction, counseling, or instruction related to the development and disorders of speech, voice, or language for the purpose of identifying, preventing, managing, habilitating or rehabilitating, ameliorating, or modifying such disorders and conditions in individuals or groups of individuals.

Similarly, an audiologist is defined as "one who practices audiology," according to this definition:

> "The practice of audiology" means the application of principles, methods, and procedures of measurement, testing, appraisal, prediction, consultation, counseling, instruction and research related to hearing and disorders of hearing for the purpose of modifying communicative disorders involving speech, language, auditory behavior or other aberrant behavior related to hearing loss; and the planning, directing, conducting or participation in programs of identification, hearing conservation, habilitation, and rehabilitation, including hearing aid recommendation and evaluation procedures such as, but not limited to, specifying amplification requirements and evaluation of the results thereof, auditory training, and speech reading.

As with most professions, legal definitions of speech-language pathology and audiology are accomplished at state, rather than federal, levels. A notable exception to this principle is found in the regulations for Public Law 94-142, usually referred to as the Education for All Handicapped Children Act. Although not actually defining the profession of speech-language pathology and audiology, it defines speech-language pathology and audiology services, which, in effect, defines the profession, at least with respect to its scope of practice within the public schools.

As summarized by Dublinske and Healey (1978), PL 94-142 defined the following as speech-language pathology services:

1. Identification of children with speech or language disorders.
2. Diagnosis and appraisal of specific speech or language disorders.
3. Referral for medical or other professional attention necessary for the habilitation of speech or language disorders.
4. Provision of speech and language services for the habilitation or prevention of communicative disorders.
5. Counseling and guidance of parents, children, and teachers regarding speech and language disorders.

Dublinske and Healey summarized the audiology services included under PL 94-142 as:

1. Identification of children with hearing loss.
2. Determination of the range, nature, and degree of hearing loss including referral for medical or other professional attention for the habilitation of hearing.
3. Provision of habilitative activities, such as language habilitation, auditory training, speech reading, hearing evaluation, and speech conservation.
4. Creation and administration of programs for prevention of hearing loss.
5. Counseling and guidance of pupils, parents, and teachers regarding hearing loss.
6. Determination of the child's need for group and individual amplification, selection and fitting an appropriate hearing aid, and evaluating the effectiveness of amplification.

Even from these few examples, it is obvious that the profession of speech-language pathology and audiology has been defined in many ways. Despite the plethora of definitions, however, it is remarkable that their similarities always outweigh their differences. Although no single authoritative definition can be proposed, there seems little disagreement as to the appropriate professional domain of speech-language pathology and audiology.

DEFINING OUR PROFESSIONAL SERVICES

Although many definitions of our profession suggest the services we provide, some classification of those services must precede later discussions of the delivery of those services. Any categorization is arbitrary. At any given moment, a clinician may pursue activities that fall into two or more categories. Nevertheless, in the chapters that follow, primary speech-language pathology and audiology services will be categorized as: *screening*, *evaluation*, *therapy*, *counseling*, and *consultation*.

Screening

This service consists of those activities carried out for the purpose of selecting people from a large population who should be studied more carefully to determine whether a particular problem is present. If the problem is distributed throughout the entire population, ideally everyone might be included in the screening procedure. For example, since all adults are at risk for hypertension, everyone should submit to blood pressure screening at regular intervals. If, on the other hand, the problem is found chiefly among identifiable subpopulations, screening devices are concentrated within the "at-risk" groups. Therefore, because sickle cell anemia is found primarily among people of African descent and Tay-Sachs disease among Ashkenazic Jews, these particular subpopulations are targeted for screening.

The field of audiology offers an excellent example of screening a general population versus identified subpopulations. At one time, there was widespread interest in screening the hearing of all newborn infants in nurseries. Various devices were developed for these screening procedures which were administered primarily by paraprofessionals or even volunteers. Gradually, it became apparent that these programs were inefficient; despite substantial time and effort, very few infants were identified who ultimately showed significant hearing impairments. Worse yet, because of logistical problems, infants with significant hearing impairments were missed.

Eventually, when mass data became available, it was evident that more than 80% of the infants who ultimately showed significant hearing impairments came from identifiable subpopulations (e.g., children from families with histories of congenital impairment, children with craniofacial anomalies, children with high bilirubin levels at birth). It was concluded, therefore, that screening programs could probably be substantially more effective and economical if they were to concentrate on these subpopulations.

Speech-language pathologists and audiologists may participate in two different types of screening programs. Either type may be directed toward general populations or may target specific at-risk groups. In the first type, screening for speech, language, and hearing problems is included among a variety of procedures carried out to identify a wide range of health and developmental problems. The second type of program focuses exclusively on the identification of speech-language or hearing problems.

The first type of program is well illustrated by the Early and Periodic Screening, Diagnostic, and Treatment Plan (EPSDT) established by Congress in the 1967 amendments to the Social Security Act. EPSDT expanded provisions of the Medicaid program for children to include payment for services aimed at the early identification of incipient health and developmental problems with a view to instituting whatever treatment was required to forestall more serious problems. EPSDT programs must include screening for a wide range of health and developmental problems. Most identify hearing screening as an essential service. Many also offer screening to identify problems in speech and language development.

The exclusive purpose of the second type of screening program is the identification of individuals who may have speech, language, and/or hearing problems. The involvement of speech-language pathologists and audiologists in such specific screening programs dates virtually from the inception of this profession. By screening the members of large populations (e.g., all children in a school district, all admissions to hospitals and outpatient medical clinics, or even as many members of a community as possible), speech-language pathologists and audiologists revealed twofold needs: they identified individuals who needed special services, and they demonstrated the magnitude of the service needs within the school district, the medical center, or the community in which they were employed.

As the demands for speech, language, and hearing services have grown, we have tended to focus screening efforts on subpopulations where the prevalence of these problems is greatest. Therefore, in many school districts, except for screening all preschoolers, speech-language pathologists now check only those children who are identified by their teachers as presenting possible communicative disorders together with children who may be at particular risk, e.g., children with low scores on reading readiness and reading achievement tests, children being considered for placement in special learning disabilities programs or children identified as mentally retarded. Although many school districts still attempt hearing screening of all children, the initial screening is often conducted by school nurses or paraprofessionals. In these instances, audiologists restrict their screening activities to children who fail the mass screening, perhaps also including other children in certain high-risk categories.

Screening progams in hospitals and outpatient medical clinics have also concentrated on high-risk subpopulations. Speech-language screening may involve only children seen for suspected neurologic or neurodevelopmental problems or adults undergoing evaluation or treatment of central nervous system lesions. Hearing screening may involve all individuals in specific age categories (e.g., children under 17 and adults over 50); or all admissions for otolaryngologic services; or individuals in such high-risk categories as children with histories of prenatal, natal, or neonatal problems, individuals with cleft palate and other craniofacial anomalies, individuals with renal disease, and individuals being treated with potentially ototoxic drugs.

The involvement of speech-language pathologists and audiologists in screening programs has changed considerably in recent years. To some extent, these changes may have decreased the total number of children and adults seen by speech-language pathologists and audiologists for direct screening services. So long as these reduced contacts reflect greater accuracy in identifying at-risk populations or more efficient use of paraprofessionals and automation, they may represent positive achievements. Nevertheless, planning, directing, supervising, and directly providing screening services continues to be one of the most important contributions of our profession.

Evaluation

Evaluation comprises those services that are provided for the purpose of describing a client's communicative disorder and for reaching decisions about appropriate management. Some speech-language pathologists and audiologists prefer the term "assessment" to describe these activities, but my thesaurus considers evaluation and assessment to be synonymous. In some usages one "evaluates" a program but "assesses" an individual enrolled in that program, but I know of no absolute basis for this usage.

Some members of our profession prefer the use of "diagnosis" as the term to describe these services. In the strictest sense, since this term derives from the root meaning "to discern" or "to distinguish," the usage is probably appropriate. Unfortunately, however, there are frequent semantic extensions of this term that may get us into trouble. "Getting into trouble" does not mean courting the ire of our colleagues in medicine who may believe that the term applies exclusively to their practices. "Diagnosis" is widely employed by auto mechanics, plumbers, cosmeticians, reading specialists, and countless other professionals, technicians, and tradespeople. It is essentially silly, therefore, for any group to claim the term as an inalienable right.

Regardless of whose services are being characterized, however, the use of "diagnosis" usually implies some assumptions that are overly restrictive. At least from a popular point of view, diagnosis describes a set of maneuvers that will lead to the exact labeling of a problem, to the specification of one or more causes for the problem, and hence to the definition of the regimen that will lead to the resolution of the problem. In idealized form, a set of symptoms is entered into a computer; momentarily, a readout emerges that identifies the problem and dictates the treatment to be prescribed. Some of our colleagues have aspired to this idealized situation in the evaluation of speech, language, and hearing problems; yet it could only be achieved through some very gross oversimplifications. Human communication is a sufficiently complex behavior that its impairments can seldom be adequately characterized by a single label. The behavior that is observed at any given moment is the result of innumerable physiologic, developmental, and experiential phenomena, so that specific causes can seldom be characterized. Even when they can be identified, those causes rarely lead to an automatic characterization of the required treatment. Therefore, although diagnosis may sometimes be an appropriate description of what speech-language pathologists and audiologists do, it too frequently carries implications that both restrict evaluation and distort the processes involved in the evaluation of communicative disorders.

Evaluations serve the following purposes:

1. An evaluation should determine whether a communication disorder is present and the degree to which that disorder constitutes a handicap to the client, his or her family, and the other people he or she encounters in daily life. When the client is a child, it may also be important to consider the likely future handicaps the disorder may impose.
2. An evaluation should describe, in behavioral terms, the manifestations of the communicative disorder—both the primary manifestations reflected in a client's proficiency as a speaker and listener and the secondary manifestations in other aspects of behavior, e.g., interpersonal relationships, learning, vocational adjustment.
3. An evaluation should lead to at least provisional conclusions about the next steps to be taken toward amelioration of the disorder. These steps may involve seeking the help of other professionals for the treatment of physiologic, psychologic, or social impediments to communication. They may involve the development of a program to help the client acquire improved communication. They may entail planning services that seek to lessen the handicaps that attend irremediable disorders.
4. An evaluation should establish baselines against which the outcomes of intervention can be determined.
5. An evaluation should suggest to other professionals concerned with the client the possible implications of the communicative disorder for whatever services they are providing. If they are engaged in the evaluation of the other problems the client presents, the results of the speech, language, or hearing evaluation may assist in the completion of that evaluation. If they are offering treatment or educational services, those services may be rendered more effective by a better understanding of the client's communicative disorders.

For practical reasons, we often distinguish sharply between evaluation and therapy. Most agencies, for example, make this distinction in their fee schedules. (Often third-party payers adopt different regulations for evaluation versus therapy, in some instances allowing payment for evaluation but not for therapy.) In reporting service statistics, most programs, whether they levy fees or not, also distinguish between evaluation and therapy.

The distinction between evaluation and therapy, however, is usually a concession to practicality with no professionally defensible rationale. Evaluation and therapy are frequently indistinguishable. A skillfully conducted evaluation can be highly therapeutic. Furthermore, the extended observations enabled by enrollment in a therapy program may offer the best opportunities for evaluation.

Therapy

Therapy comprises all activities that are carried out in an effort to modify communicative behaviors. These activities can be assigned to three overlapping categories:

1. *Activities aimed at the mastery of specific components of normal communication processes.* These activities seek to assist the client toward improved comprehension and production of the various features of language: phonologic, syntactic, and semantic as well as suprasegmental features. They may also stress more efficient communi-

cation to reduce the effort expended and the likelihood of secondary impairments (as, for instance, in assisting a client to achieve more efficient voice production, which will, in turn, reduce the likelihood of secondary physical changes in the larynx).

2. *Activities aimed at the achievement of compensation for irremediable impairments.* In many instances clients must employ alternatives to normal processes if they are to communicate. Hearing-impaired clients may learn to reinforce auditory cues with visual cues as an aid to speech comprehension. Speech-impaired clients may master compensatory strategies that will improve their communication despite irremediable deficits. When intelligible speech communication is impossible, clients may learn sign language or develop proficiency in the use of nonoral communication devices. Other clients may require assistance in the use of such prosthetic appliances as hearing aids, artificial larynxes and other speech appliances for laryngectomees, and palatal appliances for clients with cleft palate or with surgical defects following treatment for oral cancers.
3. *Activities aimed at changing attitudinal barriers to better communication.* Every clinician encounters instances in which clients present better potentials for communication than they are willing to exploit. Important therapeutic goals often relate to reducing these attitudinal barriers. Audiologists constantly work with clients who are reluctant to use the hearing aids that effect substantial improvement in their communication. Many adults with moderate aphasic disorders are so fearful of making mistakes that they overmonitor responses to a degree that seriously impedes their language expression. Stutterers commonly are so apprehensive that they withdraw from communication, even in situations where they would probably be successful. Hearing-impaired adults may impede communication by dominating conversations, avoiding lapses in comprehension by keeping expression by other talkers to an absolute minimum. All of these forms of behavior are expressions of attitudes that may be more deleterious to efficient communication than are the essential problems in speech, language, and hearing. Therefore, efforts toward the modification of such attitudes may be essential in a therapy program.

Our therapy services, then, seek broader goals than the achievement or restoration of normal communication, even assuming that such can be defined. This concept influences the selection of our clients, the approaches we employ, and our criteria for accountability.

Counseling

Counseling includes those services provided to clients and their families (our use of the term "family" is meant to include all "significant others") that seek resolution of the problems relating to or deriving from communicative disorders. The counseling we offer our clients is often indistinguishable from therapy, at least from therapy as we have defined it. Nevertheless, two types of counseling services can be differentiated from speech, language, and hearing therapy: services which help clients to recognize other areas in which they need assistance and to locate, accept, and receive such assistance; and services to clients' families that help them to assume their roles in communication and to support other therapy goals.

The first type of counseling service might be offered in the following circumstances: A child's delays in language acquisition may be only the most apparent of multiple developmental delays requiring other kinds of evaluation and intervention. A child with recurrent hearing loss resulting from otitis media may be receiving inadequate medical care. An adolescent with severe dysarthria may be pursuing unrealistic vocational objectives. Another adolescent with a moderately severe hearing impairment may be withdrawing from social contacts. An adult with a voice disorder may have serious emotional problems requiring the attention of a mental health professional. A laryngectomee may be facing such serious family problems that he is unable to benefit from a rehabilitative program.

Each of these situations requires intervention which may have major implications for the client's communication. But in every instance, the intervention required lies beyond the scope of practice of a speech-language pathologist or audiologist.

An obvious first step in providing these kinds of counseling services is recognizing the boundaries of our professional practice. Because the scope of our practice impinges on the practice of so many other professions, we can easily become confused and assume responsibilities outside our professional domain. We can become quasimedical advisors ("In my opinion, decongestants are an unsatisfactory treatment for recurrent middle ear problems"), or pseudopsychiatrists ("It seems to me that your voice problem represents an expression of unresolved conflicts that lead to excessive tension"), or sometime special educators ("Kevin should be placed in a regular fourth-grade class with supplementary work in reading, spelling, and math provided on a daily basis in a pull-out learning disability group"). In each example, the speech-language pathologist or audiologist is offering well intentioned advice (which may even be quite accurate), but the counsel offered lies outside of the scope of our discipline.

The second type of counseling we cited aims at assisting our clients' families to play more successfully their roles in communication processes. For example: The family of a child with meager and poorly intelligible communication can be assisted in setting up situations which will increase substantially the likelihood that they can decode their child's communication. The parents of a child with incipient stuttering behavior can learn to structure communication situations so that negative consequences are less likely to occur. The spouse of a hearing-impaired adult can be counseled to optimize communication by reducing ambient noise levels, avoiding such pitfalls as speaking to the client from another room, informing the client of the topic of a conversation when he or she enters, etc. Environmental management can also optimize the communication of laryngectomees and of clients with parkinsonism and other debilitating neurologic diseases.

Skillful counseling may well be one of the most important services provided by speech-language pathologists and audiologists. The ultimate effects in the amelioration of communicative disorders may often surpass the effects of therapy. But our roles as counselors are often misunderstood by other professionals and by the administrators responsible for the programs in which we work. In medical settings, treatment is usually provided by one group of professionals and counseling by another group. In schools, there is also often a clear division between what are considered teaching services and counseling services. Consequently, we encounter frequent problems in establishing counseling as legitimately within our scope of practice, problems such as scheduling time for counseling and including that time in the computation of costs for providing necessary services. Yet, when limitations are imposed on counseling services, serious limitations are usually imposed on the effectiveness of the entire speech-language pathology and audiology program.

Consultation

Consultation includes those services provided by speech-language pathologists and audiologists to assist other professionals. Such services may relate specifically to clients whom they are serving or may be directed toward the solution of problems that are not specific to one client. The single most significant indicator of our profession's growing stature and maturity may be the increasing demand for our consultative services.

The oldest tradition of such consultative services is probably found in the schools. Speech-language pathologists and audiologists consult with teachers to assist them in the management of children with communicative disorders. They may suggest approaches to maximizing participation in classroom activities; they may interpret the implications of communicative disorders for the acquisition of academic skills; they may help teachers monitor a child's use of hearing aids or other communication prostheses.

School consultation services may also address problems that are not specific to a single child. Speech-language pathologists and audiologists may help teachers to identify children with communicative disorders, to plan activities for increasing oral language proficiency, or to teach phoneme recognition as a basis for the mastery of reading and spelling skills. They may also consult with other school personnel, such as psychologists, school health workers, school social workers, and other pupil personnel specialists. Once again, these consultations may either relate to individual children or concern more general problems, such as adapting psychologic evaluation instruments to accommodate communicative disorders, improving medical follow-up on children with potentially treatable problems, or identifying appropriate community resources.

Speech-language pathologists and audiologists increasingly provide consultative services to physicians. These services may assist a physician in establishing a diagnosis and in planning treatment. For example, we may provide specific information about a client's auditory responses that will assist in localizing the site of a lesion or describe speech patterns which may be idiopathic to certain neurologic diseases. We can identify patterns of vocal abuse which will assist in planning the treatment of patients with certain laryngeal pathologies or describe the likely effects on speech of contemplated surgical approaches for clients with cleft palate. Again, consultative services to physicians may not relate to individual clients. Otolaryngologists often seek guidance on improving office procedures used to identify hearing and voice problems. Pediatricians frequently ask for advice about the recognition of developmental problems and about the educational management of children with chronic or recurrent otitis. Neurologists, and particularly pediatric neurologists, have frequent questions about diagnostic approaches that involve communication processes, e.g., tests of oromotor proficiency, screening tests for aphasia, and specialized procedures, such as auditory brainstem response measurement.

Our consultative services now extend beyond the boundaries of the education and health professions. Increasingly, we are serving consultative roles in legal matters where attorneys are involved. Speech-language pathologists are called upon to offer expert opinions about the testamentary capacity of aphasic clients. They may also be called upon to offer opinions about the possible relationships between speech, language, and hearing disorders and accidents or medical and surgical misadventures.

Because communicative disorders may have significant vocational implications, speech-language pathologists and audiologists are involved in consultations with rehabilitation counselors and with various public and private employment agencies. Again, these consultations may relate to individual clients or they may deal with more general issues concerning the rehabilitation and employment of people with communicative disorders.

Speech-language pathologists and audiologists also provide consultative services to business and industry. Occasionally, consultations may concern individual employees with communicative disorders. More frequently, however, they relate to potential hazards within the industry. The most common example is the growing participation of audiologists in industrial noise programs, where they consult regarding modifications in the environment that will reduce noise levels and regarding the protection of individual workers. However, with the increasing stringency of regulations requiring businesses and industries to offer equal employment opportunities to disabled individuals, our profession is also called upon for advice related to affirmative action programs.

Of the several areas of service we have defined, it is probably fair to conclude that consultation is the most frequently overlooked in our education and training. The cardinal requisites to effective consultations are expertise in our own profession and appreciation for the practices of other professions. In many respects, good consultation resembles any other professional service; it is valuable only if offered in a way that is useful to the recipient. The information we offer our clients in therapy and counseling is useful only when that information is understood, is acceptable, and is relevant and appropriate to their circumstances. And so it is also with consultation; consultations are useful only when the speech-language pathologist or audiologist is sensitive to the precise needs of the recipients of the consultation and provides information and advice which are relevant, practical, and applicable.

ESSENTIAL CHARACTERISTICS OF GOOD SERVICES DELIVERY

Having defined the services delivered by speech-language pathologists and audiologists, it is now advisable to define the criteria according to which the quality of those services can be assessed. Those criteria fall under five headings: *efficacy*, *coordination*, *continuity*, *participation*, and *economy*.

Efficacy

The obvious first criterion for judging any human service considers whether that service made any difference to the consumer. The efficacy of screening services can usually be judged in fairly objective terms. But the efficacy of many of the other services we provide is often more difficult to assess. It is easy to say that the efficacy of our professional services should be assessed on the basis of the insights gained by clients, families, and other concerned professionals and on the basis of overall improvement in communicative competence. However, it is frequently difficult to propose measures that will establish whether such achievements have, in fact, occurred. The problem of accountability will be discussed in a later chapter.

Coordination

Most clients with communicative disorders are served by several different professionals. Some of these professionals may provide services that are directly related to the communicative disorder, e.g., the learning disabilities specialist working with a child with problems in language acquisition, the teacher of a hearing-impaired child, the plastic surgeon treating a child with cleft palate, and the otolaryngologist treating the adult with laryngeal pathology. Other professionals provide services with only peripheral relevance to the communicative disorder, e.g., the teacher of a classroom where a young stutterer is enrolled, the social worker serving the family of a child with a communicative disorder, or the vocational counselor working with a recent laryngectomee. Whenever multiple professional services are provided to the same client, the effectiveness of any of those services will often depend on their coordination with all other services. This particularly pertains in speech-language pathology and audiology, regardless of whether the other services relate directly to the evaluation and treatment of a communicative disorder.

Continuity

Not only do most clients with communicative disorders require multiple professional services, they often require sequential services over a period of several months or even several years. Good care, therefore, demands an approximate total plan for services, with each phase of that plan staged and integrated into an uninterrupted sequence toward the ultimate goals.

Participation

Professional services were once planned and carried out with little regard for clients' wishes and with little concern for their understanding of what was going on. Not only did these attitudes abridge basic human rights, they often seriously impaired the effectiveness of services. Excellent speech-language pathology and audiology services involve the fully informed participation of clients and families at every turn. They particularly involve participation in all decision-making processes, recognizing that, in fact, the final responsibility for decisions always rests with the client and family.

Economy

A shortsighted view equates economy with spending as little money as possible.

Although limiting expenditures is one facet of economy, it is by no means the only concern. For example, although they are cheaper, services that are so infrequent that they are ineffectual or services provided by poorly prepared hence low-salaried staff members are actually wasteful because no value accrues from the money expended. In a broader sense, economy refers to the orderly management of services to avoid waste and to the achievement of efficiency through careful planning. Economy, therefore, refers not only to conservation of financial resources but to conservation of time and energy as well. In the final analysis, economy may be the single ultimate criterion in determining whether a plan for services to an individual client will ever be instituted or will continue and, indeed, whether an entire program of clinical services will survive.

It is inevitable that my value judgments as to what constitutes good practices in the delivery of speech-language pathology and audiology services pervade discussions throughout this text. Insofar as possible, however, such value judgments will derive from the five cited criteria.

SUMMARY

During the early years of development as a human services profession, speech-language pathology and audiology probably devoted more concern to refining and expanding professional services than to perfecting systems for delivering those services. We also tended to place inordinate emphasis on the settings in which we deliver our services, sometimes assuming this factor to be a primary determiner of the essential nature of our professional practices. Gradually, however, we developed a more mature sense of professional identity, defining with greater precision the scope of our practice and designating certain services as best provided by members of our profession. Simultaneous with the emergence of a stronger identity there has come a greater awareness of our place in the entire spectrum of human services professions and a stronger sense of individual responsibility for the quality and efficiency of the services that fall within our purview.

References

American Speech-Language-Hearing Association: Position paper on the single profession and its credentialing. *ASHA*, in press.

Cogan ML: The problem of defining a profession. *Ann Am Acad Polit Soc Sci* 297:105–111, 1955.

Curtis JF: Size, diversification and unity. *ASHA* 5:471–473, 1963.

Dublinske S, Healey W: PL 94–142: questions and answers for the speech-language pathologist and audiologist. *ASHA* 20:188–205, 1978.

Freund PA: The legal profession. In Lynn KS: *The Professions in America.* Boston, Houghton Mifflin, 1965.

Peterson GE, Fairbanks G: Speech and hearing science. *ASHA* 5:539–543, 1963.

United States Department of Labor: *Dictionary of Occuptional Titles.* Washington DC, United States Government Printing Office, 1979.

CHAPTER TWO

Speech-Language Pathology and Audiology in the Constellation of Human Services Professions

The figure of the superprofessional is ever popular in American folklore. Superprofessionals are most frequently embodied in the physicians featured on television series. One week he or she will diagnose a rare, but always operable, brain tumor; the next, rescue a marriage from seemingly hopeless incompatibility; the following week, motivate an autistic child to sing three choruses of "Old MacDonald Had a Farm"; and the next, teach the fundamentals of sign language to a 3-year-old deaf child. The figment of the superprofessional is also familiar in educational mythology, usually some version of the doyenne of the little red schoolhouse who is completely capable of providing comprehensive educational and counseling services to children of all ages without regard to intellectual capacity, cultural diversity, or sensory, motor, or attentional handicaps.

These fantasies can be easily dismissed as entertainment for the undiscriminating, but they often represent the ideals of people who establish policies for the delivery of human services. Too many elected officials and appointed bureaucrats would be pleased to assign most health care responsibilities to all-knowing family physicians, and all educational responsibilities to classroom teachers. It may be true that overspecialization brings negative consequences and that our human services delivery system has become too complex. Yet, in most human services fields, essential knowledge has so proliferated that honest professionals can only provide acceptable services within well described areas. This is particularly true in speech-language pathology and audiology where we daily encounter problems of almost infinite complexity. Like every provider of human services we must continually weigh the risks of overreaching our expertise against subjecting clients to such an array of specialists that they become hopelessly confused and even impoverished.

The succeeding sections of this chapter will review the professionals who are most often our colleagues in serving clients with communicative disorders. Some terms that will recur are best defined at the outset. These definitions, originally formulated by the National Commission on Accrediting, were published in the *Staff Working Papers* of the Study of Accreditation of Selected Health Professions (1971).

> *Certification* is the process by which a non-governmental agency or association grants recognition to an individual who has met certain predetermined qualifications specified by that agency or association.
>
> *Licensure* is the process by which an agency of government grants permission to persons meeting predetermined qualifications to engage in a given occupation and/or to use a particular title or grants permission to institutions to perform specified functions.
>
> *Registration* is the process by which qualified individuals are listed on an official roster maintained by a governmental or non-governmental agency.
>
> *Accreditation* is the process by which an agency or organization evaluates and recognizes a program of study or an institution as meeting certain predetermined qualifications or standards. It shall apply only to institutions and their programs of study or their services.

SPEECH-LANGUAGE PATHOLOGY AND AUDIOLOGY

Speech-language pathology and audiology are somewhat unique as human services professions. The primary development of other human services professions has usually occurred within a single system: the health care system, the educational system, or the social welfare system. Although practitioners of these professions may serve other systems—physicians and nurses may serve schools, teachers may work in hospitals, and social workers may work in both educational and health care programs—their essential professional identities remain within the system that has fostered their traditions. In the United States, the early development of speech-language pathology occurred primarily within educational programs. Yet during the past 40 years, the profession has played an increasingly important role in the health care system. Except, perhaps, for clinical psychology, no other profession has the same kind of multisystem tradition.

This tradition offers many advantages, particularly with respect to the breadth of our professional scope, the variety of contexts in which we deliver our services, and the multiplicity of professional specialists we claim as colleagues. It also incurs many disadvantages. We may appear anomalous in more conventional settings. We may seem too treatment oriented to fit comfortably into educational settings but too educationally oriented to fit comfortably into health care settings. We work very differently from other specialists concerned with the education of handicapped children. We also work very differently from other specialists concerned with the restoration of physical function.

Our multisystem tradition has also created some serious problems with respect to establishing professional standards. Because most governmental jurisdictions establish different laws and regulations to define qualified providers in their educational systems than to define providers in other settings, multiple standards have been set to define speech-language pathologists and audiologists. These sometimes conflicting standards may confuse our professional colleagues and the potential consumers of our services.

Who may practice speech-language pathology and audiology? Regrettably, the answer in many states (and, until comparatively recently, in all states) is: anyone who wishes to. This may include people who have completed two or three courses in the field, singing teachers, actors temporarily between engagements, salesmen of various communication aids and appliances, and people with communicative disorders who believe personal experience to be superior to academic degrees. Fortunately, even where no legal standards for practice exist, completely unprepared practitioners of speech-language pathology and audiology are rare. (However, their apparent natural proclivity for radio talk shows and newspaper interviews may make them somewhat conspicuous rarities.) Many extralegal controls limit the success of unqualified providers. Most speech-language pathologists and audiologists rely on referrals from other professionals, who are usually selective in making those referrals. Furthermore, we are increasingly dependent upon third-party payment, and such payment is usually available only to providers who meet established standards. Both of these factors mitigate against the survival of completely unqualified providers.

Most professions offer a single index for identifying qualified practitioners, usually licensure by the state in which one practices. Speech-language pathology and audiology, however, offer three different indices of professional qualification: (1) Certificates of Clinical Competence issued by the American Speech-Language-Hearing Association, (2) credentials or certificates issued by state education agencies, and (3) state licenses. A presumably qualified speech-language pathologist or audiologist may hold one, two, or all three.

Not only are there multiple indices of professional qualification, there are substantial disparities among the requirements for each. Most state licensure laws are consonant with ASHA certification requirements, the one national standard. State education agency certification requirements, however, often not only differ substantially from ASHA certification, but also vary widely from one state to another. Inasmuch as this situation is not likely to change in the forseeable future, all three types of provider standards must be considered in defining our professional qualifications.

ASHA Certification

Since its beginnings almost 60 years ago, the American Speech-Language-Hearing Association (first established as the American Academy of Speech Correction) has held the promotion of professional standards among its primary purposes. For the first 25 years of its history, these standards were effected through requirements for membership. Originally, the requirements were remarkably high, considering the small number of people who met those requirements and the paucity of university programs capable of providing the specified preparation. When it became apparent that the standards were so exclusionary that most providers of speech, language, and hearing services were barred from association membership, a two-category structure was adopted. These new requirements, published in 1943, designated *Professional Members* as "individuals who have completed a broad education in this field, have considerable experience and are fully equipped in the field of speech correction." *Clinical Members* were described as "individuals who have completed a minimum of experience and academic preparation, and are capable of doing speech corrective work under guidance." (A third category offered associateships to individuals who had not yet completed professional training.)

Eventually the association recognized that using membership standards to define professional qualifications was restricting and even misleading. An increasing number of people who were pursuing careers in speech and hearing, primarily related to research and academic teaching, were in no way involved in the delivery of clinical services. These potentially valuable association members were excluded when membership requirements were based entirely on clinical preparation. Therefore, in 1951, separate standards were established for membership and for clinical certification.

Those standards for clinical certification, which included the requirement of membership in ASHA, maintained the two-level concept. *Basic Certificates* were granted to applicants with relatively limited preparation, following completion of 1 year of professional experience. *Advanced Certificates* were awarded to applicants with more extensive preparation, following 4 years of professional experience. This certification program introduced for the first time recognition of concentration in speech pathology versus specialization in audiology, through the award of four different certificates: Basic and Advanced Certificates in Speech and Basic and Advanced Certificates in Hearing. Despite their differential recognition of specialization in speech or hearing, the certificates maintained a substantial core of common requirements.

Even though the two-level certification structure (Basic versus Advanced) accurately reflected diverse levels of preparation among practitioners, it created serious confusions. The members of most other professions either meet minimal standards for professional practice or they do not. There is no such thing as recognition of levels of competence.

In 1962, after adoption of the Master's degree as a requirement for ASHA membership, the association approved a new set of certification requirements which became effective in 1965. These standards eliminated the two-level structure and established two certificates: the Certificate of Clinical Competence in Speech Pathology (later changed to Speech-Language Pathology) and the Certificate of Clinical Competence in Audiology. Although requirements for these certificates have been modified subsequently, the essential two-certificate structure has remained.

A further significant modification in certification requirements occurred in 1980.

At this time ASHA membership was deleted as a requirement for certification. For the first time in the history of the program, certification became available to all qualified applicants, regardless of whether they were members of the association.

From the first institution of separate certificates in speech and hearing, a controversy has continued as to whether speech-language pathology and audiology represent one or two professions. Many who hold the single-profession view contend that the two-certificate structure inherently creates the impression of two separate professions. There are, consequently, recurrent movements toward the development of a single certificate to signify minimal professional competence in speech-language pathology and audiology.

Two widespread areas of confusion attend ASHA certification, although neither area is inherent to the certification program itself. First, although intended to signify minimal standards for independent practice, the certificates are commonly regarded as signifying a higher level of achievement. Second, in the absence of other nationally applicable criteria, the certificates have filled a pseudolicensure role.

The Principles Underlying the Requirements for the Certificates of Clinical Competence specify that they are considered as "the minimal requirements to train a general practitioner." Despite this declaration, these requirements are frequently assumed to represent more advanced preparation. Since many state education certificates accept lower levels of academic preparation, a sizeable corps of practitioners do not meet ASHA certification requirements. Consequently, it is difficult to promulgate the concept that these requirements are minimal when a substantial number of practitioners do not meet them. Furthermore, some college and university programs that purport to prepare speech-language pathologists and audiologists barely offer sufficient course work and clinical practicum to qualify their graduates for ASHA certification, and others do not even pretend to offer that amount of preparation. This situation further promotes the misimpression that ASHA requirements are optimal rather than minimal.

The second area of confusion derives from the pseudolicensure role played by the ASHA certificates. Particularly in health care fields, regulations that specify who is authorized to provide particular services use state licensure, even though the regulations apply nationally. For example, Title 18 of the Social Security Act, the legislation that established Medicare, defines "physician" as follows:

> The term "physician" when used in connection with the performance of any function or action means (1) a doctor of medicine or osteopathy legally authorized to practice medicine and surgery by the State in which he performs such function or action. . .(2) a doctor of dentistry or of dental or oral surgery who is legally authorized to practice dentistry by the State in which he performs such function. . .or (3). . .a doctor of podiatry or surgical chiropody, but only with respect to functions which he is legally authorized to perform as such by the State in which he performs them. (Part C Section 1861)

Since many states do not license speech-language pathologists and audiologists, in the same section Medicare regulations define a speech pathologist as, "a person who is (a) licensed by the state in which (s)he is practicing (in those states with licensing laws) and who is (b) eligible for the ASHA certificate of clinical competence, or who meets educational requirements for certification and is in the process of completing the Clinical Fellowship Year."

Fortunately, ASHA certification was available as a national standard when Medicare regulations were promulgated. Nevertheless, granting legal status to certification violates the essential nature of certification which, by definition, should represent something sought voluntarily from a professional association rather than a license to provide particular services. Among other problems, this pseudolicensure status opens our voluntary certification program to all manner of legal scrutiny and leads to inflexibility in attempting to alter certification requirements to reflect changing professional practices.

Despite confusions and misapprehensions, however, the ASHA certificates remain the sole nationally applicable index of professional qualification. The immediate future is not likely to see licensure in all 50 states or the achievement of essential consistency among state education credential requirements. Therefore, the ASHA certificates will continue to play an important role in defining qualified providers of speech, language, and hearing services.

School Speech, Language, and Hearing Specialist Credentials

Since the earliest days of public education in the United States, it has been assumed that teachers should complete some formal professional preparation prior to employment. Gradually, this assumption was formalized into credentialing systems to identify people who met prescribed standards to teach in the public schools. Since public education has always been considered under state jurisdiction, these standards were established separately by each state. Not surprisingly, the nature and extent of the requirements varied substantially among the various states.

As programs developed to serve children with special needs, the same practices were employed to qualify providers of these services. For example, in 1910, when the city of Chicago became one of the first to recognize the need for "speech correction" services in its schools, it implemented the plan by establishing a special 6-month curriculum at Chicago Teachers College to provide a group of classroom teachers with the supplementary education that was deemed necessary. As other school programs emerged and training requirements were formalized into credentials, similar assumptions were applied. In particular, since it was considered to be a special area of teaching competence, the requirements assumed that speech-language pathology represented an area of specialization supplementing basic preparation as a classroom teacher.

Gradually, requirements for credentialing school speech, language, and hearing specialists have increased to reflect more accurately the competencies required. Although the overall trend has been in the direction of strengthened requirements, the vicissitudes of educational fashion, personnel needs, and political expedience have also been reflected. Among the many factors that have influenced the directions of change are ASHA certification requirements, although that influence has been much greater in some states than in others. During the past two decades, changes have been particularly apparent in three areas:

1. *Requiring professional education on a graduate level.* Taylor's (1980) survey of state education agency credential requirements showed that 14 states required M.A. degrees or equivalent preparation. Twelve others required M.A.'s for speech, language, and hearing specialist credentials but also offered another type of credential in the field to applicants who held only B.A.'s. Other states exacted such extensive requirements that completion on an undergraduate level was unlikely, but did not, nevertheless, specifically require graduate education. Several still maintained requirements that could be completed easily within an undergraduate program.
2. *Specifying professional course requirements and clinical practicum requirements that approximate ASHA certification standards.* Only about one-fourth of the states included in Taylor's survey clearly specified the 24 units of professional coursework then required for ASHA certification. Although other states may well have equaled that requirement, they used terminology which made direct comparisons impossible. Other state requirements obviously fell well below ASHA standards.

   With respect to clinical practicum, Taylor found that many states specified requirements in terms that defied comparison to ASHA standards (for example, several specified completion of a given number of semester units of "practice teaching," whereas others simply specified that applicants must meet requirements established by an approved college or university training program). Of the 25 states that did specify practicum hour requirements, one exceeded ASHA's requirement, five equaled that requirement, and 19 required substantially less practicum.
3. *Reducing requirements for education courses.* As noted earlier, at the beginnings of school services,

speech, language, and hearing specialists were considered teachers with supplementary special training. In recent years, most experts on the delivery of these special services have agreed that some orientation to school practices, administration, and traditions is essential, but these courses are assigned a lower priority than academic preparation in speech-language pathology and audiology. Taylor's survey showed that only eight states did not require some coursework in education. When units were specified, in only one state did the requirement exceed 9 semester units (although some states specified combined coursework in education and psychology of 12 to 15 units). Changes in attitudes about the importance of preparation in education are readily apparent through comparisons of Taylor's data with the report of a similar survey conducted by Causey et al. in 1971. At that time, 26 states reported education course requirements exceeding 12 semester units, and 15 of those states exacted requirements of 18 units or more.

It is gratifying to study successive analyses of state education certification standards, beginning with Nelson's report in 1946. Such a review shows the growing awareness of the expertise demanded of professionals who serve school children with speech, language, and hearing disorders. Nevertheless, that review is also disheartening because of the obvious shortcomings in many state certification standards. If, as noted earlier, our profession believes that ASHA certification standards represent "the minimal requirements to train a general practitioner," it is obvious that many state requirements do not reach that minimum. Two equally untenable conclusions are likely. One is that school speech, language, and hearing specialists are subprofessionals. The other is that the delivery of acceptable and appropriate speech, language, and hearing services to students in schools is less demanding of professional competence. Since neither conclusion has any acceptable basis in fact, obviously we must continue efforts to strengthen state education agency credentialing programs.

The diversity among state requirements also generates some serious professional problems. It prevents any nationally applicable definition of our profession in school settings. It may offer insurmountable obstacles to professionals in moving from one state to another and compound the problems of personnel shortages in particular geographic areas. Furthermore, it may substantially influence the quality of clinical services children receive on the mere basis of their state of residence.

Even semantic problems are compounded by state school credential programs. Taylor (1980) found 19 different titles for speech-language pathologists in schools, including Speech and Language Clinician, Speech Correctionist, Communication Disorders Specialist, and Professional Teacher of Speech Handicapped. Little wonder that our colleagues in other professions often comment on our apparent identity crisis.

Most states offer credentials to teachers of hearing-impaired children, and several offer credentials to audiometrists or hearing conservation specialists, but only recently have a few states instituted credentials for "educational audiologists." These credentials establish qualifications for professionals providing a broad range of audiologic diagnostic and rehabilitation services in the schools. Thus far, those responsible for developing school audiologist credentials appear to have profited from recognizing the confusions and inconsistencies that characterize school speech-language pathologist credentials. Most have followed closely the established national standards in defining their individual state requirements.

State Licensure

During the 1960's, as more and more speech-language pathologists and audiologists found employment in increasingly diverse services settings, there was a growing recognition of the need for a better approach to identifying qualified professionals. Although ASHA certification standards were used in many governmental regulations, that certification remained voluntary. Uncertified individuals were excluded from treating the clients who were covered by these regulations, but they were completely free to serve anyone else. Therefore, three major motives led members of our profession in several states to seek licensure laws. First, unqualified practitioners were providing inadequate or even deleterious services to children and adults with speech, language, and hearing disorders. Second, although the practices of ASHA certificate holders were somewhat regulated by a Code of Ethics, practitioners whose certificates had been revoked because of unethical conduct, and clinicians who had never held certification, could freely engage in unprofessional practices. Third, as speech-language pathologists and audiologists became increasingly involved in interdisciplinary programs with other human service professionals, it became more and more difficult to establish their professional scope and qualifications without some form of legal definition, particularly when such definitions had long been available for most of the other human services professions.

The first licensure law for speech-language pathologists and audiologists was enacted by the State of Florida in 1969. By 1980, well over half of the states had enacted such licensure laws. In most instances, licensure requirements replicated ASHA certification standards. Depending upon the practices of the individual states, some laws referred directly to ASHA certification whereas others enumerated ASHA requirements without mentioning the association's certification program by name.

Each state established a licensure board to prepare regulations to implement their laws, to review applications, to grant licenses, and to receive and adjudicate complaints against licensees. The composition of these boards varies substantially. Some consist exclusively of speech-language pathologists and audiologists, others include members of other professions such as otolaryngologists, and some include lay public or consumer representatives. There is also considerable diversity in the administrative structure of licensure boards. Some operate under state health departments, others function under boards of medical examiners (or under the allied health divisions of those boards), and still others function essentially independently of other departments.

Some licensure laws specify that reciprocity is granted to licensees from states holding similar requirements (i.e., someone licensed by another state may be granted licensure without a complete review of qualifications). However, even when states do not openly grant reciprocity, their common basis in ASHA certification requirements usually facilitates the movement of professionals from one state to another. Thus far, at least, most state licensure programs have avoided the confusions and inconsistencies of state education agency credential programs.

Through sheer coincidence, the move toward licensure in speech-language pathology and audiology has occurred in an era of growing resistance to increased governmental regulation of our society. It has also occurred at a time of more frequent territorial disputes with members of other professions and trade groups. Therefore, the resistance to new licensure laws has increased substantially. Many years will probably elapse before speech-language pathologists and audiologists are licensed by all states. Perhaps that time will never come.

It is possible that licensure programs may be discontinued by states where they exist currently. Efforts to reduce governmental regulations have taken the form of "sunset laws." These laws require the review of all regulatory bodies at intervals, specifying that they may continue only if they yield demonstrable benefits. However, because such reviews are sensitive to all manner of political pressures, licensure boards can be eliminated even if they are making worthy contributions.

For the present, then, it is unlikely that state licensure can become the universal definition of qualified professionals in our field. Clearly, we must continue our quest for a truly effective approach to defining qualified providers of speech, language, and hearing services.

THE HEALTH PROFESSIONS

One key development in our profession during the second half of the 20th century has been its increasing involvement in the health care system. During that same interval, the health care system itself has experienced substantial changes. In earlier times, health care services models resembled primitive conceptions of "paradise" in a rigid pyramidal configuration. The "supreme being" was enthroned at the apex, and lesser luminaries occupied appropriate levels beneath. Communication took the form of pronouncements relayed from the top, although humble supplications were occasionally directed upward from the bottom. In traditional health care services models, a physician claimed the apical position and other professionals and paraprofessionals were assigned hierarchical positions beneath.

As health care has become more complex—in terms of the growing diversity of professions and professional specialities involved, of the increasing variety of health care facilities, and of the multiplication of laws, regulations, and policies—the essential models of our health care system have changed substantially. Unquestionably, the medical profession has maintained the pivotal position in the health care system, a position that is assured in all national, state, and local regulations, policies, and practices. Yet, in view of the formidable responsibilities society assigns to physicians, and the equally formidable penalties it levies for abrogations of those responsibilities, their pivotal position is probably appropriate.

Increasingly, however, our nation's health care system is characterized by multidisciplinary participation. In many areas of health care, teams comprised of physicians and other health professionals share mutual responsibilities for diagnosis and treatment. Individual physicians regularly refer their patients to nonphysician specialists for consultation. As members of one of the professions playing expanded roles in the health care system, it behooves speech-language pathologists and audiologists to learn more about the traditions, roles, and responsibilities of the other professions serving that system.

Medicine

There is an essential uniformity in qualifications for the practice of medicine throughout the United States even though each state has established its own licensure laws. Two factors affect this consistency. First, all licensure laws specify that applicants who are educated in the United States must have graduated from an institution accredited by the Association of American Medical Colleges. Second, applicants for licensure in most states must have achieved acceptable scores on an examination prepared by the National Board of Medical Examiners.

Physicians usually qualify for licensure on completion of a period of internship that immediately follows completion of the M.D. degree. (Contrary to popular belief, the degree alone does not qualify an individual to practice medicine.) At one time, many physicians entered practice immediately following completion of an internship year. Although this remains legally possible, most physicians complete further training before entering practice. That training usually leads to the completion of specialty certification.

Specialty certification requirements are defined by the appropriate component board of the American Board of Medical Specialties. Such requirements include both a prescribed training program and one or more examinations. From a legal standpoint, a Board-certified specialist holds no different qualifications than does any licensed physician. In other words, licensure grants the legal right to practice throughout the entire scope of medical practice. However, few physicians exercise that right; instead, they restrict their scope of practice to areas in which they have completed some specialized training.

With rare exceptions, the physicians in most frequent contact with speech-language pathologists and audiologists are certified specialists, usually in certain relevant fields. Although the distinctions are not absolute, medical specialists may be classified as *primary care specialists* and *secondary* and *tertiary care specialists.* Very generally, primary care specialists are concerned with general health maintenance and care, and they refer their patients to secondary care specialists for more explicit diagnosis and treatment. Tertiary care specialists provide even more discrete diagnosis and treatment. To illustrate: A person with an apparent hearing problem might discuss that problem with a family physician (a primary care specialist), who refers that patient to an otolaryngologist (a secondary care specialist). That otolaryngologist suspects, on the basis of his or her examination and the audiologic evaluation, that the patient has otosclerosis. The patient is then referred to another otolaryngologist (in this instance the tertiary care specialist) who specializes in stapes surgery.

These designations may help clarify physician roles and responsibilities, but they are not absolute. Many pediatricians and internal medicine specialists, which we will subsequently characterize as primary care specialists, have specific areas of expertise (or subspecialties) that equip them as secondary or tertiary care specialists. Similarly, many secondary care specialists have special areas of expertise that may lead them to function in specific instances as tertiary care specialists.

PRIMARY CARE SPECIALTIES

Three specialties are usually designated as principally concerned with primary care: family practice specialists, pediatricians, and specialists in internal medicine (sometimes called internists).

Family Practice

In recent years, family practice specialists have begun to replace the "general practitioners" of earlier times. The certification, established by the American Board of Family Practice, currently requires only graduation from an approved medical school, licensure, and achievement of an acceptable score on the examination the Board administers. Since residency programs in family practice, which usually extend 3 years beyond graduation from medical school, are becoming more prevalent, the eventual inclusion of a residency requirement for certification seems likely. Family practice certification is notable for its required renewal every 6 years on the basis of completion of continuing education requirements.

Although family practitioners usually do not represent a major source of referral to speech-language pathologists and audiologists, they may be important allies. They may be the first professionals to identify people with communicative disorders. They may provide important background information about clients' health problems and social situations and offer other essential information for the completion of evaluations and treatment plans. When several specialists are involved, family practitioners may coordinate diagnostic and treatment programs and integrate and interpret findings for clients and their families.

Even when clients are seen on referral from a secondary care specialist, a speech-language pathologist or audiologist may be well advised also to establish contact with the family practitioner. In the final analysis, the client is most likely to rely on the family practitioner; therefore, that practitioner's view of whatever recommendations are formulated by the speech-language pathologist or audiologist may be crucial.

Pediatrics

In many settings, pediatricians are the medical specialists most closely associated with speech-language pathologists and audiologists. Pediatricians are frequent referral sources. They are also frequent resources for helpful information about clients. Of all medical specialists, they may most nearly share the orientation of speech-language pathologists and audiologists. They usually understand child development and the implications of developmental problems. They are likely to be attuned to social, behavioral, and emotional factors rather than exclusively focused on physical pathology. They, more than most medical specialists, are usually comfortable in seeking guidance from professionals who are not physicians.

Requirements for certification by the American Board of Pediatrics specify a minimum of 3 years of hospital-based training following graduation from an approved medical school. Furthermore, the Board requires 2 additional years of practice or postgraduate training before the candidate may complete the certification examination.

Most primary care pediatricians serve children from birth to adolescence. An increasing number, however, specialize in primary care for teenagers; these physicians are usually identified as specialists in adolescent medicine. While fellowships in adolescent medicine are available and may be completed as supplemental training following the first 2 or 3 years of pediatric residency, no special certification is offered. Other pediatric subspecialties provide secondary care and will be considered accordingly in a later section.

Internal Medicine

Together with family practitioners, internists are the most frequent providers of primary care for adults. Once again, they are less likely to be sources of direct referral to speech-language pathologists and audiologists. In most communities, people with communicative disorders are referred first to secondary care specialists, who in turn refer to us. Nevertheless, it is often wise to establish direct contact with the internist who is providing primary care to a client. The internist may offer more information than is available from the referring secondary care specialist. Furthermore, when internists have the opportunity to appraise directly the contributions of speech-language pathologists and audiologists they may begin to refer their patients directly when the prior involvement of a secondary care physician is unnecessary.

Requirements for certification by the American Board of Internal Medicine specify completion of 3 years of postgraduate training in an approved residency. An examination is administered by the Board at the conclusion of that training. Many internists complete supplementary training in one or more subspecialties. The Board has established secondary certification in nine of these subspecialties, including specialization in cardiovascular disease, which will be discussed among the secondary care specialists.

Another growing primary care specialty, which as yet affords no certification, is gerontology. However, an increasing number of fellowships are becoming available in this field, and a future certification program seems likely. Because of the prevalence of communicative disorders among older people, there is an increasing alliance between physicians specializing in gerontology and speech-language pathologists and audiologists.

SECONDARY AND TERTIARY CARE SPECIALISTS

Speech-language pathologists and audiologists occasionally work with representatives of virtually all medical specialties. Radiologists may be contacted regarding cineradiographic studies of clients with velopharyngeal dysfunction. General surgeons may be consulted about clients operated for orofacial cancers. Audiologists may consult nephrologists or urologists regarding clients with associated hearing impairment and renal disease. Yet the following probably represent the medical specialties most frequently contacted. (Psychiatry and physical medicine are discussed in later sections of this chapter—respectively in the sections on the mental health professions and the rehabilitation professions.)

Pediatric Subspecialties

With the increasing complexity of pediatric practice has come a growing trend toward subspecialization. Certification has evolved in some subspecialty areas with programs supervised by sub-boards of the American Board of Pediatrics. Other subspecialties offer no formal certification; qualifications in these areas are signaled by the completion of supplementary training, usually in the form of a special fellowship. Of the four pediatric subspecialties that relate most frequently to our profession, only one, neonatology, affords certification. It seems likely, nevertheless, that certification programs may eventually emerge in other areas.

Neonatology, or neonatal-perinatal medicine, is the secondary care specialty concerned with the care of newborns, particularly high-risk newborns: premature and other low-birthweight infants, infants with congenital anomalies, infants with respiratory and vascular problems, infants with early-acquired infections, etc. The current practice of focusing on high-risk infants for the early detection of hearing impairment has brought close affiliations between neonatologists and audiologists. The growing expertise of audiologists in the use of auditory brainstem response measurement has also been of particular interest to neonatologists. Although seldom immediately involved in neonatology programs, speech-language pathologists are usually involved in the follow-up programs that emanate from neonatal intensive care units.

Genetics is another field of pediatric subspecialization with a growing relationship to members of our profession. These specialists may provide helpful clues to understanding problems presented by children with apparent congenital anomalies or other symptoms of dysgenesis. They may also counsel concerned parents about their likelihood of producing other children with similar deficits. Eventually, they may help clients with problems such as cleft palate or familial hearing impairments when questions arise about the likelihood of their parenting children with similar deficits. In return, speech-language pathologists and audiologists may provide genetics specialists with information that will assist in establishing their diagnoses.

Developmental pediatrics is a subspecialty of comparatively recent origin that evolved with the trend toward grouping mental retardation and certain congenital neurologic impairments as "developmental disabilities." The scope of practice of developmental pediatricians and pediatric neurologists may sometimes be quite similar. Developmental pediatricians serve many children with communicative disorders, hence most establish cordial working relationships with members of our profession.

Behavioral pediatrics is the newest of all the subspecialties discussed here. Its practitioners are concerned with problems in learning and development, social and school problems, and problems in family-child relationships. Specialists in behavioral pediatrics have been particularly interested in children with learning disabilities. In many instances their scope of practice may resemble the scope of practice of child psychiatry, although behavioral pediatricians usually treat less severely disturbed children. Most centers noted for their training of behavioral pediatricians include speech-language pathologists on their staffs or have established relationships with other departments providing speech, language, and hearing services. As a result, these specialists are among the most sophisticated users of our services and the most valuable resources for information about our young clients.

Cardiovascular Disease Specialists

This represents the one certified area of subspecialization in internal medicine whose practitioners are likely to have frequent contact with speech-language pathologists. Although sometimes served by neurologists, the ongoing specialty care for adults who have suffered cerebrovascular accidents is most likely to be provided by cardiovascular disease specialists. Accordingly, frequent contacts may occur with reference to adults with aphasia and certain motor speech disorders.

Certification of this subspecialty is offered by the Board on Cardiovascular Disease of the American Board of Internal Medicine following the completion of 2 years of training in the diagnosis and treatment of cardiovascular diseases. This subspecialty training follows completion of requirements for certification in internal medicine. Certification in cardiovascular disease also entails passing a subspecialty examination.

Neurology and Child Neurology

In many settings, neurologists are among the more frequent referral sources for members of our profession. Certain speech, language, and hearing disorders may be symptomatic of specific neuropathies, leading neurologists to consult speech-language pathologists and audiologists in establishing diagnoses. When neurologic disorders are irreversible, neurologists often initiate rehabilitation programs that may include speech, language, and hearing services.

Certification in neurology requires 4 years of postgraduate training. One year, usually the first, is spent in a program providing general medical care to children and/or adults (i.e., a program in internal medicine, pediatrics, or family practice). The 3 remaining years are spent in residency training in neurology. The American Board of Psychiatry and Neurology administers both written and oral examinations to candidates following completion of their postgraduate training.

Subspecialization in child neurology involves completion of 1 year in a regular pediatric residency, 1 year in a psychiatry residency, and 2 years of study of the basic neurologic sciences and of the clinical management of children with neurologic problems.

Otolaryngology and Head and Neck Surgery

Although not necessarily the medical specialty most frequently interrelating with speech-language pathology and audiology, otolaryngology has been closely identified with the development of our field. Many medical center-based speech, language, and hearing services facilities were established under the auspices of departments of otolaryngology. Audiologists are frequently employed by otolaryngology departments or groups and by individual otolaryngologists in private practice.

As the medical specialists most often involved in the diagnosis and treatment of ear disease and hearing impairment, otolaryngologists are frequent sources of referral to audiologists and are often consulted by audiologists with reference to clients the audiologists are serving. Traditionally, otolaryngologists and speech-language pathologists have cooperated most frequently in the diagnosis and treatment of voice problems. However, otolaryngologists have broadened their scope of practice in head and neck surgery and have become the major surgical specialists concerned with tumors of the head and neck. Thus, contacts have become routine in connection with the rehabilitation of laryngectomees and of other clients with postoperative deficits that impede speech production. In some communities, otolaryngologists perform primary and secondary surgical procedures on children and adults with cleft palate and other craniofacial anomalies, although this area of surgical practice is more frequently assigned to plastic surgeons.

Certification by the American Board of Otolaryngology and Head and Neck Surgery requires 4 years of training following graduation from medical school. One year consists of training in general surgery, with the other 3 years of training to be completed in an approved otolaryngology residency. An examination is conducted by the Board following completion of the prescribed training.

Neurologic Surgery

Since the first description of differential diagnostic techniques to assist in the identification of sites of lesion in the peripheral and central auditory system, audiologists and neurosurgeons have established cordial working relationships in many medical centers. Some of these audiologic procedures have been abandoned in favor of newer and more direct diagnostic techniques, such as computed tomography (CT) scans. Nevertheless, with auditory brainstem response measurement has come a new era of cooperation between neurosurgeons and audiologists.

Neurosurgeons and speech-language pathologists may also be in frequent contact. Such pathologies as brain tumors and cerebral infarcts that are treated by neurosurgeons may include aphasia and motor speech disorders among their primary symptoms. In other instances, speech and language disorders may be an unavoidable consequence of surgery.

The American Board of Neurological Surgery has established certification requirements that are among the most demanding of all medical specialties. Prior to entering postgraduate training in this field, a physician must have already completed at least 1 year of training in general surgery following graduation from medical school. Training in neurologic surgery then involves a residency of at least 4 years' duration (some residency programs extend for 5 years). A candidate must also complete 2 years of practice in neurosurgery after fulfilling the residency requirement before he or she may qualify for the Board examination.

Plastic Surgery

One of the longer histories of close cooperation between physicians and speech-language pathologists is found in the treatment of individuals with cleft palate. Some of the earliest articles about plastic surgery for cleft palate patients acknowledge that improved speech should receive equal emphasis with improved appearance. Thus, team efforts involving plastic surgeons and speech-language pathologists became an accepted principle. This tradition of cooperation has continued as surgical approaches have developed for the treatment of other craniofacial anomalies.

Certification in plastic surgery also entails extensive requirements. Candidates must first complete 3 years of general surgery before entering a 2-year approved residency in plastic surgery. The American Board of Plastic Surgery administers written and oral examinations to candidates following completion of their residency training.

Dentistry

Among the health professions, none has been more amenable to maintaining cordial relationships with our profession than has dentistry. This may relate to the well defined nature of the relationships. Although some concerns about the people served are shared, there is little overlap in responsibilities. Consequently, questions seldom arise as to where the responsibility of one profession ends and the responsibility of the other begins.

Bloomer (1971) characterized the functions of the speech-language pathologist in relation to dentistry in three areas:

1. Speech diagnosis and professional consultation with the dental specialist.
2. Referral of speech patients suspected of having dental conditions which may currently interfere with speech, general health or personality adjustment.
3. Speech therapy and consultation in connection with patients undergoing orthodontic treatment, the construction of artificial dentures or other dental prosthetic devices, or surgical corrections or restorations.

Dentists, like physicians, are always licensed by the states in which they practice. Although there is considerably less reciprocity among the different states than is found in medical licensure laws, most dental licensure laws exact similar requirements. All states require graduation from a dental school accredited by the Commission on Dental Accreditation of the American Dental Association (with special provisions to accommodate graduates of foreign dental schools). All but two states accept satisfactory performance on the National Board to meet written examination requirements, but some also administer a supplementary written examination. All states require completion of a clinical examination in which a candidate is required to carry out specified clinical procedures. Eligibility for these clinical examinations usually depends upon prior completion of the written examination.

Unlike physicians, most dentists become general practitioners. A 1977 survey showed that only about 12% of the dentists in the United States are primarily engaged in specialty practice. There has, nevertheless, been a growing trend toward specialization in dentistry, particularly in urban centers. As in medicine, specialization in dentistry is recognized by certification awarded by a specialty board. Some candidates for dental specialties complete Master's degrees at the same time they are meeting educational requirements for certification, but others do not. Currently, eight dental specialties are certified: orthodontics, pedodontics, prosthodontics, oral surgery, periodontics, endodontics, dental public health, and oral pathology. Of these, only the first four are likely to relate to our profession.

ORTHODONTICS

Questions concerning the relationships between dental occlusion and speech articulation lead to frequent consultations between speech-language pathologists and orthodontists. Even more intensive cooperation may characterize the treatment of children and adults with cleft palate and other craniofacial anomalies. Occasionally, questions about the effect of orthodontic appliances on the articulation of previously normal speakers must also be answered jointly by the members of these two professions.

Orthodontists and speech-language pathologists have also cooperated in programs directed at correcting presumably aberrant tongue patterns that have been implicated as causes of malocclusions. This area has been one of continuing controversy, and it currently does not represent generally accepted practice by either orthodontists or speech-language pathologists.

Certification by the American Board of Orthodontics requires 2 years of specialty training beyond graduation from an approved dental school. However, a candidate becomes eligible for the certification examination only after completion of 5 years of specialty practice.

PEDODONTICS

Pedodontists, as their name implies, are dentists specializing in the care of children. Speech-language pathologists may contact pedodontists less frequently than some other dental specialists, but this may relate primarily to the comparatively small number of practitioners in this specialty. Pedodontists are usually alert to various manifestations of developmental problems and may be the first to identify speech problems among the children in their care. They are also frequently found among the teams of specialists providing treatment to children with cleft palate and other craniofacial anomalies. Some pedodontists maintain particular interest in the care of developmentally disabled and other handicapped children and may, therefore, participate in the treatment of children with dysarthrias associated with such conditions as cerebral palsy.

Certification in pedodontics requires 2 years of specialized training following graduation from dental school. A candidate becomes eligible for the certification examination following 3 years of clinical experience after completion of his or her specialty training.

PROSTHODONTICS

Prosthodontists are concerned with the design, fabrication, and fitting of appliances to compensate for missing teeth or for other structural defects within the oral cavity. Maxillofacial prosthetics has been further defined as a subspecialty concerned with a broader range of prosthetic appliances, primarily designed to compensate for orofacial tissues removed in the surgical treatment of cancer or lost as the result of burns or other trauma.

Prosthodontists may occasionally refer their patients to speech-language pathologists because of speech changes occurring in conjunction with fitting dentures. Since facilitation of speech is often a major goal in designing prosthetic appliances for people with cleft palate or postsurgical defects, prosthodontists and speech-language pathologists share mutual responsibilities. Prosthodontists may also be consulted by speech-language pathologists about the construction of palatal lift appliances that may improve speech production in some patients with dysarthrias and with specific neuromuscular impairments affecting velopharyngeal closure.

Specialty training in prosthodontics also involves 2 years of postgraduate education. Thereafter, 2 years of specialty practice are required for eligibility for the certification examination.

ORAL SURGERY

Even though there are nationally applicable standards for specialty certification in oral surgery, the likelihood of cooperative efforts between these specialists and members of our profession differs among communities. In some communities, the surgical treatment of cleft palate and other orofacial anomalies may be carried out by oral surgeons. In others, such treatment is considered the province of plastic surgeons or other physicians. In many instances, plastic surgeons or head and neck surgeons work cooperatively with oral surgeons, particularly in the management of maxillofacial trauma. Occasionally, speech-language pathologists may be involved in these rehabilitative efforts.

Oral surgeons must complete 3 years of postgraduate training in their specialty. They become eligible for the certification examination administered by the American Board of Oral Surgery after 5 years of specialty practice.

Nursing

Nurses may well be the health professionals in most frequent contact with the largest number of speech-language pathologists and audiologists. Nurses may be employed in virtually all human services settings—in schools and social welfare agencies as well as in health services agencies.

Nurses are often more extensively involved with the people they serve than are most other health professionals. Therefore, they can be invaluable allies. They may provide important information about our clients and their families and communities. They may assist in developing practicable plans for evaluation and treatment. They may serve as a liaison with the other health professionals involved in a particular client's care. They may facilitate the carryover of achievements in speech and hearing rehabilitation programs into other segments of clients' daily lives.

In both legal descriptions and assigned responsibilities, the scope of practice allotted to nurses is exceeded only by the scope allotted to physicians. Most nurses discharge their responsibilities with remarkable skill, but they may sometimes be called upon to function in areas where they have little training. This situation may exist simply because the nurse is the only health professional present when the particular service is needed. On occasion, speech-language pathologists and audiologists may find nurses functioning within our areas of expertise and responsibility. This occurs most frequently when members of our profession institute new programs in facilities with well established nursing services. When conflicts arise, they can usually be resolved through open and frank discussion and through repeated demonstrations of our potential contributions to good client care.

There are three different kinds of educational programs for the preparation of nurses. Diploma programs are conducted by hospitals or proprietary schools. Associate degree programs are offered by junior colleges. Baccalaureate programs are conducted by colleges and universities. Graduates of all three types of programs qualify for licensure.

All states require nurses to be licensed. Even though each state has established its own licensure requirements, those requirements are essentially similar, so that most states grant reciprocity to licensees from other states. All states have adopted the State Board Test Pool Examination (SBTPE) as their licensure examination. Furthermore, since the majority of diploma and baccalaureate programs are accredited by the National League for Nursing, graduation from an accredited school may be used as a determiner of completion of educational requirements.

Because of the broad scope of practice covered by the nursing profession, specialization has long been characteristic. In the past, most specialization was informal and essentially achieved through experience. Gradually, however, specialty areas have been defined more precisely, and recognized specialty training programs have evolved.

A new concept in specialty training has emerged as changes in the health care system assign some nurses more and more independent responsibilities. This concept is embodied in the nurse practitioner. Areas once designated as nursing specialties or subspecialties are now defined as the province of nurse practitioners. At the present time, however, there is not always a clear differentiation between nurse specialists and nurse practitioners; therefore, the following paragraphs refer to areas of specialization rather than to titles of specialists. Six different areas of nursing specialization are especially pertinent to speech-language pathologists and audiologists.

PEDIATRIC NURSING

An increasing number of specialists in this area are qualifying for certification as pediatric nurse practitioners. These practitioners assume major responsibilities for well-child care, placing them in a crucial position for the early identification of children with suspected hearing impairment and problems in speech and language acquisition. Pediatric nurse practitioners are also being assigned significant responsibilities in the evaluation and care of children with complex physical and behavioral problems, making them important allies to all professionals who provide services to children.

Neonatal nursing is a further subspecialization of pediatric nursing. (It is also defined as an area of specialization for nurse practitioners.) Neonatal nursing specialists may provide the key for identifying infants who are at risk for hearing impairments or for problems in speech and language acquisition. They usually carry major responsibilities when hearing screening programs are carried out in newborn nurseries. In caring for newborns with cleft palate, they may participate with the speech-language pathologist in parent counseling programs and provide specific instruction when special feeding techniques are required.

PUBLIC HEALTH NURSING

These specialists may also be referred to as community health nurses. They represent one of the earliest specialties within the nursing profession. Throughout our health care system, most providers expect consumers to come to the offices or institutions where they deliver their services. Public health nurses, on the other hand, have a long tradition of going wherever their services are required: into homes, neighborhood centers, schools, or wherever they are needed. Typically, they are as much concerned with health maintenance and disease prevention as with the treatment of illness.

Public health nurses may play a pivotal role in the identification and treatment of children and adults with communicative disorders, referring them to sources of assistance, offering essential information to the professionals who will provide that assistance, and contributing whatever follow-up and follow-along services are required. In some settings, usually after completing special training in audiometry, public health nurses conduct hearing screening tests. They also work closely with the members of our profession who provide home care services, since most home health agencies assign major responsibilities to these nurses.

Public health nurses may achieve their specialization merely on the basis of work experience in a public health setting. Many, however, have completed graduate programs, often leading to a Master's degree. Recently, curricula have developed for the preparation of community health nurse practitioners; these curricula lead to certification and may also lead to a Master's degree.

SCHOOL NURSING

Of all nursing specialists, school nurses have the longest history of cooperative relationships with speech-language pathologists and audiologists. In virtually all communities, school nurses are designated as the liaison between the educational system and the health care system. Some school districts require that all contacts between speech, language, and hearing specialists and physicians or other health care providers be effected through a school nurse. Even when more direct communication is customary, school nurses often participate in these consultations. Some local education agencies also mandate, or at least recommend, the participation of school nurses in the preparation of the Individualized Educational Programs prescribed by Public Law 94-142.

School nurses have traditionally carried major responsibilities for hearing screening programs. They may conduct the tests themselves or may supervise testing conducted by audiometrists. Even when hearing screening programs involve audiologists, school nurses may coordinate referrals for follow-up evaluations and treatment.

Again, specialists in school nursing may be so designated merely on the basis of being a nurse employed in the schools. Sometimes school nurse services are provided by public health nurses, who may either be employed by the school districts or assigned by a city, county, or state health agency. Some are identified as school nurse practitioners after completing special graduate education, sometimes leading to a Master's degree. Individual states may require school nurses to qualify for special credentials offered by their education agencies.

OCCUPATIONAL HEALTH NURSING

The principal contacts between occupational health or industrial nurses and members of our profession involve audiologists. These nurses may be assigned responsibilities in industrial hearing conservation programs. They may be essentially responsible for these programs, including the conduct of hearing tests, or they may supervise the hearing testing conducted by support personnel. When programs are conducted by, or under the supervision of, audiologists, industrial nurses may provide liaison with other aspects of the occupational health program.

As with other specialties, some occupational health nurses claim that title merely on the basis of employment. Others, however, have completed special training, sometimes holding the certificate awarded by the American Board of Occupational Nurses, which signals completion of specialized studies, 5 years of experience in occupational nursing, and passing an examination.

GERONTOLOGIC NURSING

This specialty has emerged as one further facet of concern for the care of older people. Speech-language pathologists and audiologists may work with gerontologic nurses in virtually any inpatient or outpatient center that specializes in the delivery of care to senior citizens.

An increasing number of nurses are completing the graduate education required for certification as gerontologic nurse practitioners. This new specialty is a welcome addition to the field of gerontology because the needs of older people have been inadequately served by most health care institutions.

REHABILITATION NURSING

Particularly within inpatient rehabilitation facilities, nurses have developed special areas of expertise relating to the needs of disabled children and adults. They not only provide the kind of nursing care that typifies any inpatient facility, they may also coordinate treatment services, assist in the carryover of their patients' therapeutic achievements into daily routines, and participate in family counseling and discharge planning. Specialization in rehabilitation nursing has not received the formal recognition of some other specialties. Nevertheless, many rehabilitation nurses have received special postgraduate training through schools of nursing and through various continuing education programs.

Other Health Care Professions

Two other broad groups of health care providers deserve mention. The first consists of professions that are licensed to provide, independently, a wide range of primary health care services. Although states differ, some have enacted licensure laws that assign these professions scopes of practice which are similar to medicine. Osteopathy and chiropractic, although substantially different from each other in the required level of professional preparation and treatment modalities employed, are the most prominent examples of this group of health care providers.

In many respects, the diagnostic and treatment approaches employed by osteopaths resemble those employed by physicians holding M.D. degrees. Some states have even eliminated special licensure for osteopaths and granted the same licenses offered to other physicians.

Chiropractors, however, are always licensed separately on the basis of educational backgrounds that differ substantially from medical education. Many of the practices of chiropractors are unique and derive from unproven theories about physiologic processes and about the nature of disease. Speech-language pathologists and audiologists sometimes face difficult situations when clients are receiving chiropractic treatment for communicative disorders. Such situations are particularly difficult when the chiropractic treatment is administered instead of needed medical treatment.

Although speech-language pathologists and audiologists who work in most health care settings seldom interact with members of these professions, those who work in schools, in community agencies, or in private practice may see clients under osteopathic or chiropractic care. Virtually all public and private third-party payers permit osteopaths to certify the need for speech-language pathology and audiology services. Some regulations may also grant that right to chiropractors.

The second—and very different—group of health professions represents new fields of specialization that have developed out of the broadening scope of the health care system. Of this group, the one of greatest significance to our profession is industrial hygiene. Industrial hygienists conduct programs in industry to measure and help control, eliminate, and prevent occupational hazards and diseases, entailing direct relationships with audiologists who work in industry. The American Industrial Hygiene Association awards certification to individuals who have completed specified educational, practical, and examination requirements.

THE EDUCATION PROFESSIONS

It is difficult to discuss the education professions in any sort of parallel context to other human services professions since they employ such different approaches to defining professional qualifications and describing scopes of professional practice. Other professions seek national consistency, but qualifications for the education professions are defined independently by each state. There may even be major differences in the scope of practice assigned to a particular profession among communities within the same state. For example, although some local education agencies charge speech-language pathologists with responsibilities for children with severe oral language deficits, others assign those responsibilities to learning disabilities specialists.

Definitional problems are further compounded by frequent modifications in state education laws and regulations. Statements of professional qualifications, scopes of practice, and even legal designations of professional personnel are more likely to be changed at regular intervals than they are in any other area of human services. Hence, in any discussion of the education professions, the writer's terminology must be translated by readers into the terminology that is used within their own communities. In this discussion, I am using a simple two-part classification of the education professions, essentially based on the approach taken in Public Law 94-142 (recognizing this legislation as subject to change, as is any legislation).

The first group is designated as providers of instructional services, comprising the professions primarily devoted to services that emphasize student advancement within the school curriculum. The second group is designated as providers of related services. These professions are concerned with specific areas of intervention. The intervention may have substantial implications for the delivery of instructional services, but the goals need not be restricted to matters directly related to educational achievement. These related professional services may emphasize improved function in specific areas (better communication, better motor coordination, etc.), improved physical or mental health, more regular school attendance, or the resolution of social problems.

It may be ironic to use this classification of the education professions in a book concerned with the delivery of speech, language, and hearing services, since speech-language pathology is the one profession that cannot be so classified. Speech-language pathologists may provide both instructional and related services, depending upon the needs of particular children and upon the programs in which the speech-language pathologist is assigned. This peculiar characteristic of our profession leads to chronic confusion at local, state, and national levels.

Providers of Instructional Services

Providers of instructional services—classroom teachers and resource specialists—represent the education professionals most frequently contacted by speech-language pathologists and audiologists employed in school settings. These professionals, after all, carry the central burden of the nation's educational system: the preparation of students for ultimate participation in society. Therefore, their services form the core of the educational program provided for any single student.

For practical purposes, instructional services are divided into regular education services and special education services, although precise differentiations among these services are impossible. Ostensibly, regular educational services assume that, with some accommodation of individual differences, children can achieve educationally by means of curricula and teaching strategies that meet the needs of most other children. On the other hand, special educational services assume that, because of sensory, motor, or cognitive impairment, language disability, or some other special problem, a child requires different educational strategies or modifications of curricula if he or she is to achieve academically.

PROVIDERS OF REGULAR INSTRUCTIONAL SERVICES

This professional group essentially consists of "regular classroom teachers." Classroom teachers are the major source of referral to most school speech, language, and hearing specialists. Since they spend more time with children than any other education professional, they may be the most valuable source of information about children's communication and communication-related behaviors. By the same token, as the professionals most likely to be present when a child attempts communication, their understanding of his or her communicative disorders and of effective approaches to facilitating communication can be crucial.

With increased expertise in language processes and behaviors, school speech, language, and hearing specialists have expanded their consultative services to classroom teachers. In addition to consulting about individual children, they also offer advice about curriculum development and teaching strategies for all children.

The roles and responsibilities of regular classroom teachers have seen many modifications in recent years. Particularly in urban school districts, there has been a significant increase in the heterogeneity of children's social and linguistic backgrounds as a result of desegregation programs and of accelerated immigration from Third World nations. At the same time, there has been a marked shift in special education philosophy that has resulted in "mainstreaming" more and more handicapped children into regular classrooms. These trends, which have also occurred during an era of increasing class sizes, have simultaneously limited teachers' capacities for providing special assistance to individual children and increased significantly their needs for consultative services.

PROVIDERS OF SPECIAL INSTRUCTIONAL SERVICES

This group includes the professionals once referred to as special class teachers or special educators. Traditional classifications of special education teachers are based on the major disability of the children served, with disabilities defined within a medical diagnostic model. This approach is illustrated in the *Allied Health Glossary of Occupational Titles* published by the American Society of Allied Health Professions (1977). The section entitled "Health Related Teacher Preparation" contains the following occupational titles:

Teacher of the Deaf: Adapts methods and curricula in the teaching of special skills, elementary, and secondary school subjects to deaf and hard-of-hearing pupils.

Teacher of the Emotionally Disturbed: Conducts educational programs for emotionally disturbed pupils.

Teacher of the Learning Disabled: Develops and implements educational programs to assist children in overcoming or compensating for learning disabilities such as aphasia, dyslexia, or other related problems.

Teacher of the Mentally Retarded: Develops and implements educational programs for trainable or educable mentally retarded persons according to the pupil's level of learning.

Teacher of the Physically Handicapped: Develops and implements academic and recreational programs for handicapped persons after evaluating the physical limitations, abilities, and needs of the individuals.

Teacher of the Visually Handicapped: Teaches academic and practical skills to the blind or visually handicapped through the use of Braille or other specialized methods.

Teacher of Special Education—Not Elsewhere Classified: Develops and implements educational programs suited to the needs of students with physical disabilities, mental retardation, or emotional disturbances.

The serious shortcomings of this approach to professional designation are immediately apparent in the lack of parallelism of the definitions. It provides neither adequate definition of the scope of professional practice nor a reasonable basis for determining the expertise that characterizes a particular profession. In recognition of these shortcomings, some educators have proposed more rational classifications of teachers offering special instructional services. These classifications are based upon the expertise of the teachers rather than upon arbitrary categorizations of the children they serve. In some respects, however, efforts toward achieving more rational designations of special teachers were set back by the enactment of Public Law 94-142. In defining categories of handicapped children covered by the act, the authors reverted to a conventional taxonomy: mentally retarded, hard of hearing, deaf, speech impaired, visually handicapped, seriously emotionally disturbed, orthopedically impaired, other health impaired, deaf-blind, multihandicapped, and those having specific learning disabilities. Although the promulgators of this legislation insisted that it should not define the areas of professional specialization involved in the delivery of services to these children, such protestations defy our accepted national practice of assuming that definitions of areas of service simultaneously effect definitions of the professional specialists who provide those services.

An excellent example of the flaws in current classifications emerges when one attempts to answer the question, "Who is expert in providing special instructional services for children with problems in language acquisition?" Even though language problems are prevalent and may have devastating educational consequences, most classifications of special education professionals offer no answer to this question. At the present time, however, no immediate changes in the classification of special education professionals seem likely.

Speech, language, and hearing specialists relate to virtually all providers of special instructional services. Because of frequent confusions with respect to scopes of practice, two groups merit particular discussion: learning disabilities specialists and specialists in education of the hearing impaired.

Learning disabilities specialists represent one of the newer groups among providers of special instructional services. In 1967, the National Advisory Committee on Handicapped Children (NACHC) published what became the generally applied definition of learning disabilities. That definition was quoted in ASHA's *Position Statement on Learning Disabilities* (1976):

> Children with special learning disabilities exhibit a disorder in one or more of the basic psychological processes involved in understanding or in using spoken or written language. These may be manifested in disorders of listening, thinking, talking, reading, writing, spelling or arithmetic. They include conditions which have been referred to as perceptual handicaps, brain injury, minimal brain dysfunction, dyslexia, developmental aphasia, etc. They do not include learning problems which are due primarily to visual, hearing, or motor handicaps, to mental retardation, emotional disturbances, or to economic disadvantage.

The development of public and private programs for children with learning disabilities was accelerated by the inclusion of this category, defined according to the NACHC statement, in Public Law 94-142. Subsequently, virtually all states developed special education programs to serve these children.

Recognizing the shortcomings of the NACHC definition of learning disabilities, the National Joint Committee for Learning Disabilities (NJCLD), comprising representatives of six concerned organizations (including the American Speech-Language-Hearing Association), recommended adoption of a revised definition in a report written in 1981:

> Learning disabilities is a generic term that refers to a heterogeneous group of disorders manifested by significant difficulties in the acquisition and use of listening, speaking, reading, writing, reasoning or mathematical abilities. The disorders are intrinsic to the individual and presumed to be due to central nervous system dysfunction.
>
> Even though a learning disability may occur concomitantly with other handicapping conditions (e.g., sensory impairment, mental retardation, social and emotional disturbance) or environmental influences (e.g., cultural differences, insufficient/inappropriate instruction, psychogenic factors), it is not the direct result of those conditions or influences.

The learning disabilities movement again illustrates that defining a new area of human services also entails developing a profession to provide those services. At the time the definition of learning disabilities was formulated, there were no laws or regulations defining credential standards and few college or university programs for the preparation of such specialists. Most learning disabilities specialists were designated by administrative fiat ("Ms. Jones, next year you will be our learning disabilities specialist.") or on the basis of self-identification. Some of these newly created specialists had relevant training and experience, but many did not.

Gradually, state teacher credentialing programs have been developed and training programs instituted. However, at least two serious problems remain. First, the broad scope of practice implied by the fundamental definition of learning disabilities defies adequate preparation within any practicable curriculum and makes discrete definitions of credential requirements virtually impossible. Second, the field of learning disabilities has grown out of a very shallow research base. As a result, it has been inordinately influenced by faddism, cultism, and various political expediencies. This problem may ultimately be resolved by a steadily expanding body of scholarly literature.

Without denying the problems that have characterized the field of learning disabilities, one should also recognize its contributions. It has achieved virtually universal recognition that many children have specific deficits that impede their academic learning. Furthermore, the field has promulgated an awareness that children differ in their responses to different teaching-learning strategies and that no single methodology or teaching approach will reach all children.

Potential areas for cooperation—and at least equally likely potential confusions of professional responsibilities between learning disabilities specialists and speech-language pathologists—are easily recognizable in the NACHC definition. These areas come into even sharper focus in reviewing the *Competencies for Teachers of Learning Disabled Children and Youth* published in 1978 by the Division of Children with Learning Disabilities of the Council for Exceptional Children (now the Council on Learning Disabilities). This document specified that learning disabilities specialists should be competent to provide services to children with problems in the production and comprehension of oral language—services that are usually provided by speech-language pathologists. Among these competencies were, "Can develop, use and interpret informal assessment instruments in the areas of phonology, semantics, and syntax"; "Can diagnose the language impairments associated with the conditions of aphasia, hearing impairment, cerebral palsy, and brain injury"; and "Can plan and implement a remedial language program which is specifically designed for individualized use which interrelates all areas of language comprehension and production." Incidentally, these competencies were only a few items on an exhaustive list that included expertise in every segment of the academic curriculum, familiarity with all major theories of learning and child development, and expertise in behavioral management, career and vocational education, and educational planning and administration.

In specific work situations, conflicts between learning disabilities specialists and speech-language pathologists have been considerably fewer than might be expected on the basis of published statements such as the competencies inventory. In most instances, because of the formidable range of their assigned responsibilities, learning disabilities specialists are grateful for whatever assistance a speech-language pathologist can provide. The most serious problems arise when administrators and school boards assume from the outlandish claims in these published statements that learning disabilities specialists can obviate the need for other specialists, including speech-language pathologists. The learning disabilities specialist, then, can be perceived as the long-sought-after, all-purpose specialist who can provide both primary instructional services and most related services to a substantial segment of the school population.

Specialists in education of the hearing impaired may well claim the longest tradition of all special educators. This field is unique in other respects as well. Until comparatively recently, most teachers of hearing-impaired children were trained in residential schools for the deaf. Although most of these professional education programs were affiliated with colleges and universities, some were essentially autonomous. Beginning in the middle of this century, the pattern shifted so that most training programs are now conducted within college and university special education departments, with residential and day school programs offering practicum experiences. (However, some of the oldest and most respected residential school-based training programs have continued.)

A further unique attribute of this area of special education is evident in its efforts to establish national standards for professional qualifications. Although each state has established its own credential requirements, many teachers also qualify for the certificate offered by the Convention of American Instructors for the Deaf. The Convention standards have also served as a model for many state credential programs, achieving greater interstate consistency than is found in many areas of special education.

The most obvious interrelationships between specialists in education of the hearing impaired and members of our profession are found in audiology. In fact, many early leaders in the field of audiology came from this area of special education.

Joint committees representing the American Speech-Language-Hearing Association and the Conference of Executives of American Schools for the Deaf have prepared several reports addressing areas of mutual interest. These reports typically assign to audiologists such responsibilities as: assessment of children's hearing problems; selection of appropriate amplification and ongoing monitoring of that amplification; appraisal and monitoring of acoustic features in classrooms to facilitate the use of amplification; interpretation of audiologic findings and recommendations to teachers; in-service education for teachers to promote understanding of the implications of hearing levels for teaching and of the optimal use of residual hearing; and counseling parents regarding audiologic findings and recommendations.

Teachers of hearing-impaired children may, in turn, be invaluable resources for audiologists. Their observations of children may form an important basis for the formulation of diagnostic conclusions. Their evaluations of children's responses to amplification can be extremely important. Furthermore, their vigilance in discerning behavioral changes may be the best approach to identifying children who require reassessment.

As in all areas of interprofessional endeavor, problems have occurred. Kopp (1967) identified some sources of these problems in the form of "limitations," including: (1) limitations imposed by failure to delimit the role assumed either by the audiologist or by the teacher on the basis of professional preparation and experience rather than on the basis of exigencies of particular situations; (2) limitations imposed by real or assumed differences in levels of professional preparation and experience; (3) limitations imposed by geographic separation, making direct interaction difficult; (4) limitations imposed by disparities between clinical evaluation and classroom assessment; and (5) limitations imposed by failure to encourage joint evaluations of children, resulting in the problems arising from "one-shot diagnoses."

Recent years have seen the amelioration of many areas of potential conflict between audiologists and teachers of the hearing impaired. This probably reflects reductions in many of the limitations Kopp identified. As more and more audiologists have been employed in educational programs, there has been better definition of areas of separate and mutual responsibilities. Teachers of the hearing impaired have become increasingly expert in the optimal use of amplification in education. At the same time, audiologists have acquired sufficient experience to recognize that, even with the best teaching, amplification yields limited benefits for many children, and consequently they have been less inclined toward zealotry. In general, then, although some interprofessional problems still arise, they are overshadowed by a predominant atmosphere of cordiality and cooperation.

Interrelationships between speech-language pathologists and specialists in education of the hearing impaired have attracted less attention but may be no less important. Speech-language pathologists, particularly in school settings, have carried substantial responsibilities for hearing-impaired children, providing speech correction and improvement, language instruction, and aural rehabilitation services. Speech-language pathologists usually serve children primarily assigned to regular classes, hence children with mild to moderate hearing impairments. Sometimes, however, speech therapy services are provided to children placed in special classes for the hearing impaired.

Providers of Related Services

Providers of related services are essentially members of the health professions, rehabilitation professions, and mental health and social services professions discussed in other sections of this chapter. In many instances, qualifications to provide these related services are defined primarily by state licensure, even though some sort of cursory certification by the state education agency may also be required. This is true of physicians, nurses, and physical therapists serving school programs. Other providers of related services are recognized by school credentials that do not entail either state licensure or national certification. Speech-language pathologists and psychologists are usually included in this group.

Regardless of the method used for recognizing these providers of related services, their scope of practice may be essentially similar to that pursued in any setting. Therefore, no special discussion of these professions is required within this general consideration of the education professions.

THE REHABILITATION PROFESSIONS

The rehabilitation professions are among the youngest of all human services professions. Some began to emerge as areas of professional specialization during World War I, but most developed during World War II and during the years immediately thereafter. Several rehabilitation professions can be defined, but only the four major ones will be considered here.

Physical Medicine and Rehabilitation

Physicians who specialize in physical medicine and rehabilitation are sometimes called physiatrists. The American Board of Physical Medicine and Rehabilitation is among the newest of the medical specialty boards. Certification requirements include the completion of 1 year of postgraduate training that offers general experience in dealing with acute medical and surgical problems, followed by 2 years of specialty training. Following completion of this postgraduate program, a candidate may register for the first part of the certification examination. The second part may be completed after 1 year of full-time specialty practice.

Physical medicine and rehabilitation is the medical specialty devoted to the planning, supervision, and coordination of programs for physical restoration of disabled children and adults. These specialists are likely to emphasize the recovery of mobility, but they may also be concerned with other aspects of rehabilitation. Most physiatrists practice in such institutional settings as hospitals and rehabilitation centers, but some engage in independent private practice.

Our professions are most likely to work together in the treatment of children and adults with neurologic or orthopedic problems that produce limitations both in mobility and communication. These include cerebral palsy, hemiplegias following cerebrovascular accidents, quadriplegias with vocal disturbances associated with respiratory disorders, and such degenerative diseases as multiple sclerosis and parkinsonism.

Some special problems may characterize our relationships with physiatrists. Physical therapy and occupational therapy, professions with which we may be closely associated in rehabilitation settings, may offer their services on the basis of written medical prescriptions. Yet in customary practice, and indeed according to our ethical standards, we do not yield the responsibility for determining the nature of the services we provide to anyone who is not fully qualified in our field. Consequently, although we are pleased to accept the guidance and counsel of physicians within their areas of expertise, we cannot accept their prescriptions. This situation has led to misunderstandings, particularly with specialists in physical medicine and rehabilitation who are accustomed to prescribing the treatment approaches to be used by physical and occupational therapists.

Several years ago, the American Academy of Physical Medicine and Rehabilitation, or at least some members speaking for that academy, "offered" to assume responsibility for all medical supervision of speech-language pathology and audiology. Needless to say, this offer met with little enthusiasm from our profession and from several of the other medical specialists with whom we work. Fortunately, the subsequent tempest left few scars, and, at least within most individual rehabilitation programs, interprofessional relationships are cordial.

Physical Therapy

Physical therapists have the longest tradition of all rehabilitation professionals. First organized in 1921, the American Physical Therapy Association has represented this profession in the establishment of professional standards and in the definition of its scope of practice.

Physical therapists are primarily concerned with the amelioration and prevention of impairments affecting posture, ambulation, and hand and arm mobility and dexterity. These impairments may be associated with acute or chronic illness, with trauma, or with congenital anomalies.

Physical therapists are employed in a wide variety of services settings. If a health care facility employs any rehabilitation professional, that professional is likely to be a physical therapist. Increasing numbers of physical therapists are also entering private practice.

Three types of educational programs are available for training physical therapists. Some programs offer baccalaureate degrees to students who complete 2 years of preprofessional course work followed by 2 or 3 years of professional coursework in physical therapy. Others offer certificates to students who have previously completed Bachelor's degrees and have completed a 1- or 2-year curriculum of graduate training in physical therapy. An increasing number of academic programs are offering Master's degrees in physical therapy. Some of these programs are designed for students who have previously completed Bachelor's or certificate programs in physical therapy, but others offer basic professional training as a part of the graduate degree program. Virtually all training programs are approved and accredited by the American Physical Therapy Association.

The right to practice as a physical therapist is defined by licensure in all states. There is, however, a high level of consistency of requirements among the various state licensure laws. Many do not detail academic requirements, but simply specify completion of an American Physical Therapy Association-approved training program. All states use the same examination.

Of all rehabilitation specialists, physical therapists have been most successful in maximizing their professional efforts. They have developed notable proficiency in planning programs so that several patients may be treated simultaneously. Furthermore, they have refined the use of aides so that professional efforts are primarily devoted to activities requiring greater expertise.

Physical therapy was once provided only as prescribed by a physician. However, as physical therapists have achieved higher levels of professional independence, the requirement for "medical prescription" has given way to "medical referral" in many settings. Usually, physical therapists develop a written treatment plan for each patient which is countersigned by the responsible physician to signify approval.

Physical therapists and speech-language pathologists most frequently work together in inpatient and outpatient rehabilitation centers, although they may also work together in school programs serving children with orthopedic and neurologic impairments, in home care programs for stroke victims, and in nursing homes and other long-term care facilities. Developmental programs for "high-risk" infants also often include both physical therapists and speech-language pathologists on their teams.

Physical therapists may provide specific assistance to speech-language pathologists: assistance in achieving the best posture for optimal breathing support and control, in stabilizing clients to reduce extraneous movement that may impede communication, and in assessing the motor abilities and optimal range of movement for clients who are candidates for the use of communication boards or electronic augmentative communication devices. In turn, we may be of substantial assistance to physical therapists through offering clues to the establishment of efficient communication with their clients who have speech, language, or hearing disorders.

Occupational Therapy

The scope of practice of occupational therapy may be the most difficult to define of all rehabilitation professions. The practices of occupational therapy focus on the amelioration of problems that impede independent living and social adjustment. Traditionally, occupational therapists have been primarily concerned with assisting disabled children and adults to master the activities of daily living. Occupational therapists have also provided programs aimed at counteracting the deleterious effects of inactivity during hospitalization or institutionalization.

In recent years, some occupational therapists have devoted increased attention to modalities intended as direct treatment of underlying pathologies. Of these approaches, so-called "sensorimotor integration" has probably achieved the widest attention, if not the most rigorous scientific investigation.

The official designation of professional qualification in occupational therapy is the registry maintained by the American Occupational Therapy Association (AOTA). Two routes are provided to meet the educational and experiential requirements for registration. First, academic programs are available within Bachelor's degree programs, as postbaccalaureate certificate programs, or as Master's degree programs. Most of these academic programs involve from 18 months to 2 years of coursework and clinical training. Second, an experiential route is also available to occupational therapy assistants. (Like physical therapists, occupational therapists have maximized the efficient use of professional services through the use of assistants.) After 4 years of work under the supervision of a fully qualified occupational therapist, and upon completion of a 6-month professional level fieldwork requirement, an occupational therapy assistant may apply for registration by the AOTA.

Occupational therapy is one of the last human services professions to seek licensure. Thus far, they have achieved licensure or registration laws in only a few states. In each instance, these licensure laws are based on AOTA registration. Currently, all occupational therapy training programs are accredited by the American Medical Association in collaboration with AOTA.

Like physical therapy, occupational therapy was once provided only on medical prescription, although currently most settings merely stipulate medical referral. Of all rehabilitation specialists, occupational therapists are most attuned to assessing impairments in terms of impact on successful daily living. The speech-language pathologist who views his or her role as maximizing client communication in all life situations can often benefit from the advice and assistance of occupational therapists. Occupational therapists are also expert in the development of adaptive devices. Their cooperation can be invaluable in working with severely disabled clients, particularly when the speech-language pathologist is training clients in the use of conversation boards, augmentative communication devices, or other nonoral approaches to communication.

As the result of their imprecisely defined scope of practice, occupational therapists may be at the center of conflicts regarding areas of professional responsibility. These conflicts may sometimes involve speech-language pathologists. Since occupational therapists are charged with the responsibility of evaluating the impact of disease and disability on daily life functions, communication is an essential area for evaluation. They sometimes attempt more detailed appraisals of speech, language, and hearing than their expertise permits. A recent brochure outlining the contributions of occupational therapists in special education programs included "improved breathing techniques for improved speech" and "enhanced levels of auditory perception to improve academic performance" among the goals of occupational therapy services. Occupational therapists, particularly those who specialize in sensorimotor integration, are increasingly concerned with children with language disorders. Their involvement in programs for these children has created substantial interprofessional problems. Not only is their approach radically different from the approach of most speech-language pathologists, it is also incompatible with the views supported by most recent research in speech and language acquisition.

Like most questions about the appropriate scope of professional responsibilities, apportioning areas of responsibility between occupational therapists and speech-language pathologists is best accomplished in individual work settings. Each profession has unique skills and knowledge to offer their clients and colleagues. Rigid demarcations probably serve nobody well. Through mutual respect and good will, functional definitions of areas of individual and cooperative responsibility usually evolve.

Rehabilitation Counseling

Rehabilitation counselors were once primarily concerned with assisting clients with physical impairments or psychosocial problems to obtain employment. Their activities centered on the assessment of vocational potential, planning and securing vocational training, exploring employment opportunities, effecting job placements, and following clients who were placed to see that they were successful. Although these are still important activities for rehabilitation counselors, many now assume much broader responsibilities. In general, these broader responsibilities reflect concerns that are not limited to achieving gainful employment. As a result, rehabilitation counselors are serving younger clients who have not yet reached the age for entry into the work force, older clients who are no longer interested in employment, and clients who are so severely handicapped that competitive employment is unlikely.

At one time, virtually all rehabilitation counselors were employed by state departments of rehabilitation, usually called Departments or Offices of Vocational Rehabilitation. While a substantial segment of this profession is still employed by these departments, a growing number are to be found in rehabilitation centers, in various community agencies, and, increasingly, in industry-sponsored rehabilitation programs or private for-profit rehabilitation firms.

Currently, although there are fewer nationally applicable standards for professional qualifications for these counselors than for most other human services professionals, the more than 90 programs for education in this profession are accredited by the Council of Rehabilitation Education. Since most rehabilitation counselors have been public or civil service employees, such qualifications were usually defined by specific position descriptions. Formerly a Bachelor's degree was specified for entry-level positions, but, increasingly, rehabilitation counselors must have a Master's degree in their field. Certification by the Commission on Rehabilitation Counselor Certification is being increasingly specified as a condition of employment. Some states currently license rehabilitation counselors, and several are moving toward licensure, often as a part of generic counseling licenses.

Rehabilitation counselors may be major referral sources for speech-language pathologists and audiologists. Our services may be sought in connection with overall appraisals of client rehabilitation potentials, for specific services such as hearing aid selection and orientation, or, occasionally, for therapy services in connection with an overall rehabilitation program.

In return, speech-language pathologists and audiologists serving adult clients may initiate referrals to rehabilitation counselors. Our clients often seek assistance in achieving social and vocational independence despite their communicative handicaps, assistance which is best initiated by rehabilitation counselors.

THE MENTAL HEALTH AND SOCIAL SERVICES PROFESSIONS

Many of the roots of our profession lie within the mental health professions. Before the advent of graduate degrees in speech-language pathology and audiology, many members of our profession completed their degrees in such mental health fields as clinical psychology. Even today, our certification requirements identify work in mental health fields as important, both as background education and as education directly related to specific training in speech-language pathology and audiology.

Although current theories may place less emphasis on emotional etiologies for communicative disorders than was once prevalent, there is no less concern for the importance of mental health in the total management of clients with speech, language, and hearing disorders. Of all areas of our professional interests, this may well be the one with the least distinguishable professional boundaries. Consequently, it may also be the area where territorial disputes are most likely to occur.

This discussion considers only the three most readily definable mental health and social services professions: psychiatry, clinical psychology, and social service. Other professionals may play important roles in the delivery of these services, but it is impossible to establish universally applicable definitions in terms of licensure, certification, or some other specification of professional qualifications. Most frequently, these other professionals are designated as "counselors."

Some states offer licensure to marriage and family counselors. Such counselors may hold degrees and even licensure in psychology or social work, but many come from other fields. Counselors employed by school districts and sometimes by colleges and universities may also be highly competent mental health professionals. Often, however, they may be primarily concerned with providing advice as to academic requirements, career planning, and the like. Many ministers, rabbis, and priests have completed extensive preparation for working as mental health professionals, but others have received little training in these fields. In failing to discuss these various groups in greater detail, I do not mean to disparage their contributions; rather, I find it impossible to propose useful generalizations. When one is searching for professionals to assist particular clients with mental health and social problems, it is usually necessary, in the absence of some form of licensure, to scrutinize the actual preparation and previous experience of anyone who is merely designated as a counselor.

Psychiatry

Psychiatry is, of course, a medical specialty. Psychiatrists, therefore, are first licensed to practice as physicians by the state in which they work. They are additionally certified in their specialty by the American Board of Psychiatry and Neurology.

Specialty training in psychiatry may begin after a physician has completed 1 year of postgraduate training in internal medicine, pediatrics, or family practice. Specialty training in general psychiatry involves a 3-year residency in that field. Certification in child psychiatry is offered to individuals with additional special training following completion of certification in general psychiatry.

Many psychiatrists also complete formal programs centering on particular approaches to psychiatric diagnosis and therapy. A clear example is psychoanalysis, which entails completion of specialized training, usually within psychoanalytic institutes, following satisfaction of the requirements for certification in general psychiatry. (Some institutes also train psychoanalysts who are not physicians.)

In their traditional practice, psychiatrists provide intensive treatment to relatively few patients. Since this pattern of care affords limited impact on the mental health needs of our society, many psychiatrists have explored other treatment approaches. Several have experimented with intensive short-term treatment as an alternative to protracted psychotherapy. Others believe that periodic counseling sessions may afford benefits equal to prolonged intensive treatment. Many work with several patients simultaneously in therapeutic groups. Perhaps the most significant development of all, more and more psychiatrists, instead of providing direct treatment, supervise other professionals, particularly psychiatric social workers and psychiatric nurses, who are engaged in the actual treatment of mental health problems.

In the past, the most frequent contacts between psychiatrists and speech-language pathologists have probably occurred with reference to children and adults who stutter. Of all communicative disorders, stuttering has attracted the widest interest from the field of psychiatry.

Some child psychiatrists have been interested in children with delayed speech and language acquisition. At one time, most psychiatrists perceived this problem to be primarily a manifestation of emotional maladjustment. However, after more eclectic training in child development, many younger psychiatrists now take a much broader view.

A few psychiatrists have shown particular interest in functional aphonia and in other presumably emotionally based voice problems. Others have devoted special attention to the aberrant communication behaviors that may characterize certain adult psychoses and to the communication deficits of autistic and schizophrenic children.

Each of these areas of interest may bring psychiatrists into contact with speech-language pathologists. Some facilities that are devoted primarily to psychiatric diagnosis and treatment now include speech-language pathologists on their staffs. With some notable exceptions, the potential benefits of cooperative efforts between psychiatrists and speech-language pathologists remain essentially unexplored.

Instances of cooperative efforts between psychiatrists and audiologists are even less common. These professions may be mutually concerned when questions occur about possible functional hearing impairments. Furthermore, a small but deeply concerned group of psychiatrists have become especially interested in the mental health problems of severely hard-of-hearing and deaf children and adults.

Clinical Psychology

Clinical psychology and speech-language pathology share the professional characteristics of involvement in a wide spectrum of human services settings. Like those in our profession, clinical psychologists may be found in educational, health care, and rehabilitation agencies as well as in programs devoted exclusively to mental health services. Many psychologists engage in private practice; to some extent their success in this area has served as a model for speech-language pathologists and audiologists.

Psychologists have adopted official designations to identify their areas of special interest: social psychologists, experimental psychologists, physiologic psychologists, etc. These specialties have been identified in a formal taxonomy by the American Psychological Association (APA). That association offers 38 divisions, each focused on a particular area of professional interest. This model is often cited by members of our profession who believe that a similar means should be available for speech-language pathologists and audiologists to identify their areas of special interest and expertise.

All 50 states now offer licensure or certification in psychology. The majority offer licensure only to candidates with doctoral degrees in psychology, although some states offer additional special designation for M.A.-level candidates (e.g., psychological examiner, psychological examiner technician, psychological associate). These individuals must work under the supervision of a fully licensed psychologist. This pattern is based on APA's *Standards for Providers of Psychological Services*, which defines professional psychologists as individuals who have completed a doctoral degree and specifies that all other persons may offer psychological services only under the supervision of a professional psychologist. Training programs leading to the doctorate are accredited by APA.

Licensure and certification standards in clinical psychology are more variable among states than is characteristic of most professional licensure programs. Although academic requirements are similar, clinical practicum and examination requirements may differ substantially. Many states employ the test developed by the Professional Examination Service; some supplement this written test with oral examinations.

Many states, through their departments or divisions of teacher certification, have also established credentials for school psychologists, usually requiring completion of only a Master's degree. Although most state licensure laws exempt school psychologists from their provisions, some offer special licenses or certificates to school psychologists.

Specialization within particular areas of practice can be recognized by diplomas offered by the American Board of Professional Psychology. Diplomas are offered in four fields: clinical psychology, counseling psychology, industrial and organizational psychology, and school psychology.

In many settings, psychologists and speech-language pathologists work closely in the evaluation of children and adults with communicative disorders. Few evaluations of children with delayed language acquisition are complete without an adequate developmental assessment by a psychologist. Psychologists also contribute substantially to the assessment of adults with neurogenic speech and language disorders since information about cognitive functioning may be essential in the formulation of treatment plans.

Speech-language pathologists may also refer clients and their families to psychologists for therapeutic services in lieu of or in addition to speech therapy. Consultations between psychologists and speech-language pathologists may be mutually beneficial. Psychologists may offer helpful suggestions about therapeutic approaches and behavior management. Speech-language pathologists may, in turn, offer advice about the accommodation of clients' communicative disorders.

Audiologists also consult with psychologists regarding the implications of hearing impairment for psychological evaluation and treatment. In return, psychologists may make substantial contributions to the evaluation of hearing-impaired children and, occasionally, to the evaluation of hearing-impaired adults. The field of psychoacoustics, which has its roots in experimental psychology, has been closely allied with audiology, particularly in audiologic research.

Occasional territorial disputes arise between psychologists and members of our profession. Particularly in school settings, questions may arise regarding qualifications for administering certain standardized tests. Speech-language pathologists may question the qualifications of psychologists who conduct detailed appraisals of language proficiencies of children and adults with language impairments. On the other hand, psychologists may question the observations of speech-language pathologists regarding cognitive behaviors and emotional adjustment. Some psychologists, trained in such research-oriented specialties as psycholinguistics and neuropsychology, have engaged in delivering clinical services that may be indistinguishable from services usually provided by speech-language pathologists. Once again, local resolution of all of these potential conflicts is usually the best solution.

Social Service

Although scarcely a new profession—its beginnings extend well into the last century—social service has substantially broadened its scope of practice during the last three decades. In most settings, the responsibilities of social workers once focused on the practical aspects of daily existence and, particularly, on the economics of meeting those needs. While these responsibilities still remain within social workers' purview, the members of this profession have become major providers of a wide range of mental health services. Their responsibilities may differ considerably among services settings. In health and rehabilitation agencies, they may be concerned with overcoming financial obstacles to obtaining needed treatment; they may help patients and families confront and seek solutions to problems created by disease and disability; and they may formulate plans for care following discharge from the agency. In schools, social workers deal with problems in school adjustment or attendance and behavior, and they work with families toward the resolution of these school-related problems. In mental health settings, they may function almost exclusively as psychotherapists. Social workers are increasingly engaging in private practice, usually devoting their major efforts to psychotherapy. They may practice independently or jointly with psychiatrists or psychologists.

The National Association of Social Workers (NASW) has defined four different levels of professional social workers. A *social worker* holds a baccalaureate degree in social work from an accredited program. A *graduate social worker* holds a Master's degree from an accredited school of social work. A *certified social worker* holds certification awarded by the Academy of Certified Social Workers (ACSW)and is considered qualified for the autonomous self-directed practice of social work. Certification entails completion of a Master's degree, followed by 2 years of supervised professional practice and successful completion of the ACSW examination. A *social work fellow* has completed a doctoral degree or substantial practice in the field following certification by ACSW. Training programs in social work are accredited by the Commission on Accreditation of the Council of Social Work Education. Several states have instituted licensure, certification, or registration for social workers, but currently less than half of the states offer such programs.

The field of social service has been generally successful in the development of effective use of paraprofessionals. NASW defines two levels, *social service aides*, who have completed no formal educational requirements, and *social service technicians*, who have completed a 2-year junior college program in social service or a baccalaureate in another field. Paraprofessionals drawn from various minority groups, and who are fluent in other languages, have been used with particular success in many programs. All paraprofessionals must work under the supervision of professional social workers.

Social workers may be invaluable allies of speech-language pathologists and audiologists in many work settings. They may be the best single resource of important information about clients and families. They may offer a wealth of information about community resources, and, even more importantly, about available routes to securing the assistance of those resources. They may be particularly skillful in helping clients to seek whatever services are needed. Clients may more willingly accept referrals to social workers than to other mental health professions since, in the popular view, the acceptance of such a referral does not imply admission of serious psychiatric problems.

SUMMARY

As we speech-language pathologists and audiologists have extended our participation into more and more segments of our nation's human services system, our multiple professional standards have increasingly created some serious confusions. Virtually all other professions offer some single index of who is qualified to practice the professions, but we identify qualified providers of speech-language pathology and audiology services in three different ways: through ASHA Certificates of Clinical Competence, through credentials by state education agencies, and through state licensure.

Our increasing ventures into new areas of human services have also necessitated greater familiarity with the other professions with which we now interact. These include members of the health, education, rehabilitation, and mental health professions. To some extent, our success in cooperative efforts depends upon appreciation of their traditions, educational backgrounds, professional qualifications, and scopes of practice—especially the areas in which those scopes intersect with our areas of professional responsibility. Cordial and effective interprofessional relationships are often essential components of the delivery of optimal services to our clients.

References

American Board of Medical Specialties: *Directory of Medical Specialists: 1981–1982.* Chicago, Marquis Who's Who, 1981.

American Society of Allied Health Professions: *Allied Health Glossary of Occupational Titles.* Washington DC, American Society of Allied Health Professions, 1977.

American Speech and Hearing Association. Position statement on learning disabilities. *ASHA* 18:282–290, 1976.

Bankson NW: Report of state certification requirements in speech and hearing. *ASHA* 10:291–293, 1968.

Bloomer H: Speech defects associated with dental malocclusion and related abnormalities. In Travis L: *Handbook of Speech Pathology and Audiology.* New York, Appleton-Century-Crofts, 1971.

Causey LM, Johnson KO, Healey WC: A survey of state certification requirements for speech clinicians. *ASHA* 13:123–129, 1971.

Division for Children with Learning Disabilities: *Code of Ethics and Competencies for Teachers of Learning Disabled Children and Youth.* Washington DC, Council for Exceptional Children, 1978.

Downey M: Legal developments: antitrust and sunset laws. *ASHA* 21:7–11, 1979.

Grossman DB: Progress and peril; a report on the status of state licensure. *ASHA* 21:1004–1009, 1979.

Kopp HG. Attitudes of audiologists and teachers of the deaf. *ASHA* 9:214–215, 1967.

Nelson SE: Training and certification of speech correctionists. *Speech Disord* 11:205–217, 1946.

Nicolais JP: Summary of 18 state laws licensing speech pathologists and audiologists. *ASHA* 17:99–102, 1975.

Study of Accreditation of Selected Health Professions. *Staff Working Papers.* Washington DC, Study of Accreditation of Selected Health Professions, 1971.

Taylor JS: Public school speech-language certification standards: are they standard? *ASHA* 22:159–165, 1980.

CHAPTER THREE

Speech-Language Pathology and Audiology Services in Different Settings

The roots of speech-language pathology and audiology services lie in such diverse antecedents as the education of deaf children and the instruction of genteel ladies and gentlemen in the refined art of elocution. As our profession has developed, its services have become better focused and defined but increasingly diverse. A major symptom of that diversity is the variety of settings in which we deliver services.

In the United States, the initial development of our professional services occurred in the public schools. Even in those early days, however, a small corps of our profession were found in hospitals and other health agencies, in rehabilitation programs, in community and mental health agencies, and even in private practice. That corps has grown steadily until each of these settings has become an important segment of the total delivery system for speech, language, and hearing services.

Paleontologists tell us that the capacity for adapting to different environments is the best insurance for the survival of a species. Along with our proficiencies in providing essential human services, our ability to adapt to so many different settings may account for the rapid growth of our profession during the past three decades.

SCHOOL SERVICES MODELS

The major impetus for the development of speech-language pathology services in our country occurred during the early years of the 20th century. It emerged as one segment of a growing awareness of public responsibility for meeting the special needs of school children. The first programs for children with speech problems, identified as speech correction or speech improvement programs, evolved in large urban school districts. There is some disagreement as to the location of the first program, but the period between 1909 and 1916 saw the beginnings of school-based speech services programs in Chicago, Detroit, and New York City.

Gradually, state departments of education perceived the needs for such services until, by midcentury, over half of the states had enacted legislation mandating or permitting speech services in their schools. By 1974, the needs of speech- and language-handicapped children were so generally recognized that in enacting Public Law 94-142, the Congress mandated that, to comply with the provisions of this law, a state education agency must provide appropriate services for these children.

There are many popular misconceptions about school speech, language, and hearing services. Prominent is the misconception that all such services are delivered according to the single model of itinerant clinicians removing children from classrooms once or twice weekly for group therapy sessions lasting 20 to 30 minutes. Some school speech-language pathology services are delivered within this model, but it is only one of several models that are regularly employed.

Although changes were well under way before the enactment of Public Law 94-142, this legislation has further encouraged experimentation with different services models. First, its requirement that children be served within the least restrictive environment has encouraged the development of resource specialist programs to provide the supplementary assistance for handicapped children assigned to regular classrooms. Speech-language pathologists are often included among these resource specialists. Second, this law has fostered the development of school-based multidisciplinary assessment services, which usually involve speech-language pathologists and sometimes involve audiologists. Third, in mandating services to such previously underserved groups as the severely impaired and multiply handicapped, PL 94-142 has substantially broadened the populations served by school speech, language, and hearing specialists and has profoundly influenced the models for delivering those services. Finally, this legislation has increased the utilization of nonpublic schools and other community facilities by public school districts. This has enabled school speech, language, and hearing specialists to secure needed consultations and to obtain other services for children that are seldom directly provided by local education agencies. It has also involved speech-language pathologists and audiologists in the delivery of services under school agency auspices but in out-of-school settings. (Under the provisions of PL 94-142, school districts may, in some instances, purchase services for some children from nonpublic schools and agencies.)

At this writing, PL 94-142 faces an uncertain future. Nevertheless, many of its workable concepts will probably be preserved in one form or another. Some of the new services models it has encouraged will undoubtedly survive so long as they remain efficient and effective.

The clearest classification of models for the delivery of school-based speech, language, and hearing services appeared in an ASHA publication, *Standards and Guidelines for Comprehensive Language, Speech and Hearing Programs in the Schools*, first published in 1973. Although its publication predated PL 94-142, most current services models still fit within that classification. Once again, because of the variability of terminology among different states and local communities, readers may need to translate the descriptors of these models into more familiar terms.

Diagnostic-Educational Teams

Diagnostic-educational teams provide comprehensive diagnostic and assessment services and educational planning. Usually, these teams serve all children with potentially significant problems, including children with communicative disorders. All children who are served by school speech, language, and hearing specialists do not necessarily require the comprehensive services provided by diagnostic-educational teams, but such services can be important for children with attendant learning and social problems.

Speech-language pathologists, and sometimes audiologists, usually are included among the members of these teams, which may also include physicians, psychologists, and social workers as well as various educational specialists. Such teams can provide an excellent environment for speech-language pathology and audiology services by furnishing the opportunity to study children from multidisciplinary viewpoints. Furthermore, these teams may have substantial advantages over multidisciplinary teams in out-of-school agencies because they may enjoy more immediate working relationships with the programs that will provide ongoing therapeutic and educational services.

Diagnostic Centers

Diagnostic centers, unlike the teams described above, usually enroll children in diagnostic-teaching programs on a short-term basis. This provides for the longer and more intensive observations that may both illuminate the nature of a child's problems and allow for experimentation with various approaches to the amelioration of those problems. These centers also usually involve the participation of representatives from several different professions, if only on a consultative basis. Ideally, one or more speech-language pathologists should be on the full-time staff.

Current research suggests that standardized tests provide only limited information about children's speech and language competence. Because a diagnostic center affords the opportunity for ongoing observations, rather than abbreviated administrations of questionable testing procedures, it may be unequaled as a setting for evaluations. Continuing observations can also be invaluable to audiologists who are called upon to assess hearing in very young or multiply handicapped children.

Full-time Special Classes

Despite recent emphasis on mainstreaming, most special educators agree that some children can only receive the assistance they need through full-time special class placement. (Such classes usually provide some occasional contacts with children who attend regular classes.) At least during the primary grades, most children with severe or profound hearing impairments require full-time special class placement. In addition, many school districts provide such placements for children with severe language disorders.

Speech-language pathologists and audiologists commonly provide related services to children enrolled in full-time special classes. In some instances, when a class is designed to accommodate children with severe language disorders, a speech-language pathologist may serve as the full-time instructional specialist responsible for the class.

Transition or Integration Classes

As the name implies, these classes are designed to facilitate a child's transition from full-time special class placement to placement in a regular classroom with supportive and related services. Often children spend half the school day in transition classes and the remainder of the day in regular classrooms. Once again, speech-language pathologists and audiologists may provide related services to children enrolled in these classes, or, when the classes are designed to serve children with language disorders, speech-language pathologists may be in charge.

Resource Rooms

The resource room is intended to serve handicapped children who are primarily assigned to regular classrooms but who also require reasonably intensive special instructional services. Usually these programs provide for 1 or 2 hours of daily instruction and tutorial assistance based on the curriculum of the regular classroom. The services provided by speech-language pathologists for children with language disorders often assume the resource room model. Usually resource rooms for hard-of-hearing or deaf children are staffed by teachers of the hearing impaired.

This model has not been fully exploited in the development of services to children with language disorders. These children often receive only supportive services from speech-language pathologists through comparatively brief sessions two or three times a week, which is completely inadequate for the degree of assistance these children usually require.

Regular Classroom Placement with Supportive (or Related) Services

In this model, the child receives most instructional services in a regular classroom. Whatever additional services are required are provided through occasional or regularly scheduled appointments with a specialist. Such specialists may work on an itinerant basis, serving several different schools, or may be assigned to a single school site. This is the most familiar model for the delivery of school-based speech-language pathology services, and undoubtedly the one most frequently employed. Occasionally, audiologists also provide services within this model.

A variety of scheduling patterns have been used. Sometimes services continue throughout the school year. Sometimes intensive services are provided with intervening periods of no services or occasional services. In other instances services provided by speech-language pathologists are supplemented by practice sessions conducted by aides. Each scheduling pattern offers advantages and limitations, so choices must be based on practical considerations and on the particular needs of the children to be served.

Hospital and Homebound Services

The original purpose of hospital and homebound school services was to reduce the impact on school achievement of periods of hospitalization or convalescence. Occasionally, homebound services are used when children cannot accommodate their behavior to the demands of school or, in other instances, when no suitable school placement can be accomplished. A youngster with a communicative disorder who requires hospital or homebound instruction for other reasons might also be served by a speech-language pathologist. Hospital and homebound speech-language pathology services may be particularly appropriate for children who are recovering from cerebral vascular accidents or other insults to the central nervous system.

Parent-Infant Instruction Services

A discussion of high-risk infant programs is included later in this chapter. Such programs are provided by some education agencies as a part of their total special education program.

Residential Program Placement

At one time, a substantial portion of special educational services, particularly services for more severely disabled children, were provided by residential schools. Even though most educators now favor day school placement whenever possible, the need for residential schools remains. Such placement usually occurs when children live in communities where appropriate educational programs are unavailable, when families are unable to provide whatever care children require in addition to their special education, when children require such extensive special treatment that 24-hour care and supervision are required, and, sometimes, when parents are convinced that the best educational program is only available in a residential school.

Many severely hearing-impaired children are still educated in residential programs. Most residential schools for the hearing impaired include audiologists on their staffs. It would be unusual for a child to be placed in a residential school solely because of a speech and language disorder, but many children enrolled in residential schools because of other problems also have communicative disorders. Consequently, speech-language pathologists are frequently employed by these residential schools, if only on a part-time basis.

HEALTH SERVICES MODELS

The early history of our profession's participation in America's health care system is obscure. Clearly the situation was much different than in Europe, where speech-language pathology and audiology have always been closely identified with medical services, and, in some instances, are even considered as areas of specialization for physicians.

Even though, in the United States, our profession initially developed outside the health care system, some important relationships between speech-language pathology and medicine have always been assumed. Three of the 25 founding members of the organization that became the American Speech-Language-Hearing Association were physicians. The first university speech clinic, at Wisconsin, was directed by a physician, although it was administered through the college of arts and sciences. In an article published in 1941, Hawk enumerated hospitals among the settings served by speech-language pathologists, but she also noted that such programs were few and generally were staffed by volunteer professionals. Weissman (1938) surveyed 75 American medical schools and found that, of the seven that offered some speech services, six depended upon the faculty and students of their university speech clinics and one offered services provided by the local school district.

The major embarkation of speech-language pathology into the health care system began during World War II with the assignment of speech-language pathologists to rehabilitation departments in military hospitals. Their services were primarily concerned with the treatment of language impairments caused by head injuries. As the physicians who directed these military programs returned to civilian life, many developed similar rehabilitation programs in university and community hospitals and employed speech-language pathologists on their staffs. As these clinicians became established in hospitals, they soon began to serve a much wider range of clients than those typically served by rehabilitation departments. Eventually, many hospital speech-language pathology programs were reorganized as separate departments.

Audiology has quite a different developmental relationship with respect to the health care system. The two major antecedents of audiology are educational (i.e., the provision of special education to hearing-impaired children and adults) and medical (i.e., the identification and treatment of patients with ear pathologies). Articles regarding approaches to hearing measurement, the selection and fitting of hearing aids, and the counseling of individuals with irremediable hearing impairments appeared in otolaryngology journals during the 1930's. These articles were written primarily by physicians, with occasional coauthors who were educators or psychologists.

Audiology first emerged as an area of professional specialization during World War II, again as a part of military rehabilitation programs. These programs employed personnel with backgrounds in education of the hearing impaired, speech pathology, and psychology to conduct rehabilitation programs for men and women with service-connected hearing impairments. At the end of the war, many of these professionals went on to establish audiology programs that were associated with medical services. Subsequently, audiology services have generally identified more closely with health care delivery than have speech-language pathology services.

Concurrent with the increasing involvement of the members of our profession with the health care system are the far-reaching changes that have taken place in that system. These changes are particularly apparent in the development of new models for the delivery of health care. Many factors have stimulated these changes. First, there has been growing concern for overall improvement in the health care system, particularly with respect to the delivery of services to previously ill served segments of society. Second, health care costs have increased more rapidly than the costs of virtually any other commodity or service, leading to the exploration of more cost-efficient approaches to the delivery of health care. Third, federal and state governmental agencies have substantially increased their involvement in the financing and regulation of health care. Fourth, demographic changes have occurred in the major consumers of health care services; as an increasing portion of our population is found in the older age groups, there is increasing need for long-term care of the aged and chronically ill. Finally, as a result of increased out-of-home employment by all adult family members, and because of the steadily decreasing size of residential units, fewer chronically ill people can be cared for at home.

All these factors have stimulated the development of new models of health care. Such models may be established as separate free-standing agencies or institutions, or they may be component units of larger health care centers. For example, some medical centers provide only acute inpatient care, whereas others provide acute care, extended care, home care, and ambulatory care within different units of the same institutions.

Once again, there are many regional and intercommunity differences in the terminology applied to identify health care programs. In presenting these programs, the terms used are those that seem to be most prevalent, are most likely to be used in federal regulations, or are employed by such official bodies as the Joint Commission on Accreditation of Hospitals (JCAH).

Acute Inpatient Health Care Institutions

Acute inpatient health care institutions represent what most people refer to as "hospitals." They are designed for the conduct of comprehensive diagnostic evaluations (particularly when those evaluations require intricate technology or invasive procedures); for the treatment of acute illness requiring close supervision and intensive nursing care; and for surgery and immediate pre- and postsurgical care. Some, but by no means all, of these facilities also provide obstetric and neonatal care.

As the segment of the health care system that has experienced the most rapidly escalating costs, acute care facilities have been the center of the most detailed studies and the most concerted efforts at regulation. These efforts have produced stringent restrictions on admissions, so that admission is now limited to people who require the level of care and the equipment and facilities available only in this environment. There is regular scrutiny of the length of stays within these facilities, with requirements that patients be discharged as soon as acceptable care can be provided in another setting. As will be discussed in a later chapter, various health planning bodies are also encouraging specialization among acute care institutions, so that costly equipment and facilities are not duplicated in neighboring institutions. The efforts to restrict admissions to acute inpatient facilities have resulted in serious underutilization in many communities. Some have closed entirely; others have adapted these facilities to serve different functions; still others merely operate well below capacity. (Many acute care facilities currently operate with bed occupancy rates averaging 50% or less.)

Few speech-language pathologists and audiologists are employed exclusively in acute inpatient care facilities. We are more likely to serve such facilities when they are components within comprehensive medical centers. Nevertheless, we can render important services as a part of acute care.

Speech-language pathologists may participate in intensive inpatient diagnostic studies, as for example in assessing deteriorating speech and language in children and adults with various neurologic diseases. They may assess the residual speech and language abilities in those who have suffered cerebrovascular accidents, brain injuries, or surgically induced cerebral dysfunction. They may establish preoperative baselines for clients with laryngeal pathologies and craniofacial anomalies. They may provide preoperative counseling, particularly for people facing laryngectomies or other extensive excision of speech-related structures.

Within the limits of short stays in acute care facilities, speech-language pathologists may provide intensive therapeutic services. Such services may involve clients with acute aphasias, usually as an extension of the evaluation process. They may also involve services to laryngectomees, assisting them to master artificial larynxes or other speech prostheses, or introducing other forms of alaryngeal speech.

One of the most important functions of speech-language pathologists in acute care facilities is counseling families of people with newly acquired speech and language deficits. They also provide consultative assistance to other staff members participating in the care of these individuals, helping in the understanding of whatever problems are present and assisting in the establishment of serviceable systems for communication. Finally, speech-language pathologists may play important roles in discharge planning in instances where continuing speech and language services are needed. The speech-language pathologist may be responsible for ensuring that such services will be available in the facility or community where the client will receive his or her continued care, and for assisting the client and the family in solving practical problems that may be encountered in securing needed services.

Audiologists may also make unique contributions in acute facilities. They may assist with intensive diagnostic studies seeking to identify neuropathologies or the origins of sudden hearing loss. They may provide preoperative evaluations when hearing loss accompanies whatever problem is being treated surgically. Occasionally, they may even administer tests during surgery. (For example, pure-tone audiometry may be conducted during stapes surgery, or auditory brainstem responses may be measured in the course of certain neurosurgical procedures.)

Audiologists may conduct or supervise hearing screening programs in newborn nurseries, particularly in the intensive care nurseries for high-risk newborns. They may monitor the hearing levels of children and adults receiving intensive treatment with antibiotics that may be ototoxic.

Audiologists may also provide short-term therapy and counseling in instances where hearing impairment has occurred suddenly in connection with an acute illness. Occasionally, they may serve clients with preexisting hearing losses unrelated to the reason for hospitalization. Sometimes clients decide to attend to long-neglected hearing problems while they are inpatients in facilities that provide needed services.

Long-term Inpatient Health Care Institutions

The earlier noted social and economic factors—the increasing number of chronically ill and aged people, the inability of many families to care for these people at home, and the exorbitant costs of lengthy stays in acute care facilities—have led to increased emphasis on the development of long-term inpatient health care facilities. In most communities, invalids and convalescing patients who are not able to go home are transferred to long-term care facilities (sometimes referred to as extended care facilities) as soon as close physician supervision is no longer required.

The Joint Commission on Accreditation of Hospitals (1979) defines two different types of long-term inpatient facilities, essentially differentiated by the level of medical care provided:

> *Long-term Health Care Facility:* A facility for inpatient care other than a hospital with an organized medical staff, medical staff equivalent, or medical director, and with continuous nursing service under professional nurse direction. It is designed to provide, in addition to the medical care dictated by diagnosis, comprehensive preventive, rehabilitative, social, spiritual and emotional inpatient care to individuals requiring long-term health care and to convalescent patients who have a variety of medical conditions with varying needs.
>
> *Resident Care Facility:* A facility providing safe, hygienic living arrangements for residents. Regular and emergency health services are available when needed, and appropriate supportive services, including preventive, rehabilitative, social, spiritual and emotional, are provided on a regular basis.

Speech-language pathologists and audiologists may provide services within either of these types of facilities. Sometimes they are employed directly by the long-term care facility, but more frequently their services are obtained on a contractual basis.

Children, adolescents, and young adults are sometimes served in these facilities, but the overwhelming majority of patients are older. Speech-language pathologists principally serve clients with language disorders resulting from cerebrovascular accidents, head injuries, and other encephalopathies; with motor speech disorders attending diseases of and other impairments to the central nervous system; and those with speech and voice problems associated with carcinomas of the head and neck.

Audiologists serving long-term care institutions encounter the same kinds of hearing problems found in any group of older clients. They may also serve clients with hearing problems caused by chronic diseases (e.g., multiple sclerosis) or the treatment modalities used for chronic diseases (e.g., irradiation for cancer or antibiotic treatment of individuals with renal failure). Hull (1975) described an audiology program designed specifically for long-term care facilities.

The services provided by members of our profession in long-term care institutions may be of two general types. They may provide direct services in the form of evaluation and therapy for individual clients, and, at least equally important, they may provide consultative services. These services may be directed toward teaching staff members to recognize communicative impairments, and toward assisting them to communicate more successfully with speech-, language-, and hearing-handicapped patients in their care. Consultative services may also be directed toward modifying the environment to facilitate patient comfort and safety, with attention to such factors as the reduction of ambient noise and the installation of visual stimulus alarm systems. Another type of service occasionally provided by speech-language pathologists and audiologists seeks to keep the residents of long-term care facilities alert and responsive to other people and oriented to their environment. Regular sessions are organized in which group verbal interaction is encouraged. Such sessions may actually be conducted by a speech-language pathologist or audiologist or by paraprofessionals or volunteers working under the supervision of a member of our profession.

Ambulatory Care Centers

The ambulatory care center model evolved primarily from the clinics that were affiliated with medical schools or with large city, county, and other community hospitals. The primary objective of these clinics was to provide efficient and economical services to large numbers of people who could not afford to obtain health care from private practitioners. At least three factors encouraged the transformation of medical clinics so they no longer were primarily institutions providing indigent care. First, with the advent of Medicare and Medicaid, many people who previously went to clinics were now able to seek private care. Thus, if they were to continue, clinics had to reevaluate their views of the population they served. Second, new and highly specialized diagnostic and treatment procedures demanded costly equipment and facilities—equipment and facilities that independent private practitioners simply could not afford. Therefore, when these procedures could be done on an outpatient basis, private practitioners began to refer their patients to ambulatory care centers providing these services. Third, the escalating cost of inpatient care encouraged physicians and medical centers to conduct all possible diagnostic and treatment services on an outpatient basis. As a result, many medical centers developed ambulatory care centers to provide services that they had previously offered only to inpatients. In one form or another, ambulatory care centers are probably the most rapidly developing elements of America's health care system.

Virtually all types of speech-language pathology and audiology services may be delivered at ambulatory care centers. Nevertheless, certain characteristics predominate among the clients served in this setting. An obvious first characteristic is that clients are not so seriously ill or disabled that they are unable to be cared for on an outpatient basis. Yet the clients seen in these centers are more likely to present organically based or organically related communicative disorders than are the clients seen in nonmedical facilities. Furthermore, these clients are usually under the simultaneous care of other specialists and departments within the ambulatory care center; that is, few clients go to ambulatory care centers only for speech-language pathology and audiology services.

The speech-language pathologists and

audiologists who work in these centers usually spend more time conducting evaluations and counseling clients and their families than conducting long-term therapy. This situation probably relates to two different factors. First, many people come to ambulatory care centers from distant communities to receive secondary or tertiary care; therefore, extended schedules of regular therapy visits are infeasible. Second, as will be discussed in a later chapter, ambulatory care centers tend to distribute their high overhead costs over all departments, including speech-language pathology and audiology. Consequently, speech, language, and hearing services tend to be comparatively expensive in this setting. When extensive therapy programs are required, clients are referred to other facilities where services are less costly or are provided at no cost to the client. Despite their limitations, however, ambulatory care centers represent institutions within the health care system where speech-language pathologists and audiologists can make important contributions.

Day Health Care Centers

The day health care center represents one of the newest health services delivery models. This model has also developed in response to increasing costs of inpatient care and problems in maintaining chronically ill and aged people at home. These centers are designed to serve people who require long-term care or treatment, but who can, nevertheless, be maintained at home or in minimal care settings at night and during weekends. Typically, they serve people whose families are able to care for them except during normal working hours. Occasionally, they also serve people who live alone or under the surveillance of neighbors, but who require some long-term care and treatment. Clients of day health care centers, then, are transported to the centers each morning and returned to their homes each evening.

Day care health centers serve populations similar to those found in inpatient extended care facilities except that their clients are more capable of some degree of independence. Nevertheless, they present similar communicative disorders and require similar speech-language pathology and audiology services. These centers may represent optimal settings for speech-language pathologists to develop communication improvement and maintenance groups for clients who are not appropriate candidates for individual speech and language therapy. Again, these groups may be conducted by speech-language pathologists or by aides or volunteers working under their supervision. This setting may also present excellent opportunities for aural rehabilitation programs conducted by audiologists.

Home Health Agencies

Home health agencies are designed to serve two different client groups. The first consists of individuals who, although discharged from acute or long-term inpatient facilities, still require care which they cannot obtain as outpatients. Thus, home health agencies provide care during the interval between discharge from an inpatient facility and the time the client has recovered sufficiently to go to an outpatient facility. In other instances, the home health agency may serve clients until no further care is required. The second client group comprises people with severe irremediable deficits or with progressive chronic diseases who, nevertheless, can be maintained at home with appropriate professional care. In these instances, home care may be provided as long as the person lives or until he or she can no longer be maintained at home and must be transferred to an inpatient facility.

Visiting Nurse Associations pioneered the home health care system in the United States. The advent of the home care provisions of Medicare and Medicaid have, however, accelerated the development of new home health agencies. These agencies are typically of four different types: (1) They may be nonprofit community agencies such as the Visiting Nurse Association;

(2) they may represent services provided by city, county, or state health departments or other governmental agencies; (3) they may be programs sponsored by community or private hospitals; (4) they may be autonomous private or proprietary agencies.

Two excellent reviews of speech-language pathology and audiology services in home health agencies were reported by Lubinski and Chapey (1980) and by Hester (1981). The former describes a survey of 206 home health agencies. Of these, 64% provided speech-language pathology services. (This substantially exceeds the Social Security Administration data from 1976, quoted by Hester, showing speech services in only 39% of Medicare-Medicaid participating home health agencies.) In most instances these services were provided by speech-language pathologists employed on a part-time basis or retained on an as-needed contractual basis. However, some home health agencies do employ one or more full-time speech-language pathologists.

Despite the likely prevalence of hearing impairment among home health agency clients, audiology services are infrequent. Among the 206 agencies reporting in the Lubinski and Chapey survey, only 5% provided audiology services. (Thirteen employed audiologists on a part-time basis, six on a full-time basis.)

Although more fully utilized than audiology services, all data suggest that speech-language pathology services are seriously underutilized by home health agencies. One of the most important responsibilities of members of our profession who work in this setting is staff education. Typically, the first client contacts by home health agencies are established by nurses, who then exert considerable influence over the establishment of treatment plans. These nurses should receive a thorough orientation to assist them in recognizing communicative disorders and the potential benefits of speech-language pathology and audiology services. Even better, in some home health programs, speech-language pathologists screen all clients on initial referral.

Although quite different from the usual home health care model, Vaughan (1976) described an ingenious approach to providing home services, one particularly suited to clients living at substantial distances from the institution where they have received inpatient care or to those who are otherwise unable to avail themselves of continued services on an outpatient basis. This approach, called *telecommunicology*, involves services provided via telephone. Vaughan described five different types of direct client services. *Tel-check* consists of "supplementary and reinforcement sessions for the rehabilitation and maintenance of expressive and receptive communicative skills." Such checks may follow termination of regular therapy or intervene between regular but infrequent therapy sessions. *Tel-talk* provides counseling for clients and their families and may complement Tel-check contacts. *Tel-consult* calls include the client, the clinician, and a consultant. Such calls may be particularly useful when a client is being treated locally and the clinician wishes to consult the speech-language pathologist at the institution where the initial evaluation and treatment program was carried out. *Tel-rap* consists of conversations between two or more clients, either with or without the participation of a speech-language pathologist. *Tel-recheck* provides follow-up of patients discharged from conventional or telecommunicology services.

An additional device, which Vaughn calls *Tel-staff*, has been widely used by home health agencies. Here, staff meetings are conducted via telephone, reducing the time spent on travel when the various concerned specialists are located at several sites.

Mobile Health Clinics

Mobile health clinics represent another model for the delivery of services to underserved and hard-to-reach clients. These clinics usually involve specially equipped trailers or vans, which may either function independently or be attached temporarily to another health care or community facility. They have been particularly successful in providing specialized screening services. Most familiar are the mobile diagnostic chest x-ray units operated by the American Lung Association, but other organizations have established mobile screening units for such diseases as sickle cell anemia.

This model has been applied to the delivery of audiology services. Appropriately designed and equipped mobile units have been widely used for hearing screening and, sometimes, for follow-up evaluations and rehabilitation services. These units may be operated under the auspices of state or local health departments, school districts, or various community agencies. A prototype of this model for hearing services can be found in the program conducted by the Michigan Association for Better Hearing. Some audiologists in private practice operate mobile units to deliver contract services to industries and to public school districts.

Neighborhood Health Centers

Neighborhood health centers represent a concept rather than define an organizational model. Nevertheless, these centers may provide needed elements of primary care, especially well-child care, to anyone who seeks their services. In recent years, neighborhood centers have been primarily concerned with bringing services to populations historically ill served by our nation's health care delivery system. They are designed to overcome cultural and language barriers and such practical deterrents as client work schedules and transportation problems, and to focus on the prevention and treatment of diseases and disabilities that are particularly prevalent among specific groups in our society.

Neighborhood health centers may be supported directly by the federal government, by state or local governmental jurisdictions, or by community hospitals and other community agencies. Several neighborhood health centers were established by counterculture groups during the 1960's. These centers often targeted such populations as poor people living in urban tenements and public housing projects, migratory agricultural workers, Native Americans living on reservations or in large cities, newly arrived immigrants, and young people who had "dropped out" of the conventional social structure, particularly those who were also involved in drug abuse.

Thus far, neighborhood health centers have rarely employed speech-language pathologists on their staffs, although there are occasional reports of such programs. More frequently, these centers function as case-finding and referral services; therefore, in their delivery of primary health care they may identify children and adults needing speech-language pathology and audiology services and refer them to other agencies for those services.

Public Health Departments

State, county, and city health departments play diverse roles in our nation's service delivery systems. They attack such disparate concerns as immunization against communicable diseases, maternal and infant nutrition, industrial waste disposal, restaurant sanitation, noise control, and mosquito abatement. The services they provide vary widely in both nature and scope from community to community, from state to state, and from region to region.

Health departments may participate in the delivery of speech-language pathology and audiology services in three general ways. First, they may employ speech-language pathologists and audiologists to provide consultative services to various agencies. Second, they may purchase speech-language pathology and audiology services, particularly services for needy clients. These services may be secured on a contractual basis from local agencies or by the payment of fees for services provided to individual clients. (In most states, Medicaid and Crippled Children Services programs are administered by health departments.) Third, speech-language pathologists and audiologists may be employed by health departments to provide direct services to individual clients. Some health departments provide none of these services, some provide one, and others provide two or three.

Many health departments assume responsibility for school health programs, which may include hearing screening. They may sponsor diagnostic clinics to serve children with such multiply handicapping problems as cleft palate and cerebral palsy. Some provide hearing and speech-language screening services to child care centers, to Head Start programs, and to other programs for pre-schoolers.

The contributions of health departments in the identification, evaluation, and treatment of children and adults with communicative disorders are many and varied. In such states as Alaska, health departments are among the most important providers of these services (Canterbury, 1978). In other states, their contributions to the speech, language, and hearing services delivery system are very limited.

Health Maintenance Organizations (HMO's)

Another services delivery model that has attracted increasing attention in the second half of this century—and may well become even more important in the years ahead—is the health maintenance organization. HMO's may be of two general types. The *prepaid group practice* consists of a multispecialty medical group which usually operates one or more inpatient and outpatient care facilities. The *foundation for medical care* (also referred to as an individual practice association) is based on the traditional model of delivering medical care through individual practitioners and hospitals. Subscribers to the first type of HMO go to the facility operated by the medical group to receive care. Subscribers to the second type see any of the independent physicians affiliated with the HMO in much the same way they would obtain services in the typical private health care system. Both types, however, share the characteristic of prepayment, that is, subscribers pay regular membership premiums that defray the major portion of fees for all covered services.

Some HMO's, particularly prepaid group practices, have emphasized preventive care, presumably as a means of reducing the ultimate cost of caring for their clients. They have instituted multiphasic screening programs which utilize automation and paraprofessionals to provide efficient comprehensive examinations. However, many experts do not believe that these multiphasic screening programs effect ultimate savings in expenditures for health care.

Dowling (1973) wrote an excellent analysis of the HMO model, with particular reference to the potential role of speech-language pathologists and audiologists. A small corps of speech-language pathologists and audiologists are currently employed by HMO's. More frequently, however, when speech, language, and hearing services are included among the benefits available to HMO subscribers, these services are secured on contract from another agency or from a speech-language pathologist or audiologist in private practice.

Industrial Health Programs

The scope of services provided by industrial medical clinics is highly variable. Their services usually fall into two major categories. They may provide some modest primary health care for mild but acute health problems, usually in order to reduce lost work time as a direct result of the illness or from seeking whatever treatment is necessary. Their major services are, however, directed toward the prevention of and emergency treatment for job-related injuries.

Since hearing impairment is one of the more common work-related disabilities, audiologists have made substantial contributions to industrial health programs. Their services in this setting include the conduct of noise surveys to identify potentially damaging conditions; the development of suitable approaches to hearing protection; the planning, conduct, and supervision of hearing screening and evaluation programs; the planning and implementation of appropriate care for at-risk or already disabled employees; and the conduct of educational programs about hearing conservation for management and employees. Several excellent discussions of industrial audiology programs have been published, such as articles by Cluff (1973), Miller (1976), Feldman and Grimes (1977), and Melnick (1978).

REHABILITATION SERVICES MODELS

Diverse events and circumstances have contributed to the development of America's rehabilitation services. Most important have been the forces that spur the initiation of rehabilitation services in wartime. The sudden proliferation of young disabled men and women led a conscience-stricken nation to create programs to ameliorate their disabilities. At other times, the impetus has come when the lives of national leaders are touched by misadventure. This occurred in the 1930's when Franklin Roosevelt's own experiences with poliomyelitis spurred the development of rehabilitation programs for the orthopedically handicapped. Again, during the 1960's the personal experiences of the Kennedy family led that administration to focus on rehabilitation efforts for the mentally retarded.

More recently, consumer activism has become a major force in the stimulation of new rehabilitation programs. This activism was first characterized by the efforts of individual parents and local parent groups. Gradually, these parents formed state and national organizations which both initiated direct services programs and demanded governmental support for new program development.

The last decade has seen the emergence of an even more vigorous movement—consumer activism among the disabled themselves. These consumer groups have rejected many of the parent-initiated organizations as too paternalistic and have formed new groups to initiate programs and to lobby for expanded governmental support. These consumer activists have also prompted equal rights for the disabled as a civil rights issue. Their efforts in this regard have focused on overcoming architectural and other barriers to adequate housing, to higher education, to employment, to public transportation, and to the use of any public facility.

Two not always compatible motivations have undergirded governmental support for rehabilitation programs. Humane considerations are unquestionably primary, centering on the belief that all citizens, including disabled citizens, enjoy rights to life, liberty (i.e., independence), and the pursuit of happiness.

The other motivation, which cannot be ignored, is essentially economic. This motivation derives from the concept that money invested in rehabilitation reduces long-range requirements for welfare support. Crudely stated, clients for rehabilitation services may, as a result of those services, become independently employed taxpayers when they might otherwise spend their lives as public wards. Although this motivation has many merits, it can be exclusionary. Because of age or degree or type of disability, many disabled people will never attain competitive employment. Nevertheless, they deserve the opportunity to achieve whatever degree of independent living is possible. Therefore, an acceptable delivery system for rehabilitation services cannot be centered exclusively on potentially employable clients.

During the decades between 1950 and 1980, concepts of rehabilitation expanded beyond exclusive emphasis on vocational rehabilitation toward broader considerations of rehabilitation for optimal living. As a consequence, new clients, particularly older and more disabled clients, became candidates for rehabilitation services.

The essential differences between health care and rehabilitation services are often elusive. By the same token, distinctions between health care facilities and rehabilitation facilities can be arbitrary. Many rehabilitation services are provided within long-term health care institutions. On the other hand, medical and other health care services may be delivered in rehabilitation facilities. If distinctions can be defined, they probably derive from focus and perspectives. Whereas health care institutions seek the restoration of physical wellness, rehabilitation facilities seek the achievement of higher levels of functional independence.

Although this discussion will consider only institutional models for the delivery of rehabilitation services, such services are also provided by private practitioners. Private practitioners representing different professions often work together in team efforts to effect coordinated rehabilitation programs for individual clients, even though these professionals are not located within a single institution.

As in health care, two or more models can exist within a single setting. For example, many rehabilitation facilities provide services to both inpatients and outpatients.

Inpatient Rehabilitation Facilities

Inpatient rehabilitation facilities generally provide intensive multidisciplinary services for clients with severe, and frequently multiple, physical disabilities. Because of the high cost of care, these facilities usually admit clients with reasonable potentials for eventual physical independence, but who require the coordinated services of several different specialists—services that can best be provided in an inpatient setting. In some instances, clients may also be admitted to these facilities because they require intensive nursing care or more extensive rehabilitation services than are typically available in extended health care institutions.

The cost of establishing and maintaining inpatient rehabilitation facilities has led to centralization, usually in larger urban areas. Consequently, some clients are admitted who might otherwise be served on an outpatient basis if facilities were available in their home communities.

Most inpatient rehabilitation facilities primarily serve adults. Furthermore, their clients, because of the emphasis on favorable rehabilitation potential, tend to be somewhat younger than those who are typically found in extended health care facilities.

Children and adolescents may sometimes be admitted to inpatient rehabilitation facilities. There are, in fact, a few centers devoted exclusively to serving children. Most children are admitted to these facilities for the treatment of acquired disabilities, but youngsters with congenital disabilities may sometimes be admitted after surgery or for the trial of some new treatment regimen.

Most inpatient rehabilitation facilities employ or contract for the services of speech-language pathologists. Fewer employ audiologists, but many arrange for their consultative services as needed.

Although these facilities are sufficiently different that generalizations are risky, they all share some features that dictate the character of their speech-language pathology programs. Clients usually present fairly serious disabilities. Occasionally, their speech and language disorders may be milder when other disabilities have led to their admission. Clients are most likely to present language disorders or motor speech disorders relating to encephalopathy or other central nervous system deficits. Young adults with traumatically induced speech and language disorders are more frequently treated in these facilities than in any other setting.

Another likely characteristic of speech-language services in this setting is intensiveness. Since all efforts are directed at achieving maximum rehabilitation in the shortest possible time, daily, or even twice daily, speech-language therapy sessions are not unusual. Again, because of the cost of maintaining clients in this setting, speech-language pathologists share with every other specialist the requirement to demonstrate objectively, at regular intervals, the effects of their services.

Outpatient Rehabilitation Facilities

Clients who do not require, or no longer require, the level of care or intensiveness of services provided by inpatient facilities may be served by outpatient rehabilitation facilities. Occasionally, these facilities concentrate on a limited range of disabilities (e.g., paraplegics, amputees, severely visually impaired), but most admit any client who may potentially profit from the range of services provided by the facility. Even in these outpatient facilities, the need for multidisciplinary services usually holds as a requisite for admission, but a few clients may be admitted for services from only one specialist. Usually, therefore, speech-language pathologists who work in these facilities serve clients who are simultaneously receiving other rehabilitation services.

Children, adults, or both may be served. Typically, more older adults are served than in inpatient facilities. Because outpatient care is less costly, these facilities admit more clients who require long-term services, clients with poorer prognoses for independent living, or even clients with little potential for rehabilitation who may, with optimal treatment, maintain current levels of function.

Since they usually offer broader programs than typify inpatient centers, outpatient rehabilitation centers often provide both speech-language pathology and audiology services. The communicative disorders served may be quite diverse, although disorders associated with neuropathies again predominate. Outpatient rehabilitation facilities may serve a wide range of clients, from the standpoint of the severity of their communicative disorders. Although they may serve clients with milder deficits than are usually found in inpatient facilities, they may also serve more severely disabled clients with poorer rehabilitation potential. In most outpatient facilities, clients receive speech-language therapy once or twice weekly, although occasionally more intensive programs are possible.

Rehabilitation Workshops

Although a wide range of services may be provided by rehabilitation workshops, this model emphasizes vocationally related independence. These workshops usually provide detailed assessments of clients' vocational aptitudes, interests, and abilities. They may offer training in specific vocational skills, with particular emphasis on adapting these skills to accommodate disabilities. They provide counseling related to vocational objectives, job-seeking skills, and vocational and social adjustment. They may provide work experiences within the workshop and through field placements in business and industry. Some provide long-term employment in sheltered workshops for clients who are unlikely to succeed in competitive employment.

The predominant age group served by these workshops ranges from school-leaving age to the early fifties. Although older clients may sometimes be admitted, the basic emphasis on ultimate vocational placement inevitably favors admission of younger people to most workshops. (When sheltered workshop programs are available, more older clients may be admitted.) Some rehabilitation workshops provide prevocational services for teenagers, sometimes in cooperation with local education agencies. Certain rehabilitation workshops serve specific disability groups (e.g., the visually impaired, the mentally retarded, people recovering from mental illness), but many admit clients with all types of disabilities.

Few rehabilitation workshops employ full-time speech-language pathologists and audiologists. They may, however, retain members of our profession as consultants. Most frequently these professionals participate in client evaluations, addressing questions about the vocational implications of clients' communicative disorders and about their potentials for improved communication. Therapy services may also be provided, but these services are usually limited in scope and aimed at specific short-term objectives. Some rehabilitation workshops refer all clients needing speech, language, and hearing services to other agencies or to individual practitioners. Most refer those clients who will require long-term services.

Independent Living Centers

Independent living centers represent a model that has developed during the last decade, primarily as an outgrowth of the consumer activist movement among disabled people. These centers emphasize solutions to the practical problems that thwart the independence of disabled people—problems in self-care, housing, and transportation. They attack these problems directly through seeking acceptable specific solutions for individual clients and through advocacy of more general remedies. Their activities range from training and referring attendants for the severely disabled, to operating alternative transit systems, to counseling clients about legal rights and representing them in hearings that appeal decisions about those rights, to counseling disabled clients about problems in sexual adjustment.

In keeping with the spirit of consumer activism, independent living centers stress the concept of disabled people helping other disabled people. Many of them feature peer counseling, either on a one-to-one basis or in groups. Wherever possible, professionals are employed who are themselves disabled. Able-bodied professionals are not, however, excluded from employment when they can contribute to center programs. It is too early in the history of independent living centers to assess their ultimate effectiveness or to predict their future growth or distribution. Nevertheless, they represent a healthy trend toward disabled, and even severely disabled, people taking charge of their own destinies. Whatever the future of independent living centers, it is certain that disabled people will continue to assume more dominant roles in planning, building, and conducting rehabilitation programs and services.

At their current stage of development, it would be unlikely for an independent living center to employ a speech-language pathologist or audiologist. This unlikelihood relates to the nature of their programs rather than to the nature of our profession. Thus far, these centers have not offered the kinds of specific evaluation and therapeutic services we provide. When such services are required, clients are usually referred to other agencies.

Independent living centers may represent an important referral resource for speech-language pathologists and audiologists who serve severely disabled clients. Often, they emphasize the self-reliance that so many clients with communicative disorders need.

MENTAL HEALTH AND DEVELOPMENTAL DISABILITIES SERVICES MODELS

Many people would disagree with the inclusion of models for mental health services and models for services to the developmentally disabled in a single category. Combining them does not imply that mental health facilities and developmentally disabled services facilities accommodate similar populations, provide identical services, or share common philosophies. These areas of service do have a common history, and any clear differentiation is a comparatively recent development. Furthermore, while programs now usually direct their services either to clients with mental health problems or to clients with developmental disabilities, the models employed for the delivery of those services are often essentially similar.

Until well into the middle of this century, the psychiatric hospital was the primary model for delivering long-term care to both the mentally ill and the developmentally disabled. Larger states often developed separate hospitals for serving the two groups. Other states housed these diverse groups in different wards of the same institutions. Still others, fortunately few, did not differentiate between the two populations in providing care.

Major changes began during the 1950's, changes that eventually revolutionized concepts of what services were needed as well as approaches to delivering those services. Previously, clients were designated as either mentally ill or mentally retarded, implying significant commonalities between these categories. Clear differentiation between these populations was finally effected through the Mental Retardation Facilities and Community Mental Health Centers Construction Act of 1963 (PL 88–164). Subsequently, the term mentally retarded was supplanted by the term developmentally disabled in referring to that broad category of clients. This usage was formalized in 1970 by the enactment of Public Law 91-517, the Developmental Disabilities Act, which expanded the scope and purpose of PL 88-164. The concept of developmental disabilities was further formalized in 1975 by the enactment of PL 94-103, the Developmentally Disabled Assistance and Bill of Rights Act. In this law, developmental disability is defined as a disability attributable to mental retardation, cerebral palsy, epilepsy, or autism, which originated before the age of 18, which has continued or can be expected to continue indefinitely, and which constitutes a substantial handicap to functioning normally in society.

Once again, it is impossible to distinguish arbitrarily between mental health and developmental disabilities services models and models described in other sections of this chapter. Particularly elusive are the differences between several educational services models and other models for serving developmentally disabled and mentally ill children. In practice, most residential or full-day programs for these children are labeled "schools," whereas essentially similar programs serving older clients are called hospitals, treatment centers, or residential or day care programs.

Inpatient Treatment and Care Facilities

As has already been noted, the dominant model for providing treatment and care to mentally ill and seriously developmentally disabled children and adults once called for placement in inpatient facilities. Most familiar are the large institutions established by all states. Despite increasing emphasis on other services models, inpatient centers still play an important role. Large state institutions remain most typical of this model, but many smaller private and community facilities have been established.

Just as major changes in patterns of care for the developmentally disabled were initiated by the Developmental Disabilities Act, historic changes in the pattern of care to the mentally ill culminated in 1963 with the enactment of the Community Mental Health Centers Act. To a large extent, this act merely reflected changes that had been under way since the early 1950's. These changes were manifest in three areas. First, through discoveries in psychopharmacology, dramatic changes were effected in the problems faced by the mentally ill and by the professionals responsible for their care. Second, the philosophy of the *therapeutic community* revolutionized concepts of inpatient care. This philosophy envisioned the psychiatric hospital as a community of patients, professionals, and support staff working together toward the solution of problems. Third, there was a growing trend toward decentralization of mental health facilities, away from large state institutional models. Out of these developments, then, emerged the programs specified in the Community Mental Health Services Act. The major thrust of this legislation was the facilitation of care within the client's home community. An essential characteristic of the centers funded through this legislation was that each must provide emergency and short-term inpatient care. As a result, increasing numbers of small inpatient mental health care centers have been established in local communities. Most operate in conjunction with general hospitals, but some are components of centers exclusively devoted to mental health care.

Inpatient centers, both those serving clients with mental health problems and those serving clients with developmental disabilities, have changed drastically in recent years. No longer is their primary mission long-term, even lifelong, custodial care. Many now provide excellent diagnostic centers where children and adults are admitted for short-term diagnostic studies to define the nature and extent of their problems and to plan further treatment. In most centers, when a client is admitted for residential placement, it is assumed that all efforts will be directed toward his or her eventual return to the home community.

A notable outcome of the reorientation of these facilities is the involvement of a wider variety of specialists, including speech-language pathologists and audiologists. Most large inpatient centers for the developmentally disabled now employ speech-language pathologists. Because of the prevalence of hearing impairment among the developmentally disabled, and because of the all too common misdiagnosis of mental retardation among children who are actually severely hearing impaired, audiology services are also important.

Inpatient facilities for mentally ill children may also offer speech-language pathology services; however, they are seldom provided in facilities serving mentally ill adults. Surveys have been reported describing the prevalence of communicative disorders in adult psychiatric hospital populations (Jeter, 1976), but, for the most part, this essentially remains a seldom explored setting for speech-language pathology and audiology services.

Day Treatment and Care Centers

Two factors led to the growing importance of day treatment and care centers in the delivery of services to the mentally ill and the developmentally disabled. First, long-term placement in large institutions may not only exacerbate their existing problems, it may also create additional problems. Second, like all inpatient care, the cost of maintaining clients in these institutions is great. Wherever possible, therefore, these clients are maintained at home or in small residential units. Those who require substantial special attention are also admitted to day treatment and care centers. Some of these centers may offer rehabilitation services, and some may even provide sheltered workshop employment.

Typical day treatment and care programs tend to accommodate limited numbers of clients; therefore, speech-language pathologists or audiologists are not usually employed on a full-time basis. However, many programs do arrange for such services, particularly speech-language pathology services, through agreements with school districts, other community agencies, or private practitioners.

Outpatient Mental Health and Child Guidance Centers

The development of outpatient mental health centers was also spurred by provisions of the Community Mental Health Services Act, since outpatient care was a mandated component of all qualifying community facilities. Typically, outpatient mental health services provide initial assessment, followed by therapeutic services when necessary. Although traditional individual psychotherapy is provided, other treatment modalities, such as group therapy and conjoint family therapy, are widely used. These centers usually emphasize preventive care, admitting clients with less severe mental health problems—problems in personal adjustment, parent-child problems, and other family problems—than those who would typically be served by inpatient or day treatment facilities. Most provide crisis intervention and other forms of short-term evaluation and treatment. In recent years, many centers have been particularly concerned with the delivery of mental health services to impoverished clients and to members of Third World cultures.

The child guidance center model actually predates the outpatient community mental health center model. Child guidance centers were established at the beginnings of the mental health movement in the 1930's. In their broad concepts, they essentially resembled the community mental health centers that were to develop later. They provided evaluation and therapy services for children with manifest behavioral problems. Such services involved individual and group programs for these children and their families.

In 1970, a series of amendments to the Community Mental Health Services Act included specific extensions in services to children. Subsequently, although some communities continued to maintain separate child guidance centers, many discontinued these separate programs and integrated services for children into their outpatient community mental health centers.

Interestingly, in an article published in 1941, Hawk enumerated child guidance clinics among the then relatively few settings for the delivery of speech-language pathology services. Although never a major employment setting for speech-language pathologists, some continue to work in mental health centers, particularly in centers emphasizing services to children. More frequently, however, members of our profession see clients from these centers on referral. In turn, these centers may be excellent resources for referral by speech-language pathologists and audiologists of clients who require mental health services in lieu of, or in addition to, the services that fall within the purview of our profession.

Centers for Information, Referral, and Coordination of Care

A further consequence of the movement away from full-time institutional care has been the establishment of community and regional centers devoted to providing information, referral, and coordination of care. Once again, the essential philosophy is that with appropriate support children and adults with mental health problems or with developmental disabilities can be maintained in their home communities. Furthermore, these centers assume that individual needs can often be met by utilizing existing community resources rather than by the development of new facilities exclusively devoted to these clients.

Such centers inform clients and families about the sources of needed services, effect appropriate referral, and assist in coordinating the services provided to individual clients by multiple agencies. They may also directly administer state and federal funds for the purchase of services, or they may merely assist the client to qualify for funding through such third-party payers as Medicaid and Crippled Children Services. Occasionally, these centers may provide some direct services, particularly when those services are unavailable elsewhere in the community.

Since few of these centers provide direct services, few employ specialists like speech-language pathologists, except as occasional consultants. However, they may be invaluable resources to members of our profession who are seeking appropriate referrals for developmentally disabled clients who require diagnostic, treatment, or rehabilitative services from members of other professions.

High-risk Infant Programs

The development of special programs to serve high-risk infants derives from two assumptions. One assumption is based on evidence that the majority of developmentally disabled children are identifiable through factors in family and prenatal histories, or through conditions at birth or during neonatal life (low birthweight, intrauterine growth retardation, hyperbilirubinemia, respiratory distress, etc.). The other assumption holds that healthier development can be encouraged, and secondary handicaps prevented, with early intervention through family counseling, physical therapy, speech and language stimulation, and other special services.

High-risk infant programs generally serve children from birth to 3 years of age. They may be sponsored by public agencies (occasionally including public schools) or by various private nonprofit community agencies. They usually employ teams of specialists including nurses, social workers, physical and occupational therapists, and speech-language pathologists. Services may be provided within centers or by specialists going into homes.

Since hearing impairment may also result from many of the same risk factors, most of these programs have established relationships with individual audiologists or audiology centers. When hearing losses are identified among these children, audiologists or teachers of the hearing impaired may join with the other specialists in providing regular therapy and parent education.

Child Development Centers

Child development centers represent another model for the delivery of services to children with developmental disabilities, particularly in the younger age groups. These centers are often components of comprehensive medical facilities, although some have been established in conjunction with other programs. In rare instances these centers may operate independently. This model also emerged from recognition of the need for multiprofessional participation in the evaluation and treatment of developmentally disabled children. Therefore, although nearly always under medical direction, child development centers usually employ multidisciplinary staffs.

In addition to their diagnostic and treatment programs, many child development centers offer special nursery school programs. As public school districts have expanded their programs for early childhood education of handicapped children, some child development centers have abandoned their nursery schools, while others have continued them in cooperation with or under contract to local school districts.

Virtually all child development centers employ speech-language pathologists to assist in their diagnostic programs, to provide direct therapy services, to counsel families, to consult with other professionals, and to assist in educational planning. Some also employ audiologists, but most arrange for audiology services on contract or by referral.

Facilities for Juvenile Offenders

It may be overly optimistic to categorize facilities for juvenile offenders among mental health services models. Nevertheless, the presumed focus of these programs is assisting young people to achieve the level of adjustment essential for independent living and acceptable conduct in our society. Toward those ends, then, most such programs offer some special education and rehabilitation services.

Speech-language pathology services in facilities for juvenile offenders are of recent origin. They have usually developed out of concern for the high rate of poor academic achievement among their wards. Although many factors contribute to that failure, language problems figure prominently—problems that may originate in deviant early language acquisition, in difficulties in mastering English as a second language, or in culturally based language differences. Speech-language pathologists employed by facilities for juvenile offenders, therefore, may serve clients with all types of communication disorders, but language problems usually predominate.

OTHER COMMUNITY AGENCY MODELS

One of our nation's oldest traditions is that members of a community are responsible for assisting other members of the same community when help is needed. Although this philosophy is most evident in governmental programs, it also characterizes the voluntary agencies found in most communities. Typically, such community programs are incorporated as nonprofit agencies and are governed by volunteer boards of directors. Their services may be partially supported by city, county, state, or federal funds, but most rely heavily on private contributions. Funds may be solicited through appeals to the general public, to individual philanthropists, to businesses and corporations, or to private foundations. Many are supported through united givers' campaigns (e.g., United Way, Catholic Charities, United Jewish Appeals). Others receive assistance from voluntary health agencies such as the United Cerebral Palsy Association, American Cancer Society, American Heart Association, etc.

Understandably, since these agencies have developed to meet specific needs in individual communities, they differ substantially from community to community and from region to region. Commonly, however, founders of new programs study already established programs in other communities. Consequently, many common features are discernible.

Community Speech and Hearing Centers

The community speech and hearing center model is a product of the late 1940's and 1950's. Few new community centers have been established in recent years, but many older centers continue to flourish, albeit usually with substantial modifications. These agencies are generally independent, free-standing programs, deriving their support from local united givers' campaigns, from individual benefactors, or from private foundations, as well as from fees for services. Many initially received federal funds in the form of establishment or demonstration grants which served as the basis for instituting and expanding programs. Often affiliated with universities or housed within large medical centers, they were, nevertheless, essentially independent financially. Many community speech and hearing centers grew out of local chapters of the American Hearing Society.

Probably the oldest, and certainly the best known, of these community agencies is the Cleveland Hearing and Speech Center. Its origins, concepts, and pattern of operation were described by Chapin (1947) and later by Fortune (1958), who was its first director.

These early community centers not only represented an innovative model for the delivery of services, they also expressed what was then an innovative philosophy: that speech, language, and hearing services are essential within a community's human services delivery system, and that such services should be available to all members of the community regardless of age or financial circumstances. For the first time, then, speech, language, and hearing services provided outside of the public schools became an integral part of the total human services delivery system of many communities.

Many factors account for the decreasing use of this model in the establishment of new programs, but two are probably paramount. First, inherent in the model was centralization of services to the communicatively handicapped within a single, and usually separate, facility. Some centers even actively discouraged the development of other speech and hearing programs in their communities. Yet, it has become increasingly apparent that many speech, language, and hearing services can be delivered most efficiently within facilities where a wide range of multidisciplinary services are available. Thus, there has been a trend toward decentralization of speech-language pathology and audiology services rather than toward the development of new free-standing agencies devoted only to serving clients with communicative disorders. In recognition of this trend, many established community speech and hearing services created satellite programs in other institutions and developed contractual relationships to provide their services within other human services agencies.

The second motive for changing the typical community speech and hearing center model has been the increasing importance of third-party payment programs. As the cost of providing speech, language, and hearing services has grown, programs have become increasingly dependent upon third-party payment. Most such payment is intended to cover health care services. Therefore, although third-party payers may cover speech-language pathology and audiology services, their regulations may require, or at least strongly encourage, those services to be provided within a health care institution or medically based rehabilitation facility. As a result, in order to qualify for third-party payment, many community speech and hearing centers have strengthened their alliances with medical centers and other health care agencies. Some have even abandoned entirely their free-standing status to become component units of comprehensive medical centers.

Typically, community speech and hearing centers provide the broadest possible range of speech-language pathology and audiology services. In their services for children, they have tended to focus on preschoolers, although school-age children who do not qualify for school-based services or who require supplemental services may be included. Many provide early childhood education programs for children with hearing impairments or with delayed language development. However, with the increased definition of public responsibility for special education programs for very young children, some of these programs have been transferred to the aegis of public school districts.

Community speech and hearing centers provide diagnostic services on referral from virtually all professionals in a community. Many accept self-referrals. Some centers have established multidisciplinary evaluation programs by retaining other professionals as consultants. They provide a wide range of therapy services involving both individuals and groups of clients. Often, parents of children with similar problems meet regularly in groups for education and counseling. These centers often conduct screening programs within their facilities or out in the community—at health centers, in nursery schools, in senior centers, etc.—to identify individuals who may need further services.

Undoubtedly, the community speech and hearing center model will change even further in future years. It seems likely that such centers will continue toward increasing integration with other human services agencies and programs. Nevertheless, well established community speech and hearing centers will remain an important force in the delivery system of speech, language, and hearing services.

Child Care and Other Early Childhood Programs

No other element of community services has received greater attention during the last two decades than has child care. In a large measure, this interest has been spurred by the many factors that have led more and more women to seek out-of-home employment. Another important catalyst has been emphasis on efforts to "break the poverty cycle" by freeing women who might otherwise be welfare recipients to enter the workforce, and by offering children early learning experiences, better nutrition, and preventive health care with a view to lessening future educational failures and consequent social problems.

Child care centers are often virtually indistinguishable from early childhood education programs. These two program models may differ only in licensure and in funding sources, except that child care centers normally offer early and late day care. In other instances, child care programs function only as the name implies, to provide care with no planned educational experiences. Occasionally, different components are identified within the same program; thus some children merely attend a "nursery school," whereas others remain beyond the end of the school day for child care.

Child care centers are a frequent target for various speech, language, and hearing screening efforts. Sometimes other speech, language, and hearing services are also provided. Chapey et al. (1978) reported surveying a sample of 160 child care centers throughout the nation. Slightly more than half reported that speech and hearing screening tests were conducted in their centers. About one-third reported more extensive services, including speech and hearing evaluations and speech therapy. Fewer offered hearing therapy. Approximately one-third of the centers employed speech-language pathologists. Of these about half were employed full time. The other centers arranged for services from various community agencies.

A massive effort in the area of early childhood services that merits special mention is Project Head Start. (At this writing, the program's future is sufficiently uncertain that the verb may soon change from "is" to "was.") Project Head Start was a product of the "Great Society" movement of the 1960's and was viewed as an approach to lessening the negative impacts of poverty and deprivation. The program first came into existence as a component of the Economic Opportunity Act of 1964. That act provided federal funds for local programs serving disadvantaged preschoolers when those programs met specified standards. The first programs were conducted to serve children during the summer before school entrance. Later programs provided year-round services.

From the outset, speech-language pathologists and audiologists provided screening services to many Head Start programs. [Monsees and Berman (1968) described a typical early Head Start screening program.] As these programs grew, many employed speech-language pathologists to deliver more extensive services. Although fewer employed audiologists, many established relationships with audiology facilities.

In 1972, the Head Start law was amended so that it substantially increased the involvement of our profession. Those amendments specified that at least 10% of the enrollment opportunities in Head Start programs in each state be allocated to handicapped children, defined as "mentally retarded, hard of hearing, deaf, speech impaired, visually handicapped, seriously emotionally disturbed, crippled, or other health-impaired children."

Insofar as our profession was concerned, the primary effect of this mandate was to increase substantially our participation in Head Start programs. A secondary effect was also noteworthy. After this mandate had been in place for 2 years, the data revealing how states met the requirement were analyzed on a national level, revealing that 35% of the "handicapped" children were classified as speech impaired. Officials soon charged that too-broad criteria were used in defining speech impairments and that the majority of these children presented "cultural-ethnic dialects," "foreign language influences," or "developmental articulation errors consistent with the level of intellectual functioning." The alleged overuse of diagnoses of speech impairments led Congress to define, for the first time, what was meant by speech impaired. Although this definition was no worse or no better than most, it is always regrettable when the bases for professional judgments are defined by political bodies. Unfortunately, the fundamental problem remained unsolved, i.e., evaluation by a speech-language pathologist was still not required to classify a child as speech impaired.

The ultimate impact of Head Start and similar early childhood programs remains a matter of controversy. Evidence supporting the contention that graduates of these programs are significantly more successful in their later school years is equivocal at best. Nevertheless, some specific justifications of speech-language pathology and audiology services seem reasonable. Whatever the ultimate effects of early speech and language intervention may be, better future education planning is probably facilitated by early identification. The urgency of early intervention for children with hearing impairments rests on even more substantive evidence.

Priorities assigned to child care and other services to preschoolers wax and wane with vicissitudes in social pressures and political priorities. Nevertheless, it is unlikely that these programs will be discontinued entirely. Therefore, although the level of involvement of speech-language pathologists and audiologists may vary considerably from time to time and from community to community, these programs will surely remain an important setting for the delivery of speech, language, and hearing services.

Senior Centers

The growing number of active older citizens in our society has led to the development of special recreational and educational programs in virtually every medium- to large-size community. Usually these programs are designated as senior centers. They may be sponsored by adult education divisions of the public schools, by city recreation departments, by churches and other religious organizations, or by diverse other civic, fraternal, voluntary, or ethnic groups.

Senior centers may be a particularly effective environment for the delivery of audiology services. Hearing screening programs are often conducted in senior centers, sometimes supplemented by aural rehabilitation programs and other counseling services. Audiologists also offer consumer education programs since clients of senior centers represent the age group frequently targeted by unscrupulous hearing aid salesmen.

Except for occasional special programs for aged clients with communicative disorders that may involve speech-language pathologists as consultants or group leaders, few speech and language services are provided in senior centers. However, speech-language pathologists may use them as a frequent referral resource for older clients who need social contacts to preserve gains made in the recovery of speech and language and to forestall the deleterious effects of isolation.

Self-help Groups

People who share similar problems may benefit from the experience of meeting together. This concept has been repeatedly substantiated by the success of such organizations as Alcoholics Anonymous and Synanon. Various self-help groups have also been organized by and for people with communicative disorders. The oldest of these organizations probably were local affiliates of the National Association for the Deaf and the American Hearing Society (established initially as the American Federation of Clubs for the Hard of Hearing), both founded early in this century. Although the latter organization disbanded, the former continues. Both organizations included family members and professionals in their membership, but their major emphasis was self-help. The Alexander Graham Bell Association for the Deaf is also a pioneer organization; it has been particularly effective in sponsoring self-help groups for parents of hearing-impaired children.

People who share the problem of stuttering have also frequently joined in self-help groups. Sometimes these groups originate in college and university or community speech and hearing clinics, but others are affiliated with no single clinical program. The National Association of Councils of Stutterers and the National Stuttering Project have met with some success in stimulating the organization of self-help groups in different communities.

Lost Chord Clubs and the International Association of Laryngectomees have been particularly effective as self-help organizations for people who have undergone laryngectomies and related surgical procedures. In many localities Lost Chord Clubs function under the aegis of chapters of the American Cancer Society. These clubs may offer educational programs for teaching communication skills, group counseling programs for laryngectomees and their families, and various social activities.

Recently, groups for adults with aphasia have been organized in several communities. Some function under the aegis of rehabilitation centers. Some are affiliated with chapters of the American Heart Association. Some function as special groups within senior centers. Others are independent of other organizations or programs. Meek (1974) described the development and operation of such a group in Cincinnati.

Other self-help groups accommodate people with a variety of physical disabilities that may also include communicative disorders. There are several local, state, and national organizations for the physically handicapped that include self-help programs among their activities. As mentioned earlier, several of these groups have led in consumer activism. Many communities have groups devoted to people with similar diagnoses, for example, groups of people with Parkinson's disease.

The involvement of professionals varies considerably among different self-help groups. Some insist that professionals be present at all times to conduct any educational programs, to provide counseling, to lead discussions, etc. Others involve professionals only by invitation: as members of advisory boards, as consultants, or as guest speakers. Some avoid all professional involvement.

The essence of a self-help group is that members help each other. It is essential, therefore, that leadership derives from the group and that members be primarily responsible for defining programs and activities. When a group is organized and directed by professionals, it is no longer a self-help group. On the other hand, the mere presence of a disability does not qualify a person as an authority on that disability, or prepare him or her to deliver expert services to people with similar disabilities. Therefore, most successful self-help groups profit from some professional involvement. When communicative disorders are the focus of the group, those professionals may well be speech-language pathologists or audiologists.

Self-help groups may be most important to our profession as referral resources for clients needing additional support and reassurance, both while they are receiving professional services and after those services are terminated. Family members may also benefit from the opportunity to meet, through these groups, other families who share their problems.

Special Summer Camping Programs

Summer camps can be a particularly effective approach to the delivery of speech, language, and hearing services. They may be established either as day or residential programs and may extend from 2 weeks to an entire summer. Some camps are designed exclusively to serve children and young adults with communicative disorders. Of these, some accommodate clients with all types of disorders; others specialize in serving such limited groups as children with hearing impairments or children with cleft palate and other craniofacial anomalies. Still others serve clients with a wide range of physical handicaps, but include special services for clients with communicative disorders.

Shady Trails Camp (Clancy and Prins, 1963) is undoubtedly the best known prototype of a special camp for clients with communicative disorders. This camp has been in operation for over 30 years under the aegis of the University of Michigan. Other camping programs have been sponsored by such voluntary health organizations as the Easter Seals Society and United Cerebral Palsy Association, by fraternal organizations, by community speech and hearing centers, and, occasionally, by school districts. A few special camping programs have developed as private ventures.

Camps may afford a unique opportunity for intensive therapeutic and counseling services in an efficient and pleasurable context. Since many young clients with communicative disorders find it difficult to establish independence from their families, camps may also provide an ideal blend of supportive understanding and stimulation of assertiveness.

COLLEGE AND UNIVERSITY SPEECH AND HEARING CLINICS

Predated by public school speech and hearing programs, college and university clinics constitute the second oldest American model for the delivery of our professional services. College and university speech and hearing clinics probably represent a unique phenomenon in the human services delivery system. Although college- and university-sponsored services provide health care, psychological, special education, and other human services, in no other field do college- and university-sponsored services play as dominant a role as in the delivery of speech-language pathology and audiology services. Clinical services accredited by ASHA do not necessarily represent a typical cross-section, but the importance of college and university clinics can be surmised by noting that approximately one-fifth of all accredited programs are of this type.

This situation has many salutary effects. The close ties between service programs and research efforts have spurred the development of new approaches to evaluation and treatment. Subsidies from the parent institutions may cover all requisite equipment and facilities as well as administrative services, so that costs borne by clients remain modest. Less experienced clinicians may have immediate access to consultations from experts, and they are usually closely supervised, again because of subsidies, without additional expense to clients.

It must also be noted, however, that there are many negative features. Furthermore, because of the dominant role of college and university clinics, these negative features may have inordinate impact on our entire delivery system. These features are most apparent in three areas. First, the primary purpose of most college and university clinics is to provide clinical practicum opportunities for students. Most programs recognize that such opportunities should never involve exploitation of the communicatively handicapped, and that only well prepared and thoroughly supervised students should provide clinical services. Nevertheless, training students rather than serving clients remains the principal objective. Admissions policies are determined primarily on the basis of the need for representative samples according to age, type of communicative disorders, etc. (Thus, clients may wait for weeks or months for diagnostic studies only to discover that, because they do not qualify according to the clinic's current needs, no services are available when the studies are completed.) These clinics usually adhere to academic schedules; consequently, services may be interrupted or even terminated, not on the basis of client need, but, rather, on the basis of academic schedules. Continuity of care is further affected by frequent changes of clinicians and by reconsiderations, at intervals, of whether particular clients are still needed for the student training program. Since most are admitted at the beginning of a semester, most must wait to begin treatment programs; this can be extremely difficult for those in need of immediate care (people recovering from cerebrovascular accidents, recent laryngectomees, children who are beginning to show stuttering behavior, etc.).

Second are economic factors. Although the fundamentally subsidized character of college and university clinics may benefit clients, it also has detrimental impacts. The inordinate share of clinical services delivered in this setting has led public and private agencies and other referral sources to rely too much on these programs, and, inevitably, to undervalue the essential worth of speech-language pathology and audiology services. Not only is this situation difficult for neighboring agencies and private practitioners, it also sets an unrealistic economic standard that can have broad consequences.

Employers also complain that college and university clinics give students an unrealistic orientation to the economics of professional practice. This complaint may frequently be justified.

The third problem area relates to the disproportionate share of professional services that are provided by inexperienced clinicians. Since the presence of such a clinic in a community may discourage the development of other clinical facilities—again attributable to economics—clients may have no choice but to seek services there. In many instances, therefore, if they are to receive any services, clients must obtain those services from immature and inexperienced clinicians. Most of us would never accept a situation in which we would receive all our health care from medical students, our dentistry from dental students, or all of our children's education from student teachers. Yet a comparable situation has prevailed within the speech, language, and hearing services delivery system.

The growing concern over these problems has led many college and university programs to initiate changes. In recognizing their failure to provide real-life educational experiences, some have reorganized their programs so that the primary focus is on quality client care rather than on accommodating student needs. In an effort to improve their financial base during an era of declining support for all higher education, some clinics have reoriented their services to qualify for third-party payment; this has entailed substantial participation by fully qualified clinicians. Many colleges and universities have established satellite centers or other cooperative programs in conjunction with medical centers, speech and hearing centers, or other community programs. These efforts may both strengthen their training programs and enhance the scope and quality of services in the affiliated clinical facilities.

Another college-based model of recent origin deserves special mention: the community college program. The roles of community colleges vary widely in different parts of the country. Most were originally established to provide greater access to the first 2 years of college education and to provide terminal, vocationally oriented educational programs. In recent years, however, many community college programs have assumed the functions once assigned to public school district adult education programs. These include both day and evening programs that are primarily diversionary—arts and crafts, physical education, conversational foreign-language instruction, creative writing, literature, dramatics, etc. But they also include such important programs as education for citizenship naturalization, English as a second language, basic academic skills instruction, and specific technical education for vocational advancement.

During the past decade, several states have encouraged community colleges to initiate special programs for disabled students. In some instances, these programs primarily offer adapted, vocationally oriented instruction to improve employability. Others have taken a wider view, offering comprehensive special services to adults of all ages with diverse disabilities.

Many community colleges now offer speech-language pathology and audiology services. These may consist of courses in the pronunciation of American English for speakers of English as a second language, courses in communication skills for people with hearing impairments, or sign language instruction for newly deafened adults and for the families of children and adults who use sign language. Some community colleges offer special courses to teach alaryngeal speech to laryngectomees, and offer programs for adults with chronic aphasias. Some have even established speech and hearing clinics. Ostensibly, such clinics serve students already enrolled in these colleges, but with liberalized definitions of what constitutes enrollment, they may accommodate virtually any adult resident of the district they serve.

PRIVATE PRACTICE

It has often been claimed that a telling index of a profession's maturity is the number of its members who engage independently in private practice. Success in private practice depends on some exacting criteria. Successful private practitioners must attain high levels of professional competence and be sufficiently confident to offer their skills in the world of free enterprise. They must be able to project that competence and confidence to their clients to encourage the investment of the time and money required to secure whatever services are needed. They must also be skillful in maintaining relationships with the other professionals and community agencies that provide the referrals on which most private practitioners depend. Finally, they must master a level of business acumen that will enable them to operate efficiently and economically.

Despite the changes that have occurred in our service delivery system in recent years, most speech-language pathologists, and many audiologists, still work in settings where services are delivered at no cost or at negligible cost to the client. This has led to an erroneous perception that private practice is synonymous with any practice involving fees for services. The distinguishing characteristic of private practice, however, is that services are delivered *for profit.* A private practitioner's livelihood derives from the difference between fees paid by or in behalf of his or her clients and the total costs involved in providing those services (office rental, equipment purchase and maintenance, clerical salaries, supplies, etc.).

It is also important to distinguish between being *engaged* in private practice and being *employed* by a private practice. The former constitutes the situation we have just described. The latter obtains when a speech-language pathologist or audiologist is employed by another speech-language pathologist or audiologist who is actually engaged in private practice or by a private practitioner of another profession. (For example, audiologists are frequently employed by otolaryngologists in private practice.) Such employees may either be paid a salary or paid a percentage of fees collected, but they bear no direct responsibility for overhead expenses. Their situation, therefore, is essentially similar to that of a professional employed in any clinical services setting.

Speech-language pathologists and audiologists in private practice may practice alone or in groups. These groups may involve other individuals in the same profession or involve members of other professions such as psychologists, social workers, physical or occupational therapists, or, in rare instances, even physicians. Sometimes these groups are organized into legal partnerships; in other instances, less formal agreements are effected, involving proration of expenses, scheduling of office space, use of clerical personnel, etc. In some states, both solo and group practices may derive substantial advantages from establishing themselves as professional services corporations.

Although direct fees for services form the economic base of most private practices, other sources may also be important. As will be discussed later, several third-party payment programs (particularly Medicare) proscribe payment to independent practitioners for speech-language pathology services. Therefore, private practitioners frequently become suppliers of services to other facilities (acute hospitals, extended care facilities, day care centers, etc.) who are authorized providers of services. The provider then bills for the services delivered by the supplier.

Private practitioners may not depend entirely upon fees for individual client services. Many provide broad consultative services through agreements with health care facilities, early childhood programs, mental health facilities, schools, industries, rehabilitation facilities, and other public and private agencies.

Clients served by speech-language pathologists in private practice may represent the entire range of people with communicative disorders. Nevertheless, some characteristics predominate. In communities with extensive school-based speech and language services, school-age children are often less frequently represented in private practice caseloads than are other age groups. (This may not obtain when public programs serve few private school students or when they contract with private practitioners for the delivery of certain services.) Because of the financial limitations of individual clients and the restrictions imposed by many third-party payers, clients requiring long-term therapy are less likely to be seen by private practitioners. Typically, these clients are seen for evaluation, and sometimes for an initial period of therapy aimed at completion of the evaluation or at accomplishment of specific therapeutic goals, and are then referred to a public or other community facility for further care. Individual private practitioners may gain recognition from referral sources for particular areas of expertise. In these instances, caseloads may consist primarily of preschoolers with delayed language acquisition, adults with voice disorders, adults with aphasia, or some other restricted client population.

Audiologists in private practice may serve the same cross-section of clients served by any audiology program. Again, however, because of economic factors, few become involved in the delivery of long-term rehabilitation services. An increasing number of audiologists in private practice are including hearing aid dispensing among the services they provide.

Although precise differentiation is difficult, a distinction should be made between full-fledged private practitioners and professionals who augment their incomes by offering occasional independent services to clients on the basis of fees for services, which may either be paid by the clients themselves or by third-party payers. Particularly in smaller communities, these professionals may play an important role in the speech, language, and hearing services delivery system. However, since they do not depend on private practice for their essential livelihood, occasionally they are less scrupulous in client selection, less conscientious professionally, less attentive to interprofessional relationships, and less likely to establish fees that reflect fairly the cost of truly professional services. The essential professional and ethical responsibilities of private practitioners are no different whether they are engaged in practice 1 hour a week or 40 hours a week.

SUMMARY

One of the clearest indices of our success as a human services profession is the diversity of settings in which we now practice. Even though there are many common elements among the services we provide in these varied settings, there are also typical differences. These differences may relate to the demographic characteristics of clients, to the types and the severity of the communicative disorders represented, and to the pattern of services provided (e.g., frequency and duration of services and amount of interdisciplinary cooperation). There are also significant differences in administrative practices that may determine the level of authority and the degree of professional autonomy of individual speech-language pathologists and audiologists.

In all probability, the continued success of our profession will also depend on our ability to persist in extending our professional services into even wider varieties of programs and institutions and to adapt approaches to delivering our services to new models for the delivery of all human services.

References

American Speech and Hearing Association: *Guidelines for Comprehensive Language, Speech and Hearing Services in the Schools.* Rockville, MD, American Speech-Language-Hearing Association, 1973.

Canterbury DR: Public health audiology in rural Alaska: an interagency approach. *ASHA* 20:887–894, 1978.

Chapey R, Lubinski R, Salzberg A, et al: The availability of language, speech, and hearing services in day-care centers. *ASHA* 20:1030–1033, 1978.

Chapin AB: Community speech and hearing clinics. *J Speech Hear Disord* 12:331–333, 1947.

Clancy JN, Prins D: Speech therapy in a camp setting: the growth and development of a speech habilitation center. *ASHA* 5:823–826, 1963.

Cluff GL: Professional services relative to conservation of hearing in industry. *ASHA* 15:339–342, 1973.

Dowling RJ: Health maintenance organizations: new arenas for health-service delivery. *ASHA* 15:591–593, 1973.

Feldman S, Grimes CT: Review and referral of industrial audiograms: a professional dilemma. *ASHA* 19:231–234, 1977.

Fortune GJ: Essential elements of speech and hearing center operation. *J Speech Hear Disord* 23:213–218, 1958.

Hawk SS: The year 1938 in speech correction. *J Speech Disord* 4:87–95, 1939.

Hawk SS: The speech clinician and community service. *J Speech Disord* 6:131–136, 1941.

Hester EJ: The status of speech-language pathology

in the home health setting. *ASHA* 23:155–162, 1981.
Hull RH: A community wide program in geriatric aural rehabilitation. *ASHA* 17:33–48, 1975.
Jeter IK: Unidentified hearing impairment among psychiatric patients. *ASHA* 18:843–845, 1976.
Joint Commission on Accreditation of Hospitals: *Accreditation Manual for Long-Term Care Facilities.* Chicago, Joint Commission on Accreditation of Hospitals, 1979.
Lubinski RB, Chapey R: Communication services in home health care agencies: availability and scope. *ASHA* 22:929–934, 1980.
Meek SD: The Cincinnati Communications Club—a community solution to needs of the chronic aphasic. *ASHA* 16:739–740, 1974.
Melnick W: Industrial hearing conservation. In Katz J: *Handbook of Clinical Audiology.* Baltimore, Williams & Wilkins, 1978.
Miller MH: The audiologist's role in occupational hearing conservation. *ASHA* 18:846–849, 1976.
Monsees EK, Berman E: Speech and language screening in a summer Head Start program. *J Speech Hear Disord* 33:121–126, 1968.
Vaughan GR: Tel-communicology health-care delivery system for persons with communicative disorders. *ASHA* 18:13–17, 1976.
Weissman SM: Courses in speech pathology and correction in the American medical colleges. *J Speech Disord* 3:215–222, 1938.

Supplemental Readings

Black ME: The origins and status of speech therapy in the schools. *ASHA* 8:419–425, 1966.
Chapey R, Burke JP, Schiavetti N, et al: Survey of language, speech, and hearing services at community colleges. *ASHA* 19:470–472, 1977.
Dublinske S: New opportunities for speech-language pathologists and audiologists. *ASHA* 21:998–1002, 1979.
Fox D: *Private Practice: Guidelines for Speech Pathology and Audiology.* Danville, IL, Interstate Printers, 1971.
Garrard KR: Consideration of the speech pathologist's role in early childhood education for the handicapped. *ASHA* 17:90–92, 1975.
Garrard KR: The changing role of speech and hearing professionals in public education. *ASHA* 21:91–98, 1979.
Haller RM, Sheldon N: *Speech Pathology and Audiology in Medical Settings.* New York, Stratton Intercontinental Medical Books, 1976.
Joint Committee on Audiology and Education of the Deaf: Guidelines for audiology programs in educational settings for hearing impaired children. *ASHA* 17:17–20, 1975.
Knight PD: Private practice in speech pathology. *ASHA* 10:436–441, 1968.
LaBorwit L: Speech and hearing services within a local county health department. *ASHA* 5:822–823, 1963.
LaVor M, Harvey J: Head Start, Economic Opportunity Community Partnership Act of 1974. *Excep Child* 42:227–230, 1975.
Lawrence CF: Communicative disorders and public health. *ASHA* 8:35–36, 1966.
Lloyd LL: The establishment of standards for speech pathology and audiology services in facilities for the retarded. *ASHA* 13:607–610, 1971.
Neidecker E: *School Programs in Speech-Language: Organization and Management.* Englewood Cliffs, NJ, Prentice Hall, 1980.
Oglesby A, Harrington DA: *Proceedings, Workshops on Speech Pathology and Audiology in Public Health.* Berkeley, CA, University of California, School of Public Health, 1971.
Rittmanic PA: A state-wide speech and hearing program for the mentally retarded and mentally ill. *ASHA* 8:182–187, 1966.
Rolnick MI: Speech pathology services in a home-health agency: the visiting nurse association of Detroit. *ASHA* 11:462–463, 1969.
Siegenthaler BM, Owsley PJ: Audiologists in schools for the deaf. *ASHA* 10:471–472, 1968.
Smith CR, Fay TH: A program of auditory rehabilitation for aged persons in a chronic disease hospital. *ASHA* 19:417–420, 1977.
Strandberg TE: A national study of United States hospital speech pathology services. *ASHA* 19:160–163, 1977.
The Developmental Disabilities Act. *ASHA* 13:391–393, 1971.
Van Hattum RJ: Services of the speech clinician in the schools: progress and prospects. *ASHA* 18:59–63, 1976.
Walle EL, Newman PW: Rehabilitation services for speech, hearing and language disorders in an extended care facility. *ASHA* 9:216–218, 1967.

CHAPTER FOUR

Referral Patterns and Procedures

Every clinician has a collection of true tales that illustrate the paradoxes of our human services delivery system. A particularly choice specimen from my chamber of horrors concerns a young man who came to a large comprehensive medical center seeking treatment for his stuttering. Medical center policy directed that clients could be seen in the speech and hearing clinic only on referral from a physician. Since the young man had no personal physician he was referred to the comprehensive primary care clinic to obtain the necessary referral. The resident physician in that clinic had never before dealt with the problem of stuttering and had no idea what to do, so he proceeded with a conventional physical examination. During that examination he learned that the stutterer had a history of allergies and observed several allergic symptoms. Accordingly, he referred the young man to the allergy clinic. Since the stutterer was rather passive and had been offered no opportunity to ask any questions, he accepted the referral. In fact, since he had come for help with his stuttering, he concluded that some link must exist between his allergies and his speech problem.

The allergy clinic began exhaustive studies to determine the agents that precipitated allergic reactions. As each agent was identified, they instituted desensitization therapy. But after many months of allergy treatment, the young man became discouraged because no changes occurred in his stuttering. He finally gained enough courage to complain that his major problem was not responding to the treatment. The resident then treating him was dismayed at the young man's naïveté and could not understand how he could have assumed that the stuttering was in any way related to the allergies. Even so, that resident still had no idea of what treatment was needed and concluded that speech problems must fall within the province of the ear, nose, and throat (ENT) clinic.

The ENT resident who examined the young man had never before dealt with a stutterer either. Therefore, he proceeded with a standard ENT examination, noting that the young man's nasal airway was seriously restricted. After further examinations and consultation with a staff otolaryngologist, the resident recommended that a submucous resection (SMR) be performed to improve the nasal airway. Again, since no one clearly explained why the surgical procedure had been recommended, the stutterer assumed that the SMR might somehow alleviate his speech problem.

Not surprisingly, after the surgery, the stuttering remained unchanged. The young man was becoming increasingly discouraged and finally made a vehement complaint to a new ENT resident who was providing postoperative care. (The resident who had performed the surgery had rotated to another hospital.) The new ENT resident, although nonplussed by the stutterer's hostility, was anxious to be helpful. Since he remembered the mention of stuttering during a course in psychiatry he had taken during medical school, he referred the young man to the adult psychiatry clinic.

Because of its waiting list, the stutterer was not seen in the adult psychiatry clinic for 3 or 4 months after the referral. Eventually, however, a psychiatric resident initiated a diagnostic study that involved several testing sessions and interviews. When the study was complete, the psychiatric resident recommended that the young man be enrolled in a regular program of psychotherapy. There were, however, no openings for psychotherapy in the clinic's schedule, and they were not even accepting names for their waiting list. A social worker met with the young man and offered a list of possible resources of psychotherapy in the community, suggesting that he contact each of them to determine whether they were currently accepting clients. The social worker offered to send reports of the diagnostic study to any agency that might accept the young man for psychotherapy.

Understandably, the young man was very perturbed at this outcome of his efforts to seek assistance for his stuttering. He was so preoccupied that in leaving the medical center following this final appointment in the psychiatry clinic, he slipped on the front steps and fell to the sidewalk. Although uninjured, hospital regulations required that, because of potential liability, he must be examined immediately in the emergency room.

Through sheer coincidence, the orthopedic resident covering the emergency room that day was himself a stutterer who was a regular participant in a group therapy program for stutterers conducted by the medical center's speech and hearing clinic. In the course of examining the young man, the resident asked whether he had ever thought about getting help for his stuttering. As a result of this chance encounter, then, the young man was referred to the speech and hearing clinic—almost 2 years after he first came to the medical center seeking help for his stuttering.

This story is unique with respect to specific details, but it could be retold with almost infinite variations to describe the experience of countless clients—and potential clients—in our human services delivery system. This particular client experienced all of his misadventures in seeking assistance within a single, albeit a gargantuan, institution. His experiences would have been even more bewildering had he been referred from one agency to another. In many communities and institutions, the services system has become labyrinthine. When the referrals that are intended to initiate those services are inept, clients and their families can wander aimlessly within or among institutions like the lost souls in *Outward Bound*.

SOME FUNDAMENTAL CONSIDERATIONS

Expertise in the management of referrals is as important as any other aspect of clinical competence. Being a proficient maker and receiver of referrals may be as demanding of knowledge and skill as being a proficient therapist, diagnostician, counselor, or consultant. Effectively managed referrals may have as much influence on the outcome of services to a particular client as any other assistance we can provide.

Referrals can accomplish two related purposes:

1. *Referrals can lead to the determination of what services a client requires.* The development of a plan is usually the first step in any human services process. Many factors will determine the structure of that plan: the precise nature of the client's problems and needs, the strategies that are most likely to be effective in helping the client overcome those problems and meet those needs, the source or sources available for whatever services are needed, and the client's ability and willingness to avail himself or herself of those services. The first purpose of referrals, therefore, is to gather whatever information is needed to formulate that plan.
2. *Referrals can ensure that the client receives the services he or she requires.* After the plan has been drafted, the obvious next step is instituting the components of that plan. Referrals should expedite the initial receipt of whatever services are called for, enable the client to receive additional services as new needs and circumstances arise, and facilitate the continuation of services for as long as they are helpful.

Regardless of the purposes to be served by referrals, one precept remains: A client must always have a coordinator—a primary care provider, a staff member at a familiar facility, or a concerned specialist—who remains available to guide the client through the referral process, to offer alternatives when referrals go awry, to provide ongoing guidance and encouragement, to interpret and integrate findings and recommendations as they emerge, and to plan next steps when services are completed or otherwise terminated. As professional services have become more specialized, this coordinator is often elusive. Yet, of the elements of a human services system, effective coordination is most likely to determine success or failure when multiple services are required and multiple providers are involved.

Speech-language pathologists and audiologists usually consider themselves to be providers of specialized services rather than case managers. But sometimes a member of our profession properly functions as the coordinator of all services provided to a single client. When the client's major problems center on communication, the professional most expert in the area of communicative disorders, i.e., the speech-language pathologist or audiologist, may best serve as the focal point as clients move through the referral process. Clearly, this may be antithetical to the traditions and policies of many health care, education, and rehabilitation programs. Even in these settings, however, a member of our profession may play this role quietly, deferring at times to whomever is assigned the role of case manager on organizational charts. As often as not, the manager is quite willing to share those responsibilities so long as his or her ultimate authority is not challenged.

Whether speech-language pathologists and audiologists serve as case managers or not, they must understand what is involved in making and receiving referrals. Furthermore, they must be thoroughly familiar with the referral policies and procedures of the institutions and agencies in which they are employed and of the other institutions, agencies, and private practitioners who may serve their clients. Clearly defined referral policies and procedures are not mere bureaucratic trappings; they may be the best insurance that referrals will be managed efficiently and economically with the fewest risks to clients and concerned professionals.

Referral policies should always strike a reasonable balance between efficient client management and appropriate protection for the client and the agency and its staff. Referral policies should impose the fewest possible obstacles. When too many prerequisites are involved, clients become discouraged and professionals seek other resources for their referrals.

When referral policies and procedures that have been established by administrators, boards of directors, or medical staff executive committees with no input from other professionals prove inflexible, a wise professional learns to adapt his practices as congenially as possible within those policies. In other instances, although policies may be equally inflexible, they may have been established and can be modified more democratically, with the participation of an entire professional staff. In still other instances, policies may be as flexible as could be hoped for by any case manager. Large institutions, particularly when primarily supported by public funds administered according to governmental regulations, tend to be most rigid in referral policies. In contrast, the policies of small independent facilities may be extremely flexible.

Speech-language pathologists and audiologists may have varying degrees of influence on referral policies and procedures. At one extreme, a speech-language pathologist in a rehabilitation department of a large city or county hospital, or an audiologist in a Veterans Administration Medical Center, may have virtually no discretion as to the procedures to be followed in making or receiving referrals. At the other extreme a speech-language pathologist in a small community agency, or an audiologist in private practice, may be free to establish whatever referral policies seem appropriate. Between these extremes are the situations in which most members of our profession work.

Regardless of how referral policies are established, certain criteria must usually be considered in making and receiving referrals. These criteria fall into two different areas: *eligibility criteria* and *procedural criteria.*

Eligibility Criteria

Many human services programs are established to accommodate particular client populations; therefore, their eligibility criteria specify who may be consumers of those services. Eligibility criteria customarily fall into five different areas:

1. *Age.* Programs may define eligibility within specific age ranges (infants, children below age 3, preschoolers, school-age children, teenagers, adults from 18 to 55, older adults, etc.). Other programs may define broader age categories (ages 3 to 21, from 21 to 65, etc.).
2. *Residency.* Some programs stipulate that clients must reside in a particular neighborhood, city, county, school district, state, or other geographic area.
3. *Economic status.* Programs may provide services only to clients who can pay for the services or have available third-party coverage. (This criterion is sometimes applied without being clearly stated.) Other programs may admit only clients on welfare, clients whose income falls below a specified level, or clients who meet other economic criteria defined by means tests. (Means tests usually consider such factors as family income, family size, fixed expenses, debts, and total assets.)
4. *Group membership.* Admission may be restricted to clients who represent certain groups; for example, members of the armed forces or their dependents; veterans, veterans of a particular war or wars, or veterans with service-incurred problems; members of particular religious or fraternal groups; subscribers to health maintenance organizations or other health plans; and members of particular ethnic or national groups or speakers of particular languages.
5. *Diagnostic and other problem categories.* Programs may limit eligibility to clients within specific diagnostic categories (orthopedic or neurologic handicaps, visual impairments, hearing impairments, developmental disabilities, etc.), or they may define eligibility on the basis of problem areas such as low academic achievement, drug or alcohol abuse, recent discharge from penal institutions, recent discharge from psychiatric hospitals, etc.

Eligibility criteria may not only determine whether a client can be served by a particular agency, these criteria may also define the way in which the client is served following admission. For example, in some medical centers, clients admitted on a part-pay basis—that is, clients who cannot afford full fees but have no third-party coverage—may become "staff patients." In this status they are treated by resident physicians (i.e., licensed physicians completing requirements for specialty Board certification), while a full-pay patient at the same medical center will be treated by a physician who is both licensed and certified. Other human services agencies, including agencies providing speech, language, and hearing services, have comparable procedures, so that clients paying adjusted fees or no fees are served by students or by recent graduates discharging internship requirements in such fields as social work, psychology, rehabilitation counseling, and physical and occupational therapy.

Various eligibility criteria may also be imposed to define admission to special programs within institutions. For example, sometimes children with the diagnosis of cerebral palsy qualify for services that are not provided to other developmentally disabled children. Or, children from welfare-recipient families may qualify for special screening programs offered by some medical centers under provisions of the Early and Periodic Screening, Diagnosis and Treatment Program (EPSDTP), while other children from other low-income families do not. Some agencies provide specialized programs geared to such restrictive categories of clients as children of migrant laborers, wives and children of imprisoned felons, recent refugees from Southeast Asia, and severely hearing-impaired adults suffering from chronic alcohol or drug abuse.

Procedural Criteria

Many human services programs also establish procedural criteria that govern referral procedures. Some criteria may seek consumer protection, that is, ensuring that the client needs the services, can profit from the services, and should not receive other services instead of, or in addition to, the service or services mentioned in the referral. Other criteria may be based on economic considerations, again ensuring that a client requires a particular service—for which the client or someone else must pay—and that the service cannot be provided more economically in another way by another facility. Still other criteria, unfortunately, are simply based on outworn traditions and institutionalized pecking orders.

Procedural criteria may be grouped into two categories:

1. *Stipulated professional points of entry.* These criteria usually stipulate that referrals must come from members of particular professions. Most often physician referral is stipulated, but some facilities may specify members of other professions.
2. *Process stipulations.* Many agencies impose procedural criteria on referrals by stipulating that certain processes must be completed prior to admission. These processes may be necessary to certify that a client qualifies according to specified eligibility criteria (e.g., certified as disabled, declared a ward of the court, or registered to attend school within a particular district). Some criteria relate to definition of financial responsibility for the services to be provided (e.g., registered as a Medicaid beneficiary, as accepted for coverage by Crippled Children Services, or as a member of a union health plan). Some agencies require that a set of diagnostic procedures be carried out before a referral is effected. For example, schools and clinics for children with learning disabilities may require prior evaluations by physicians (sometimes specifying neurologists) and psychologists. Regrettably, some agencies impose procedural stipulations which, in effect, demonstrate that a client has been considered ineligible for services by all other agencies as a requisite to admission. Such stipulations can be both frustrating and demeaning.

   Comprehensive services agencies may establish in-house procedural stipulations for referral to individual departments. Such stipulations are common in medical centers where referral for any service by nonphysician providers (such as speech-language pathologists and audiologists) requires prior diagnosis or treatment by a medical department. This may obtain even when the client has been referred by a physician outside the medical center specifically for speech, language, or hearing services. In some community agencies, referral to any department must be preceded by an evaluation by a social worker to determine a client's eligibility for services. Unfortunately, in some large facilities, referral from one department to another may involve as many, or even more, procedural contingencies than would referral for the same service to an outside agency.

In virtually all settings, speech-language pathologists and audiologists participate in referral processes. The successful completion of referrals often depends on awareness of eligibility and procedural criteria. This obtains whether a clinician is receiving referrals or making referrals.

RECEIVING REFERRALS

Speech-language pathologists and audiologists depend upon other professionals and agencies to refer most of the clients we serve. Correctly or incorrectly, we are identified within the human services delivery system as providers of secondary or tertiary care. Children with communicative disorders are enrolled in school, assigned to whatever classes seem appropriate, and then referred to speech-language pathologists. When clients or their families become concerned about communicative disorders, they may first consult their family physicians, who then may either refer them directly to a speech-language pathologist or audiologist, or, perhaps more frequently, to another medical specialist, who may then refer the client to a member of our profession. People with multiple handicaps which include communicative disorders are first referred to rehabilitation facilities which, in turn, refer for speech, language, or hearing services. And so it is in virtually every setting. In industry, workers with hearing impairments go first to industrial physicians or nurses; in mental health facilities, clients with communicative disorders are first seen by psychiatrists, psychologists, or social workers; in home health agencies, our clients are seen first by physicians or nurses.

Our professional organizations and individual members of our profession have attempted to alter these patterns, to eliminate some of the hurdles between us and potential consumers of our services. Radio and television public service announcements and articles and public service advertisements in newspapers and magazines have urged people to establish direct contacts with speech-language pathologists and audiologists in their communities. But none of these efforts has altered substantially the essential position of our profession with respect to referral patterns.

Despite all the changes in our human services delivery system, many traditions that determine our receipt of referrals seem impervious to change. Not only are referral patterns ingrained in traditions, they are also institutionalized in governmental regulations, in agency policies, in accreditation standards, and in regulations that determine payment for services. Adherence to these traditional referral patterns may be wasteful of time and money. Some clients may even abandon efforts to secure our services when too many obstacles are imposed. Others may be short-stopped by professionals who fail to recognize the existence and significance of communicative disorders. Still others may be referred for treatment procedures that will have no effect on communicative disorders. However, disregard for or defiance of customary referral patterns may either restrict the participation of speech-language pathologists and audiologists in the human services delivery system or exclude them entirely from many parts of that system. This situation benefits neither our profession nor the clients who need our services.

If changes are to occur, they will not be effected by public service announcements or newspaper publicity heralding the accomplishments and contributions of our profession. Instead, such changes begin among individual professionals in local institutions and communities. As our competencies and contributions gain recognition from our colleagues in other professions, obstacles begin to disappear.

The Responsibilities of Receivers of Referrals

Playing effectively the role of a receiver of referrals involves more than installing a telephone that is supported by an answering service, or having a mailbox in which prepared referral forms can be deposited. The manifold responsibilities of this role can be characterized within five functions.

1. *To help referral sources select appropriate clients for referral.* Most speech-language pathologists and audiologists, whether employed by institutions or engaged in private practice, invest substantial energy in interprofessional education. Although a major intent of that education may be encouragement of more referrals, of even greater importance may be the encouragement of more *appropriate* referrals. Once clients present themselves to be served, a professional or agency must either provide services or propose alternatives. This obtains whether the original referral was appropriate or inappropriate.

   The management of inappropriate referrals can be time consuming and expensive and can lead to frustration for the client, for the maker of the referral, and for the receiver of the referral. Some inappropriate referrals are inevitable, but they can be diminished by active efforts toward educating referral sources.

2. *To ensure, insofar as possible, that a client receives promptly whatever services he or she requires and wishes to obtain that fall within the purview of the receiver of the referral.* Many providers of human services assume that their professional responsibilities begin with the initial contact between a client and the provider. Actually, however, some degree of professional responsibility begins at the moment a referral source recommends that a client seek services from the provider. Throughout the early history of our profession, our situation resembled what would be described as a "seller's market" in the world of commerce. Because of personnel shortages and limited facilities, we were never able to keep up with the demand for our services. Consequently, we assumed little responsibility for potential clients during the crucial interval between the date a referral was effected and the date he or she received the first service. If clients got lost in the process, found the wait for the initial appointment intolerable, or spent weeks or even months on a waiting list, it worried us little because there were always more clients than we could serve. However explicable, such practices constituted unacceptable professional conduct. Fortunately for our clients, as speech-language pathology and audiology services become more available, this situation is changing rapidly.

   As stated, the second responsibility of referral receivers has two elements: The services for which the client is referred must be available, and those services should be available as soon as possible. Few situations create more serious problems with referral sources and with the clients they refer than accepting referrals which cannot be fully accommodated. For example, clients who are referred for therapy may be subjected to an evaluation which in turn leads to a recommendation of therapy which is not available. Occasionally, when the nature of the client's communicative disorder was unclear initially, or full information about financial circumstances was unavailable, complete services cannot be provided. But these instances should be infrequent. To avoid them, initial contacts with clients and referral sources must be managed with consummate skill so that obviously ineligible and unlikely clients can be forestalled and appropriately referred elsewhere before the first appointment is made.

The objective of promptness in the delivery of services may be difficult to achieve. The economics of many services programs directs that sufficient professional time is seldom available for immediate scheduling of all referrals. This situation presents a quandary. Should some sort of intake appointment be provided immediately, even though a delay will occur before additional services can be provided? Or should a client wait for the initial appointment until he or she can proceed immediately into whatever program is needed? These alternatives must be weighed on the basis of several factors. The first of these factors is the nature of the referral. Often, the likely scope of services can be deduced in advance. For example, an otolaryngologist's referral for a hearing evaluation of an 8-year-old with serous otitis is usually more predictable than a pediatrician's referral of a nonspeaking 3-year-old. Similarly, a referral from another speech-language pathologist or audiologist is usually more predictable than a referral from a social work aide. Predictable referrals can be scheduled as soon as the required services can be provided. Less predictable referrals, however, may best be scheduled for a preliminary intake-screening appointment. In some instances, such an appointment may reveal that no further services are needed. Sometimes, the client would be better served by another program. If continued services are needed, their urgency can be determined, their likely extent estimated, the reason for the delay in providing services explained, and any immediately available sources of assistance can be proposed.

Second, one should consider the urgency of the services recommended by the referral source. Too many speech-language pathologists and audiologists manage referrals so democratically that they become insensitive to individual client needs. Adults with recently acquired aphasias, new laryngectomees, children and adults with suddenly acquired hearing loss, and young children with incipient stuttering behavior are likely to require urgent attention. Yet these referrals often go on the same waiting lists as clients with less exigent problems. In addition to the urgency inherent in the nature of the communicative disorder, one must also consider urgencies deriving from the interrelatedness of different professional services. When a speech, language, or hearing evaluation comprises one part of a comprehensive work-up by a team of professionals, it must be provided in a timely fashion. Preoperative counseling of a client scheduled for a laryngectomy, or a preoperative audiologic evaluation of a potential candidate for middle ear surgery, cannot wait. When the assessment of a child's language competence must be completed before his or her educational placement can be decided, that service must be provided immediately. Each of these instances demands flexibility in scheduling procedures.

Finally, the wishes and attitudes of the client must be considered. Many clients and their referral sources are frustrated when they are merely informed by a clerk that their name will be entered on a waiting list to be advised when an appointment is available. Often, by the time the client's name reaches the top of the waiting list, he or she will have lost interest or sought other sources of assistance. Whenever services must be delayed, clients must be fully informed, optimally through a telephone conversation with a member of the professional staff, as to the reason for and the likely length of the delay and as to any available options (e.g., being seen for an immediate screening appointment versus waiting until complete services are available versus seeking other sources of assistance). It may even be possible to provide some initial counseling during that telephone conversation which will lessen the client's anxiety during the waiting period.

3. *To coordinate services with whatever other services are being provided to the client.* In many settings, a significant portion of clients referred for speech, language, or hearing services are either concurrently receiving other professional services or are being simultaneously referred for those other services. The referral source may assume some responsibility for coordinating those services, but each referral receiver must also assume some responsibility in order to ensure a well integrated program of services.

Effective coordination involves two aspects: logistical and programmatic. Logistical aspects relate to scheduling, arranging for payment, arranging transportation, etc. Programmatic aspects relate to coordinating the goals of all professional services so that a total, integrated program is achieved. This coordination may be more easily realized when all services are provided within the scope of a single facility than when several individual practitioners or multiple facilities are involved.

4. *To keep referral sources informed about whatever services are being provided.* Virtually all human services providers initially acknowledge referrals in some manner, most often by reports following the initial intake or evaluation appointment. Too frequently, however, no further information is offered to the referral source. Unless the referral source anticipates no further contact with the client, intermittent reports should be rendered throughout the course of whatever services are provided. The major objective is the best possible coordination of services. Nevertheless, an important secondary consideration is that such reports offer optimal opportunities to provide information about the services we can provide, which, in turn, may increase the likelihood of more and more appropriate referrals from that source.
5. *To ensure continuity of care after the purpose of the referral has been accomplished or services have been terminated for other reasons.* Professionals may become so focused in their own areas of specialization that they forget that termination of their services does not necessarily mean the client needs no further services of any type. Acceptance of a referral not only implies acceptance of the responsibility to provide services, it also implies assumption of the responsibility to guide a client appropriately when those services terminate. Sometimes, this merely involves referral back to the original referral source along with whatever recommendations for continued care seem appropriate. In other instances, clients are referred to other professionals or agencies, but always with the knowledge and participation of the original referral source (unless that source is no longer involved in any way in the client's care). In instances where no further professional services of any type are required, it may be sufficient merely to propose potential sources of assistance should further need arise.

Receiving Referrals in Different Settings

Even though the principles just outlined apply in every setting served by speech-language pathologists and audiologists, specific practices related to receiving referrals differ. Despite wide individual differences, there are likely commonalities among settings. These commonalities may derive from the kinds of services provided, the types of clients served, or the patterns of financial support. As often as not, however, referral practices are also determined by the traditions that have evolved within specific segments of the human services delivery system.

RECEIVING REFERRALS IN HEALTH AGENCIES

Nowhere is the influence of sheer tradition more apparent than in the health services system. The classic referral procedures of that system were described in an earlier chapter: A primary care physician refers a client to a secondary care physician specialist, who may then refer the client to a tertiary care physician specialist. When the services of a nonphysician provider are required, the secondary or tertiary care physician usually makes the referral.

The rationale underlying these procedures is essentially meritorious. If the primary care physician is to play the role of initiator and coordinator of all health care services, he or she is the logical point of entry for these services. Since the scope of modern health care far exceeds the expertise of any single physician, the involvement of secondary and tertiary care specialists is also sensible. If the assistance of a nonphysician provider is needed to establish a diagnosis, that referral should probably be made by the physician charged with the responsibility of making the diagnosis. If the nonphysician provider is to offer treatment services, presumably medically remediable deficits should first be ruled out or undergo concurrent treatment. These completely logical assumptions, then, undergird the referral patterns of the health care delivery system.

Health care program referral concepts are not just philosophic, they are usually cast firmly into rules and regulations. Physician referral is commonly required for any services by nonphysician providers in health care programs. Sometimes direct referrals from any physician are acceptable, but in some institutions a prior evaluation by a staff physician is required.

Our profession has been the target of recurring efforts to dictate a particular medical specialty as the sole route of entry to our services. (The most frequent example is mandating that all audiology clients be first seen by otolaryngologists.) Such restrictions have been imposed within individual programs and institutions. They are generally regrettable on at least two bases. Routine specialist evaluations, conducted solely to meet procedural requirements, subject clients to unnecessary expenditures of time and money. Furthermore, many physicians themselves find these restrictions unacceptable because they prefer to refer directly for speech, language, or hearing services without prior specialist evaluations. Such restrictive referral policies sometimes seriously limit referrals to the programs that impose them.

It is also important to distinguish between physician *referral* and physician *prescription.* Referral implies directing a client to another professional who will provide whatever services are needed according to that professional's best judgment. Prescription implies specifically directing what services are to be provided and even defining the approach to be taken in providing the services. Since few physicians have sufficient information about our professional practices to equip them to make explicit prescriptions, this practice is intolerable. It is addressed in the Code of Ethics of the American Speech-Language-Hearing Association: "Individuals must not provide clinical services by prescription of anyone who does not hold the Certificate of Clinical Competence."

Requirements for physician referral are imposed by virtually all public and private third-party payment programs covering speech-language pathology and audiology services. Ostensibly these requirements are imposed to ensure that a client receives all needed medical services and to prevent claims for unnecessary services ("necessary" is defined as deemed necessary by a physician). In reality, however, members of the medical profession play a dominant role in writing the regulations and policies of third-party payers so that physician control is assured.

Other referral practices must usually be followed by members of our profession in the health care system:

1. When a client requires services beyond the scope of an original referral, the speech-language pathologist or audiologist should consult the referring physician before recommending or instituting those services. For example, therapy should not be instituted for a client referred for evaluation without an intervening contact with the referring physician. Similarly, such services as hearing aid evaluations or aural rehabilitation services should not be recommended without the participation of physicians referring for initial hearing evaluations. Among other reasons for adhering to this procedure is the likelihood that a client's third-party coverage may be invalidated when services are instituted without physician participation. Except when required by third-party carriers, specific physician authorization for added services may be unnecessary; it may be sufficient to inform them of plans, indicating that those plans will be instituted unless the physician considers them to be contraindicated.
2. No further referrals should be instituted without the participation of the referring physicians. This applies especially to further medical referrals, but it may apply to other referrals as well. For example, members of our profession often see clients for evaluation and then refer them to other programs for therapy. This may represent good practice. When, for instance, a medical center program finds that a child requires speech therapy, and that child attends a school where appropriate services are provided conveniently and at no cost to the family, referral is obviously in order. Yet, when the physician who originally referred the child is not appraised of the basis for further referral, some serious misunderstandings can arise.
3. An earlier discussed principle becomes particularly important in health care programs: *When services are completed, always refer a client back to the referring physician or, if preferred by a referring specialist, to the client's primary care provider.* Failure to adhere to this traditional practice, which can lead to physicians losing their patients, has led to the downfall of many speech-language pathologists and audiologists working in the health care system.

Every speech-language pathologist and audiologist who works within the referral traditions of the health care delivery system recognizes the abundant incongruities. When screening services are provided through health departments of industrial hygiene programs, audiologists may be required to demand medical evaluations of clients who will in no way benefit from those evaluations. Medical center-based speech, language, and hearing services programs may insist on routine prior medical examinations when it would be more economical and efficient first to see a client for speech, language, or hearing evaluations and then to pursue whatever medical examinations may contribute to understanding the client's problem.

Often, as members of our profession become well established in health care programs, and particularly as they demonstrate the value of their contributions and the judiciousness of their recommendations, traditional referral restrictions gradually disappear. Even though restrictive policies remain, they are interpreted so generously that few restrictions actually exist. Neophytes in the health care delivery system are well advised to adhere rigidly to all stated referral policies until they achieve sufficient acceptance to question those policies.

RECEIVING REFERRALS IN SCHOOL PROGRAMS

In many school programs, referral has gradually replaced other approaches to identifying children who require speech, language, and hearing services. Some school districts have discontinued wholesale screening efforts, relying entirely on referrals. Others limit screening programs to kindergartners or first graders.

Classroom teachers usually represent the single most frequent source of referrals. Several years ago, a study of services provided by a representative sample of 252 school speech, language, and hearing specialists in California showed that classroom teachers were responsible for referring between 50% and 100% of the children served by each clinician. Parents, although a relatively infrequent referral source, were cited as second in frequency, with other school personnel—guidance counselors, psychologists, administrators, etc.—much less frequent referral sources. Referrals from out-of-school agencies and professionals were extremely rare. Data are unavailable to determine whether similar surveys in other states would reveal comparable referral patterns, but it seems likely that they typify many school programs throughout the nation.

School program referral patterns may have changed, at least superficially, to conform to the provisions of PL 94–142. Frequently, an assessment step involving several professionals now intervenes between the initial classroom teacher referral and the receipt of the referral by the speech, language, and hearing specialist. In most school districts that specialist participates in the preliminary assessment, but, regrettably, this practice is not universal.

In at least one important respect, school speech, language, and hearing specialists are in a different position in receiving referrals than are their colleagues in other settings. In most settings, the nature and extent of whatever services are provided are planned jointly by the speech-language pathologist or audiologist and the client and his or her family. This situation may be different in school programs. The principle that every child in our nation has the right to a free and appropriate education has been generalized into an assumption that every child has a right to whatever services are provided by public education agencies. If, therefore, a parent wishes a child to be enrolled for speech, language, or hearing services, it may be assumed that those services must be provided whether or not, in the considered opinion of the speech, language, and hearing specialist, the child needs or can profit from those services. In actual fact, this position is not supported by legal requirements. In practice, however, local agencies accede to militant parents and sometimes require speech, language, and hearing specialists to provide services they did not recommend.

A further feature of school programs with respect to receiving referrals is that specialists may be severely restricted in the referral qualifications they may impose. In other settings, speech-language pathologists and audiologists may insist that various medical examinations, psychological evaluations, etc., be completed prior to admission for their services. Furthermore, they may insist that the results of those examinations and evaluations be available before instituting any program. School speech, language, and hearing specialists may not enjoy these privileges, particularly when out-of-school agencies and professionals are involved. However desirable, it may be unreasonable to expect families to secure such evaluations for their children. Furthermore, it can be contended that under the terms of PL 94-142, if these evaluations are essential to providing appropriate special services, the local education agency is financially responsible for their procurement.

The stimulation of appropriate referrals is at least as important in school programs as in any other services setting. If a program is to thrive, there must be a steady flow of referrals, particularly from classroom teachers. However, a proliferation of inappropriate referrals may lead to more undesirable consequences in school programs than in other settings. Admonishing school speech, language, and hearing specialists to seek every opportunity to guide classroom teachers and other school professionals toward making informed referrals has become an equivalent of saluting motherhood and apple pie. In a very real sense, however, no other pursuit by school specialists may be more crucial in determining the ultimate success or failure of their programs.

RECEIVING REFERRALS IN PRIVATE PRACTICE

However important to the success of our professional services in other settings, in no other setting is immediate survival so directly dependent upon successfully eliciting referrals as in private practice. In fact, a private practitioner's skill in eliciting and managing referrals is probably the single most significant determiner of whether he or she will ultimately succeed or fail.

Most private practitioners, particularly during the time they are building a new practice, encourage referrals from all possible sources. Nevertheless, ultimately successful practitioners tend to concentrate on particular referral sources. These sources are usually characterized by three features. First, successful private practitioners usually establish relationships with a core of referral sources that serve many clients with communicative disorders. Although most private practitioners welcome occasional referrals from virtually any reputable source, a smaller corps of frequent referral sources is virtually essential. This involves the establishment of cordial relationships with medical specialists and other professionals and with community agencies, schools, and other institutions most likely to serve children and adults with speech, language, and hearing problems. Concentrating on fewer, but potentially more productive, referral sources may also enable the operation of a more efficient private practice. Familiar referral sources are more likely to make suitable referrals. Furthermore, when contacts between a private practitioner and a referral source are more frequent, less complex reporting systems may suffice. Both of these factors may reduce overhead expenses, a matter of great concern since cost containment is another essential key to success in private practice.

Second, private practitioners must establish relationships with referral sources serving clients who can pay fees for the services they receive, either independently or with the assistance of a third-party payer. Most communities are amply supplied with referral agencies that are constantly seeking services for indigent clients. No matter how deserving, these clients cannot be served by private practitioners.

Third, private practitioners must establish relationships with referral sources who are themselves delivering services of good quality within their areas of expertise. When clients are receiving inadequate services, the role of the private practitioner becomes precarious. Private practitioners are usually under pressure to achieve maximum results within the least possible time. But when a client is inadequately served by other professionals or agencies, timely progress is often unlikely. Under these circumstances, private practitioners may have little choice but to seek other sources for whatever ancillary services are required to coordinate those services and to counsel the client regarding the necessity of the services, while, at the same time, trying to avoid alienation of the original referral source. However important, such activities usually yield little financial return.

Private practitioners confront other problems in establishing referral policies. For example, should a private practitioner see clients only on medical referral? Such restrictions may mitigate some of the problems just described. Furthermore, in some communities, physicians may be more likely to refer to private practitioners who only accept medical referrals; this may often obtain when the practitioner is an audiologist. Problems in securing third-party payment may also be reduced when referrals come only from physicians.

Yet, private practitioners may seem overly exclusive when they only accept physician referrals. Whatever the practical benefits of such a referral policy, it can create problems in relating to other professionals and agencies. Furthermore, that policy may restrict potential clients to people whose problems led them to consult a physician before seeking some other form of assistance. As with most other problems that face private practitioners, referral policies must usually be established through reasonable—and practical—compromises.

RECEIVING REFERRALS IN OTHER COMMUNITY AGENCIES AND PROGRAMS

Speech-language pathologists and audiologists who serve community agencies may confront a unique combination of the problems faced by clinicians in all other settings with respect to receiving referrals. On the one hand, like school clinicians, they are employed in programs that must serve the widest possible segments of society. On the other hand, community agencies must increasingly rely on fees for services and third-party payments if they are to survive. As if both these circumstances do not create enough conflicts, community agencies must also respond to pressures created by various professional groups, by social activists, by conservative philanthropists, and by other community agencies. For example, county medical societies or the medical advisory committees of community speech and hearing centers often urge adoption of policies requiring medical referral. These same community centers are, however, also under considerable pressure from other community agencies and groups to impose the fewest possible obstacles to the acceptance of any and all referrals.

With due recognition of the political and social realities of their communities, every agency must develop referral policies that make services available to the widest possible population, but at the same time permit the agency to serve clients as efficiently as possible. When an agency opens its doors to every person who chooses to establish contact with that agency, it courts many problems. Inevitably, the agency assumes some responsibilities from the moment the contact is established. If, as often happens, the client is not an appropriate candidate for the services provided by that agency, it must usually invest substantial staff time in finding and directing the client to appropriate sources of assistance. Therefore, some restrictions are usually needed to reduce the frequency of clearly inappropriate referrals.

Unfortunately, the most seriously underserved people are often those who encounter the greatest difficulties in satisfying referral requirements. Securing a medical referral can involve hours of waiting in a city hospital clinic for a brief cursory contact with a house physician or medical student. Collecting reports of previous agency contacts may be hopelessly confusing to clients who are unfamiliar with agency policies and procedures, particularly when those clients have limited facility in the English language. Establishing financial responsibility for services can entail demeaning contacts with welfare departments. Therefore, however sensible agency policies seem to be, they can constitute virtually insurmountable hurdles to people in dire need of services.

Most community agencies are best served by flexible referral policies and procedures. Information obtained on initial contact can usually determine the procedure to be followed. If a potential client is under a physician's care, particularly for a condition directly related to the communicative disorder, it is logical to ask for referral information from that physician. If a potential client is receiving or has previously received relevant services from community agencies, it is reasonable to seek their participation in the referral process. When the client has been served or is being served by another speech-language pathologist or audiologist, their participation in the referral process should also be encouraged. But when no such relationship exists, no referral prerequisites should be imposed. However, in these instances, some preliminary screening must precede a commitment to accept a client for services.

Developing New Referral Sources

In virtually all settings, we must be continually developing new referral resources if speech-language pathology and audiology programs are to flourish. Many approaches have been used. The following are most familiar.

ANNOUNCEMENTS, NEWSLETTERS, AND BULLETINS

Although these are useful devices for keeping current referral sources informed of activities and new program developments, they are unlikely to elicit substantial numbers of referrals from new sources. Unless professionals are already interested in a particular program, they will probably not devote time to reading such printed material. At best, these publications may create an awareness that a particular program exists; subsequent reinforcement by other means may then create genuine interest.

PERSONAL CONTACTS

The demanding schedules of most professionals who are potential new referral sources limit the effectiveness of personal contacts as an approach to eliciting new referrals. Telephone contacts are virtually worthless when established for the sole purpose of soliciting referrals. In-person contacts may be more promising, but most brief visits with harried private practitioners or agency directors are little more effective than telephone contacts.

PUBLICITY AND ADVERTISING

Publicity approaches, like newspaper articles, radio talk-show appearances, and radio or television public service announcements, may elicit some self-referrals, but they have little influence on the development of new professional referral sources. The essential conservatism of most professionals leads them to suspect other professionals who court publicity in the popular media. These attitudes undoubtedly discourage honest attempts at public education; nevertheless, they must be reckoned with. In many communities, publicity efforts can actually discourage potential referral sources.

Recent legal actions at both federal and state levels have led most professional groups to remove prohibitions against advertising, since these prohibitions were considered both detrimental to the public interest and as attempts at restraint of trade. Nevertheless, as with publicity, many professionals regard as suspect other professionals who advertise and are disinclined to use them as resources for their referrals. Potential consumers of professional services may also be indoctrinated to believe that reputable professionals do not advertise.

Since they have been widely used by all professionals, yellow page telephone directory listings are not included among the unspoken proscriptions against advertising. Traditionally, these listings may include references to the scope of services offered and the name, address, and professional credentials of the individual professional or agency personnel. Yellow page listings may conceivably elicit some self-referrals, but few professionals are likely to refer clients on this basis.

SCREENING PROGRAMS

A timeworn approach to simultaneously identifying potential clients for speech, language, and hearing services and establishing an individual or agency as a potential referral resource for those services is the conduct of screening programs. This may be a mass screening effort directed toward an entire community, a more restricted effort involving such special groups as preschoolers in child care programs or oldsters in programs for senior citizens, or very specialized efforts targeting such limited populations as patients in long-term health care facilities or clients of home health agencies. Referral-seeking screening programs are delimited at the outset by the fact that further services do not automatically follow identification. Once identified, clients are encouraged to contact the program providing the screening service, or a responsible professional is encouraged to facilitate the referral of identified clients.

When well planned and well managed, screening programs can encourage new referrals. There are, nevertheless, some inherent hazards. Once again, these programs may be viewed skeptically by other professionals as a form of "ambulance chasing." Potential clients may also be suspicious. Hearing-impaired people may be particularly wary since they are often victimized by hearing aid sales practices that bear surface resemblance to professionally directed screening programs. ("Free hearing tests" is one of the most popular come-ons used by hearing aid salesmen.)

Screening services are usually offered at no cost to the client, a source of further problems. Other professionals, and the clients themselves, may be wary of what can lurk behind free services. More importantly, the borderline between screening services and other professional services can be elusive. Most parents who bring their children to be "screened" for speech and language problems are already aware that problems may be present. Similarly, many people who appear for hearing screening programs already recognize that their hearing is impaired. Consequently, many people who are seen in screening programs expect more than mere recommendations for further evaluations. Furthermore, when the screening program is "free" they may be dismayed to discover that the services they are actually seeking may entail substantial expense. (Some may regard this as a version of "bait and switch" advertising.)

Regardless of its purpose, every screening program should be planned with careful attention to the way services are to be provided when problems are identified. Insofar as possible, the purpose of the program should be clear to clients, preferably before they present themselves for the screening services.

CONTINUING AND IN-SERVICE EDUCATION PROGRAMS

Virtually all professions and human services institutions and agencies conduct continuing or in-service education programs. Whether they consist of meetings of professional societies, staff conferences, or regularly scheduled courses, these activities can offer unequaled opportunities for stimulating new referral sources.

Education programs should never be used as mere forums for promoting referrals to a particular professional or agency; nor should they be used as a "star turn" to dazzle other professionals with the erudition and accomplishments of our profession. Presentations should be aimed specifically at the needs, interests, and concerns of the participants, helping them to gain sufficient information to play their roles more effectively. An in-service program for classroom teachers might focus on recognizing children with communicative disorders and helping them to participate successfully in classroom activities; or it might consider the implications of problems in language acquisition for the mastery of written language skills. A program for hospital nurses might focus on alternative modes of communication with patients with severe speech, language, or hearing disorders. A program for pediatricians might consider such topics as identifying children who are at risk for communicative disorders, approaches to differential diagnosis, and resources for speech, language, and hearing evaluations and therapy. In each of these instances, an audience may acquire information that is applicable in daily practice. At the same time, however, they may identify a member of our profession as a readily available resource for assistance with clients needing expert management.

All in-service education does not occur in sessions scheduled for that purpose. Informal conferences about clients' requests for information, entries in client records, and casual encounters in corridors and lunchrooms may offer the most important teaching opportunities. The speech-language pathologist or audiologist who can exploit each of these contacts in a professionally creditable manner is also likely to be successful in stimulating new referral sources.

REFERRALS MANAGEMENT

In the final analysis, the most effective approach to stimulating new referrals is the skillful management of current referrals. Professionals should take particular precautions in managing the first referrals from new sources. Each well managed client substantially increases the probability of further referrals from the same source. Furthermore, a satisfied referral source is likely to recommend a professional or agency to colleagues. Such recommendations surpass any other means of developing new referral sources.

Current referrals may be further used to develop new sources. For example, with the knowledge and consent of a referral source, one may establish contacts with the other professionals and programs that have served the client or may subsequently provide services the client requires. When well managed, such contacts not only benefit the client but also establish the speech-language pathologist or audiologist as a potential resource for future referrals.

The old chestnut claiming "nothing succeeds like success" was never more applicable. With rare exceptions, the professionals and programs most frequently used by referral sources are those that provide clients with the best services.

MAKING REFERRALS

The circumstances in which speech-language pathologists and audiologists initiate referrals to other professionals and agencies fit into three broad categories: referrals for other professional services which must be completed first, referrals for ancillary services that may complement our services, and referrals to other speech-language pathologists and audiologists.

1. *Referrals for other professional services which must be completed before speech-language pathologists or audiologists can begin or continue their services.* In these instances, our services can only be offered if one or more other services have been completed.

   The most obviously essential referrals occur in instances in which a communicative disorder could be symptomatic of a grave or even life-threatening health problem. For example, clients with persistent hoarseness should never be scheduled for voice therapy without adequate medical examinations to rule out laryngeal carcinoma. Similarly, clients with symptoms of retrocochlear hearing impairment should be examined carefully by physicians for further symptoms of eighth nerve tumors or other neuropathies. These referrals are not only mandatory because of concerns for client welfare, they also may have significant legal implications. A speech-language pathologist or audiologist might well be subject to substantial malpractice claims if he or she failed to make appropriate referrals when symptoms of potentially serious pathologies are apparent.

Referrals may also be essential when further services from a speech-language pathologist or audiologist cannot proceed until more information is available. For example, a speech-language pathologist may be able to complete the assessment of a child with apparent velopharyngeal incompetence only if a series of medical evaluations is conducted, and speech therapy might not be instituted until the results of those evaluations are available. Or, in providing services to a client with conductive hearing impairment, an audiologist would probably consider hearing aid selection and other rehabilitative services only after an adequate otologic examination was completed. Such referrals require sensible delineations of what other services are actually required before we may proceed. Contrary to recurring allegations from some members of other professions that we frequently overstep the boundaries of our professional expertise, members of our profession more often err on the side of over-referral. Before considering a referral to be essential, one should first inquire, "How might my management of this client be changed by the outcomes of this referral?"

Unfortunately, in daily real-life clinical practice, the indications for essential referrals are not always as obvious as in these examples. We once advocated the principle, "when in doubt, refer." However, that principle can now have expensive consequences. Speech-language pathologists and audiologists—particularly those who work in settings that do not charge fees for services—may forget that each referral they effect can result in substantial expense to the client, to the family, or to whatever agency must cover the cost of the referral.

2. *Referrals for ancillary services that may complement our services or provide additional elements of a total rehabilitation program.* These referrals may be requested by the client or family or be proposed by the speech-language pathologist or audiologist. Although these referrals may complement our services, they are not prerequisite to those services. To illustrate, some children with problems in language acquisition come from chaotic families. Although the child's problems may not be directly attributable to the family problems, they are obviously related. The speech-language pathologist may, therefore, guide the family to accept a referral for counseling. Or a client with a significant hearing impairment of sudden onset may be unable to return to his or her previous employment, leading the audiologist to recommend referral for vocational counseling and rehabilitation. Or an elementary school-age stutterer may have specific learning problems that have been obscured by reticence to participate in classroom activities. When such problems become apparent in the speech therapy program, referral for special educational assistance may be in order.

   In each of these instances, a speech-language pathologist or audiologist might initiate one or more referrals. Nevertheless, these referrals are not integral to the speech, language, or hearing services.

3. *Referrals to other speech-language pathologists or audiologists, either for consultation or for continuation of services.* The commonest instances of intraprofessional consultations arise when a speech-language pathologist questions a client's hearing and refers for audiologic evaluation or when an audiologist refers a client for speech-language evaluation. Intraprofessional consultation may also be useful when a client is making insufficient progress in therapy and another professional perspective can be helpful, when the opinion of someone with special expertise is needed, or when evaluations yield equivocal findings. In settings where several speech-language pathologists and audiologists are employed, such consultations may be arranged informally. In other settings, when a client must be referred to another facility, it may be necessary, once again, to consider whether the potential benefits justify the expense.

   Sometimes, referrals to other speech-language pathologists or audiologists are necessary if services are to continue. Current services may be available only so long as a client remains in a particular setting: in a hospital, in an extended care facility, in a home health program, or in some special education facility. Sometimes, services can continue as long as resources, usually in the form of third-party payment, are available to cover fees. Sometimes a client's situation will change so that he or she can no longer be conveniently served by a particular agency or individual professional. Each of these instances may require referrals if speech, language, or hearing services are to continue.

   Some special considerations obtain when one member of our profession refers to another. Although these may seem mere matters of professional etiquette, they actually characterize good service delivery. Intraprofessional referrals should be explored as carefully in advance as referrals to members of other professions. Often, when we refer to our colleagues we make erroneous assumptions about the nature and extent of services available and about the circumstances under which those services are provided. We overgeneralize the modus operandi of the settings in which we work to all settings in which our professional services may be delivered. For example, when we work in a setting where services do not involve fees, we may forget that some settings can only serve clients when fees can be covered. Or when we work in a setting that provides intensive therapy programs, we may forget that such programs may be unavailable in many facilities.

Most importantly, a referral to another member of our profession should imply no more than a commitment that the client will be considered for services; it should never imply a guarantee to the client that services will indeed be provided. Every professional has the right to determine whether, in his or her view, a client requires services, what services are required, the approach that should be taken to providing those services, and whether the services fall within the purview of that professional.

Problems in intraprofessional referrals often occur when members of our profession working in out-of-school settings direct clients and families to seek school-based services. All manner of recommendations may be made without prior consultation with the specialist who presumably must carry out those recommendations. For many quite legitimate reasons, a child may not be an appropriate candidate for the recommended services (even assuming the services are available), placing the school clinician in the untenable position of appearing obstructive. We encounter enough problems in dealing with inappropriate referrals from the members of other professions without being confronted by similar problems from members of our own profession.

Responsibilities of Referral Makers

Making good referrals involves more than advising clients, "You should have a thorough throat examination," or "You should have your child's ears examined by a doctor," or "You ought to talk to someone about your family problems," or "You should get a tutor to help your son with his learning problems." Referral-maker responsibilities can be characterized by posing six questions to be asked—and answered—when making referrals.

1. *Does the referral resource actually provide the services the client requires?* There may be significant disparities between the services that might be assumed to be offered by a particular facility and those that are actually available. Agencies that imply the delivery of comprehensive diagnostic, rehabilitative, or special education services do not necessarily offer the specific services needed by a particular client. Even when such services are legally mandated or required for accreditation or licensure, they may actually be unavailable. (I recall an instance in which a client requiring continued speech therapy was to be discharged from an acute hospital to an extended care facility. When the speech-language pathologist contacted the facility to ascertain the availability of speech therapy—incidentally, a local requirement for licensure of extended care facilities—she was assured that it was certainly available. When she asked who provided those services, she was given the name of a speech-language pathologist who had died 5 years previously.)

   Furthermore, the programs of most human services agencies change from time to time in response to available funding, the interests and expertise of individual staff members, and other similar factors. Therefore, even though a particular service was once available, it is not necessarily currently available.

   The preparation of community directories of referral resources is a popular project for various agencies and professional groups. Although these directories may be useful in identifying the names of potential services providers, they are usually outdated soon after publication. Therefore, their contents must usually be verified before using them as a basis for specific referrals.
2. *Does the client meet the eligibility criteria of the referral resource?* Final decisions about the eligibility of a particular client must always be made by the referral resource. Nevertheless, the maker of a referral should determine in advance that the client meets the most obvious criteria.
3. *Can the client cover the costs entailed in the referral or does he or she have available third-party coverage?* In making a referral, a professional need not, and usually should not, become deeply involved in determining the exact costs entailed in the referral or in helping a client with whatever financial planning is involved. Nevertheless, a client should be informed when a referral has financial implications and should be advised how to secure estimates of those costs, how to determine what third-party coverage may be available, and how to arrange for that coverage.

   When speech-language pathologists and audiologists work in facilities where social work staff is available, that staff may assist the client in securing this information. If such assistance is unavailable, greater responsibilities must be assumed by the professional who initiates the referral.
4. *Are there restrictions with respect to location, hours of service, and other such matters that will make the referral impractical?* Regrettably, most human services agencies locate geographically and establish working schedules with more consideration for their staffs than for the clients they serve. These factors often culminate in de-

scribing particular client populations as "hard to serve." (In some communities, an employed single parent must be absent from work at least six or seven times between the time a child is identified by a school hearing screening program and he or she is equipped with a hearing aid paid for by Crippled Children Services or some other public program.) Even the most conscientious clients and families may be completely unable to pursue referrals that pose serious logistical or secondary economic problems (lost wages, cost of transportation, etc.). Once again, although a speech-language pathologist or audiologist need not become involved in solving each of these practical problems, clients must understand these ramifications of our referrals and, when available, be directed toward assistance in solving attendant problems.

5. *Is the client likely to follow through on the referral, or is he or she merely being agreeable?* Many clients may appear to accept referrals willingly when they actually have no intention of pursuing those referrals. Their failure to follow through on referrals obviously impedes the delivery of needed services. But these failures are also wasteful and ultimately add to the cost of providing services.

   When referral makers actually make appointments for a client, they may assume implied responsibility that the appointment will be kept. In all but unusual instances, appointments should be made by clients themselves. Clients who cannot be trusted to make appointments are not apt to keep appointments made in their behalf.

6. *Is the purpose of the referral clear to the referral resource?* Often, when clinicians complain that their referrals yield little that was helpful, they actually reveal their ineptitude as referral makers. It is virtually impossible for the receiver of a referral to be helpful when he or she has no clue as to why the referral was initiated.

Making Referrals in Different Services Delivery Settings

Once again, policies and procedures governing the making of referrals differ, depending upon the setting in which the speech-language pathologist or audiologist works. Even though each program may have its own idiosyncracies, there are some similarities within settings of the same type.

MAKING REFERRALS IN HEALTH CARE PROGRAMS

Many health care programs impose rigid restrictions as to which staff members may initiate referrals. Often, referrals may be made only by physicians. Sometimes, within comprehensive medical centers, even referrals to other departments within the center must be made by physicians.

Some health care programs are less restrictive, but still specify who is authorized to initiate referrals, extending the privilege to nurses or social workers. Such nonphysician referrals may require countersignature by a physician.

Other health care programs impose few restrictions, permitting any staff member to make appropriate referrals. Even in these more liberal settings, however, it is wise to keep the responsible physicians informed when referrals are made. As I emphasized earlier, regardless of program policies, only in highly unusual instances should a speech-language pathologist or audiologist initiate a referral to another physician without the knowledge of the physician primarily responsible for the client's care.

Restrictive policies in health care programs are not merely intended to preserve physician control. Physicians face frequent dilemmas with respect to making referrals. Too many referrals, particularly those that their colleagues consider unessential, can lead to negative consequences from utilization reviews (reviews primarily aimed at uncovering wasteful practices within health care programs). On the other hand, a physician's failure to make a referral later judged to be required for a client's care can lead to charges of malpractice.

MAKING REFERRALS IN SCHOOL PROGRAMS

Most school agencies also have defined policies for making referrals. These policies usually differentiate between referrals for services provided by other school personnel and referrals to out-of-school professionals and agencies. Depending upon local procedures, referrals for such within-school services as psychological evaluations, reading evaluations, or consultations from counselors or school social workers may be made directly, through the principal of the school the child attends or through a coordinator or supervisor of special education or pupil personnel services. Direct referrals for out-of-school services may also be permitted by some school agencies, although they may more often require coordination by school nurses, school social workers, or a designated administrator or supervisor. Sometimes policies are differentiated; for example, referrals for health-related services must be made by school nurses, whereas responsibilities for other referrals are assigned to other professionals, such as counselors or school social workers.

In the instance of out-of-school referrals, the ultimate responsibility for follow-through usually rests with parents. Nevertheless, the likelihood of their pursuing the referral may depend on the information offered by the professional making the referral—information as to why the referral is advisable, information about what will be entailed by the referral, and information about the referral resource—all of which usually involves more than "sending a note home" with the child. School speech, language, and hearing specialists may be able to turn to other school agency professionals to assist in interpreting referral needs to parents, but often they must assume the responsibility themselves.

Earlier alluded to were the implications of PL 94-142 with respect to referral procedures in schools. If referral made by a school speech, language, and hearing specialist were ruled a contingency for receiving special services, hence integral to those services, it might be argued that the local education agency must assume financial responsibility for the referral. In most instances, unless they are absolutely essential, recommendations for out-of-school referrals are probably best omitted from written evaluation plans and from Individualized Educational Programs.

Professionals in school programs often have less access to information about their clients than professionals working in other settings. Consequently, they may be less aware of the other professionals and programs currently serving a particular child. Prior to making any referrals, it is always advisable for school clinicians to determine whether a child is currently under professional care and then contact whoever is providing that care. We who work in out-of-school facilities are placed in awkward positions when school clinicians refer clients who are already under the care of other individuals or agencies. Furthermore, when a school clinician initiates a referral for health-related services, prior contact with the child's primary health care provider is essential—once again in the interest of continuity of care.

MAKING REFERRALS IN PRIVATE PRACTICE

For most private practitioners, the dependency on referrals for their survival mandates scrupulous management of whatever referrals they make. No private practitioner is likely to receive future referrals from any professional he or she slights in any way, particularly by making some further referral without first involving the original referral source (unless previous experience has shown that the referral source prefers to yield all such responsibilities).

Particularly among physicians, it is common to refer clients primarily to those professionals who refer clients to you. At first blush this may seem nepotistic, but it may actually represent good practice. Professionals tend to develop good working relationships when they work together frequently. Actually, then, the use of a restricted number of referral resources, which are, consequently, frequent referral resources, may result in better client care. Furthermore, as outlined earlier, the responsibilities of referral makers can be time consuming, hence expensive, for a private practitioner. Therefore, the more he or she limits referrals to familiar resources, the more economical the referral process becomes.

Private practitioners often face the need to refer clients who can no longer afford private care. This can be trying to a professional who is more attuned to the delivery of essential human services than to the economic realities of free enterprise. Obviously, however, the private practitioner who cannot deal with such situations will not long be available to serve anybody. It is merely one of life's realities that must be discussed openly with clients, with the professionals who refer to private practitioners (who, incidentally, are usually engaged in the private practice of their own professions), and with the agencies to which the client is referred for whatever services the private practitioner cannot provide.

Unfortunately, with only a small segment of our profession engaged in private practice, most speech-language pathologists and audiologists have little understanding of this setting. They may, therefore, resent referrals from private practitioners and even voice their resentment to clients. Clearly, this represents unprofessional conduct in someone whose livelihood does not depend on the ability of clients to pay fees that accurately reflect the cost of delivering services.

MAKING REFERRALS IN OTHER COMMUNITY AGENCIES AND PROGRAMS

More than any other setting, community agencies are concerned with assuring continuity of services to the widest possible client population. Consequently, community agencies have devoted considerable attention to every aspect of the referral process, often making particular staff members responsible for exploring referral resources, effecting referrals, and following through to ensure that referrals are completed. Speech-language pathologists and audiologists in this setting are, therefore, more likely to be supported in effecting referrals than in most other settings. By the same token, however, members of our profession may also be restricted from direct participation in the referral process, limiting direct communication with referral resources.

Community agencies, since they rely on the community for support, may also be in a sensitive position with respect to selectivity in making referrals. For example, although a speech-language pathologist may know that only one or two otolaryngologists in a community are interested and skilled in conducting laryngeal examinations of children, the agency may adhere rigidly to a policy of offering, in evenly rotated order, three names of Board specialists for all medical referrals. Thus it becomes difficult to obtain the expert guidance that is actually needed. In practice, however, professionals in community agencies have learned to outwit such policies unobtrusively.

Clients of community agencies are more likely to receive whatever services they need from other public community agencies than from private practitioners. This can complicate referral procedures. It is usually more difficult to obtain a specific service from an agency than from an independent professional. For example, unraveling the bureaucracies of large city and county hospitals to obtain a medical opinion in response to a specific question can be a formidable task. Once again, community agency staff members must learn short cuts to expedite referrals, even referrals to gargantuan institutions.

SOME REFERRAL QUANDARIES

Unfortunately, in daily professional practice, issues related to making and receiving referrals are not always as neat as the earlier sections of this chapter may imply. The following examples typify some of the quandaries we face. Although possible solutions are proposed, there are no absolutes.

A Quandary of Conflicting Professional Opinions

Since we are engaged in the practice of a profession that usually entails dealing with professionals of different backgrounds, referral quandaries often stem from conflicting professional opinions, as in this first example:

A 4-year-old was recently evaluated by a speech-language pathologist in a community speech and hearing center because of his parents' concerns about slow speech and language acquisition. Hearing screening at the time of the speech and language evaluation strongly supported the need for a more detailed hearing evaluation. When seen by one of the center's audiologists, all findings were consistent with a 35 to 45-dB bilateral conductive hearing impairment.

Following the hearing evaluation, the parents were urged to consult immediately the primary care physician identified as the referral source at the time of the first contact with the center. The results of the hearing evaluation were also sent directly to that physician.

On returning to the center to formulate final plans for speech and language therapy, the parents reported that the physician had denied the possibility of any significant hearing impairment. They admitted that the physician had been opposed to their contacting the center originally and that they had given his name as the referral source because they assumed the child would not be seen without a medical referral. They further reported that the physician had reiterated his opinion that the child was perfectly normal and that, if anything, he was the victim of overanxious parents. The physician was also extremely critical of the center and stated that the staff was simply capitalizing on the family's anxieties.

The next example is a variation of the same theme:

George Karnoff is a speech, language, and hearing specialist in a large urban school district. His schedule was recently changed so that he was for the first time assigned to Lincoln Elementary School. Among the children served by the previous specialist was a fourth-grader with severe speech problems related to cleft palate. This 10-year-old boy had been treated previously through four different surgical procedures. The most recent, carried out 2 years previously, involved creation of a pharyngeal flap.

The boy presented all the classic symptoms of a severe rhinolalia. Mr. Karnoff's review of the previous clinician's records showed little change in the child's speech during the previous 2 years. After working with the youngster on a twice-weekly basis for 3 months, he confirmed his initial impression that the velopharyngeal closure was so inadequate that any significant progress through speech therapy was virtually impossible. Mr. Karnoff then contacted the plastic surgeon responsible for the youngster's care to discuss these concerns and discovered that the surgeon adamantly held the position that the pharyngeal flap surgery had been highly successful and that the youngster's speech would improve with sufficient motivation.

These two situations have obvious commonalities. In each instance another professional supported a position in direct conflict with the considered opinion of a speech-language pathologist or audiologist. In the first instance, the physician is impeding further referrals to secure needed treatment. In the second instance, the physician is insisting on services that are not likely to be beneficial.

An inescapable fact of life is that professionals disagree. Anyone who strives to be a mature and independently responsible professional must deal with controversies which often involve members of the most prestigious, influential, and authoritative professions. Above all, it is essential first to be assured that one's position is correct, or at least completely reasonable. Once so assured, the client's best interests become the primary determiners of the course to be pursued.

In all instances, whether interprofessional controversies exist or not, it is the responsibility of a professional to offer clients and their families whatever information and support are needed to reach whatever decisions must be made. It is never good practice to tell clients what to do. Instead, seek to assist clients to make wise decisions. One cannot protect clients from interprofessional controversies. Instead, one must assist them in dealing with whatever controversies arise.

Within this context, then, it becomes the responsibility of the speech-language pathologist or audiologist to communicate as clearly as possible his or her findings, recognizing openly that these findings may differ from the findings of other professionals. Insofar as possible, opinions and recommendations should be distinguished from the professionals holding the opinions and making the recommendations. Disparaging the qualifications of other professionals, directly or indirectly, is seldom helpful. Even when, as in the illustration of the child with a hearing impairment, members of other professions disparage our qualifications, the most effective antidote is a quiet demonstration of thorough competence and scrupulous professionalism.

In the first example, the audiologist and speech-language pathologist should help the family understand the basis for concluding that the child has a hearing impairment, perhaps including demonstrations of testing procedures. The family should also understand the potential implications of hearing impairment for the child's speech and language acquisition and for his future education. They should also be informed of available resources for the needed medical care. In this instance, recommendations for a speech-language therapy program would probably not be contingent upon securing needed medical care, because an effective therapy program might well be conducted despite the hearing impairment.

In the second example, continuation of the speech therapy program may actually be deleterious. A fundamental ethical issue is involved in continuing services beyond the point a clinician believes the client is likely to benefit from these services. Furthermore, even though the clinician announces to the client and his family that further improvement is unlikely in view of structural deficits, the clinician negates that conclusion when therapy continues. (Why would a clinician persist unless some benefit is likely?) Thus, a clinician may interfere with optimal care by forestalling a client from seeking whatever help is actually needed. In this instance, the client should explore other approaches—surgical, prosthetic, or whatever—to improve the potential for better speech. The goal of the speech-language pathologist, then, is to lead the client and his family to inquire about other alternatives and to identify resources for whatever consultations are needed.

In both illustrations, the pursuit of the client's best interests may lead to antipathy from other professionals—antipathy that may elicit complaints to administrators and supervisors. Yet a client's best interests are always the foremost consideration. If serving those interests alienates individual professionals, this is a necessary consequence of ethical practice. Furthermore, if clients ultimately obtain the services they need, for every professional who is alienated, at least one professional will have the opportunity to observe the contributions of a skilled practitioner of the profession of speech-language pathology and audiology.

A Quandary of Limited Experience

Considering the scope of our profession, it is impossible for any single clinician, regardless of the extent of his or her education or the length of his or her experience, to be prepared to serve all clients. The following illustrates the quandaries that derive from this inevitability:

Jean Bosch was beginning her third year of professional experience as the speech, language, and hearing specialist in a rural school district. The school district employed one other clinician who was returning for her second year of employment following completion of her training.

Within the first week of the new school year, Ms. Bosch received an urgent call from a kindergarten teacher, seeking help with Eddie, a child who was entering school for the first time. On investigation, Ms. Bosch discovered that the youngster had, at age 3, sustained severe injuries. One day, when he was playing in the kitchen, his mother had left him alone to answer the telephone in another room. In exploring a cupboard he found an improperly sealed can of caustic drain cleaner and proceeded to ingest some of it, sustaining severe burns to the oral cavity, pharynx, and larynx. Several surgical procedures followed which left him with considerable scar tissue and a permanent tracheotomy. At the time he entered school, then, Eddie had no means of producing speech. A year or so earlier, someone had provided him with an electrolarynx, but he was given no instruction in its use.

Ms. Bosch was understandably overwhelmed when she saw Eddie for the first time. Although he unquestionably needed some form of serviceable communication system, she had no previous experience to draw on to formulate an appropriate therapy program. She recalled a series of lectures in a voice pathology course concerning the rehabilitation of laryngectomized adults, and she had observed two or three sessions with a clinician teaching esophageal speech. She had seen demonstrations of various augmentative communication devices but had never seen one in use by a child. She also had some general familiarity with various sign systems but had no proficiency in teaching or using any of them.

Ms. Bosch faced a serious dilemma. On the one hand, she recognized Eddie's crucial need for communication. On the other hand, she had no specific information about the approaches that might help him. Although she would have been pleased to make a referral, the nearest potential source of assistance was 60 miles away at the state university medical center.

The injunction in ASHA's Code of Ethics that clinicians should not provide "services for which they have not been properly prepared" is meritorious. But sometimes there must be a choice between less than expert services and no services at all. Ms. Bosch could quite properly decide that she is unable to assist Eddie. Every clinician must recognize instances in which he or she cannot be helpful, even though a client may desperately require some form of assistance.

Ms. Bosch might also reasonably conclude that, qualified or not, little would be lost by a learn-as-you-go approach in providing a therapy program for Eddie. When confronted with a client who appears to differ dramatically from our previous encounters, we all tend to fixate on the unique features, forgetting that there may well be essential similarities to other clients we have served. In this instance, Ms. Bosch probably knew a great deal about helping children acquire spoken language, even though she knew little about adapting those approaches for a client whose peripheral speech mechanism was so severely impaired that oral communication might be infeasible.

Although the state university medical center was too distant to be a practical referral resource for a therapy program, it might well be a practical resource for consultation. First in order would be an appraisal of the child's potential for the various alternatives for communication: the electrolarynx, another form of alaryngeal speech, sign language, or one of several augmentative communication devices. Some combination of two or more of these alternatives might well prove useful, or one might be employed immediately while others were being mastered. Such an initial appraisal of alternatives could probably be accomplished—hopefully with Ms. Bosch's direct participation—during an intensive series of daily appointments at the medical center.

Once initial approaches were identified, Ms. Bosch could devote her regular therapy sessions to experimental teaching—experimental for both the client and the clinician. She might seek continued support through consultation with the medical center and by means of occasional visits, reinforced with intervening telephone contacts.

Presumably, Eddie might progress more rapidly if he were receiving regular help from someone more expert than Ms. Bosch. However, with her help, his progress would be infinitely superior to his progress under the only available alternative: no help at all.

When more expert services are unavailable, clinicians must often learn as their clients learn. It is, after all, also a truism that every provider of expert services became such after considerable experience providing less than expert services.

A Quandary of Economics

This example illustrates the quandaries that can derive from conflicts between humanistic and practical concerns:

During the many years she has been engaged in the private practice of speech-language pathology, Margaret Evans has achieved wide recognition for her skill in working with clients with voice disorders. The high regard for her abilities in this area is shared by other speech-language pathologists in her community and by several otolaryngologists, who frequently refer clients to her for evaluation and therapy.

Recently, on referral from an otolaryngologist, she saw a vocal music student from the local conservatory of music. The student had recently developed vocal fold nodules. Ms. Evans and the otolaryngologist agreed that, regardless of the effects of singing, the student's phonation for speech was characterized by obvious hyperfunction, and that any approach to treatment of the nodules must include a period of speech therapy to begin immediately.

Since the student was covered by a health insurance plan, the otolaryngologist assumed that his referral to Ms. Evans as a private patient was appropriate. It soon became apparent, however, that speech therapy was not covered by the health insurance. Furthermore, the student was attempting to support herself and cover all of the cost of her music studies from meager earnings as a part-time clerk in a clothing store. She was, therefore, incapable of paying fees for private voice therapy.

Although details vary, this quandary is repeatedly confronted by every successful private practitioner and by other clinicians who work in programs primarily supported by fees. However gratifying, achieving the reputation as the best resource for particular services can create many problems for private practitioners. Referral sources can neglect to consider whether the clients they refer can afford private fees, even when the referral sources are themselves engaged in private practice.

In this instance, Ms. Evans must weigh the consequences of various alternatives. If failing to provide the needed therapy program might alienate a valuable referral source, she may be well advised to provide the services as a courtesy to the otolaryngologist, making it clear that she is granting the courtesy in special recognition of the client's particular needs and circumstances.

A second alternative might be to recommend a program to be carried out by a less experienced clinician in another program in the community that allows adjusted fees for services, Under this plan, Ms. Evans might see the client for one or two sessions as a basis for formulating therapy recommendations, then provide consultations to the other clinician, perhaps with occasional brief follow-up visits to assess progress and formulate modified recommendations.

As another alternative, Ms. Evans might simply complete the evaluation and effect a referral to the best available and feasible resource for the therapy program, sharing her expertise by making whatever therapy recommendations seem appropriate and offering to discuss the case further as needs arise. This offer should be made both to the agency toward which the referral is directed and to the referring otolaryngologist.

Learning to accept the practical limitations of one's practice is always a painful aspect of acquiring professional maturity. The need to restrict services primarily to clients who can pay for them is an overriding limitation for private practice, but it should be no more devastating than the inherent practical limitations confronted by any practitioner in any setting.

A Quandary of Intraprofessional Relationships

This quandary may well be the commonest of all:

Eric Schneider is the only speech-language pathologist on the staff of a community child guidance clinic. One of the clinic's social workers initiates a referral for evaluation of a 7-year-old with an articulatory disorder. During his preliminary review of the child's record, Mr. Schneider notes that the child is currently enrolled in a speech therapy program at school.

This example is so commonplace that some might wonder why it is cited as a paradoxical situation. It clearly indicates an instance where a professional is asked to intervene when a client is already in the care of a member of the same profession. Unless managed carefully, such instances cause intraprofessional conflicts. More importantly, they can create confusions for clients and families that can interfere with the delivery of appropriate services.

Every client has the inalienable right of a second opinion. Furthermore, every professional should encourage clients to pursue that right when questions arise. Seeking a second opinion does not necessarily denote dissatisfaction with whatever services have been provided or with the professionals providing those services. Nevertheless, the person who provides that second opinion bears a responsibility both to the client and to the professionals already serving that client.

As a first consideration, then, there is no reason why Mr. Schneider should hesitate in accepting that referral. If possible, he should establish contact with the concerned school speech, language, and hearing specialist before seeing the child. Of course, this contact can occur only with the family's consent. Occasionally, clients prefer that other professionals not be involved when seeking a second opinion, which is clearly their privilege. If the school clinician is consulted, he or she should not only be asked for information about the client, but also asked for recommendations as to how the second clinician can best facilitate the child's care and communicate most effectively with the family. Although Mr. Schneider is not obliged to agree with the school clinician, if, as usually happens, they essentially agree, he is in an excellent position to support and reinforce the child's therapy program.

Once the evaluation is complete, Mr. Schneider should again contact the school clinician, summarizing his findings and recommendations. If the family persists in refusing to authorize such a contact, despite urging, he would have no alternative but to report only to the family and to the referring social worker.

If Mr. Schneider and the school clinician differ substantially in their opinions, and these opinions cannot be reconciled through discussion, he must apprise the family of those differences as objectively as possible, interpreting the possible bases of their disagreements. Once again, differences in professional opinions are a fact of life whether they occur between members of different professions or between members of the same profession. No skilled clinician should incite these differences, but he or she should not conceal them from clients when they occur.

SUMMARY

Proficiency in receiving and making referrals may well be one of the most important accomplishments of speech-language pathologists and audiologists. In virtually all settings, a substantial portion of the clients we serve come to us on the referral of other professionals or agencies. Furthermore, since many clients present complex problems, requiring the expertise of several professionals, we often must effect good referrals if they are to receive the help they need. Referral traditions, policies, and practices differ substantially in different settings. Therefore, the quality of care any client ultimately receives may well depend upon the skill of speech-language pathologists and audiologists in receiving and making referrals in the myriad settings in which they work.

Despite the critical importance of well managed referrals, there has been only the most superficial regard for this topic in the literature. This situation accounts for the absence of references at the end of this chapter. I found no material that I could urge readers to review.

PART 2

Clinical Information Management

CHAPTER FIVE

Clinical Reporting

I once read a letter to the editor of *Lancet*, the eminent British medical journal, that recounted observations made by an English physician during a tour of the United States. Among the strange practices he commented on was a tribal rite carried out at the nursing stations of hospital wards. As he described it, nurses clustered in a corner while physicians entered their observations and orders in patient charts. As soon as the physicians completed their notes, they retired to a neutral corner while the nurses materialized to read those notes and then duly enter their responses and observations. When the nurses' entries were completed they vanished, and the physicians once again descended to see what the nurses had written. The English physician concluded that in America direct conversation among health care professionals was a lost art and that communication was now carried out exclusively by notes hastily scrawled in official records.

However exaggerated, the British physician's observations may have some merit. Communication among human services providers may have become less direct than we might wish. Nevertheless, there are good and necessary reasons for written reporting of all essential aspects of clinical services, regardless of the amount of direct oral communication that has transpired. When misunderstandings occur, memories fail, or challenges arise, every clinician is grateful to discover that all salient details are covered by written records. Furthermore, as the specter of litigation over the adequacy and appropriateness of services haunts us ever more frequently, adequate clinical records are no longer merely desirable, they are now mandatory.

TYPES OF CLINICAL REPORTS

Clinical reports serve three basic purposes: (1) to transmit information to other professionals; (2) to preserve information so that it can be retrieved by the recorder at some point in the future; and (3) to document whatever services are provided and characterize the nature of those services to comprise a legal record. Although relative emphasis on one or another of these purposes may differ in different settings, in no setting can any of the three be completely disregarded. Discussions of the second two have been largely relegated to Chapter 6. The present chapter focuses on clinical reports as media for inter- and intraprofessional communication.

Clinical reports may take two different forms: they may be entered into a client's clinical record, or they may be prepared for direct transmittal to one or more other professionals. In the first instance, the record may be consulted exclusively by the person who entered the information (as in the case of a single private practitioner), it may be consulted only by other speech-language pathologists or audiologists (as in a group private practice or a community speech and hearing center), or it may be consulted by several different professionals (as in school programs, rehabilitation centers, or comprehensive medical centers). In the second instance, reports may be prepared specifically for transmittal to one professional (e.g., the referring physician, a classroom teacher, or a speech-language pathologist or audiologist who is already serving a client or to whom a client is being referred), or all-purpose reports may be prepared for distribution to all professionals concerned with a particular client.

All of these factors—whether a report is merely prepared for entry into a client record or is to be sent out, the readership for whom the report is intended, etc.—may influence the form, content, and language of reports. Furthermore, as we will see in the next chapter, the context and form of reports, particularly reports prepared for direct entry into client records, may differ depending upon the record-keeping system adopted by the particular program. Nevertheless, some principles and practices of good communication obtain regardless of these factors.

A further reality must be considered in the preparation of all clinical reports. Clinical reports were once for the eyes of professionals only. Whatever reports were read by clients and families were especially prepared for that purpose. But now, in most instances, clients and families may invoke the right to read any and all reports whenever they choose.

Typical clinical reports may be classified into five different categories: *referral acknowledgments, reports of initial evaluations, therapy plans, progress notes and summaries, and discharge or transfer summaries.* A single report may sometimes serve two or more of these purposes.

Referral Acknowledgments

Continuity of client care and the maintenance of cordial relationships with referral sources are best served when referrals are acknowledged promptly. If the client is seen for some initial service soon after the referral ("soon" can be defined as within 3 or 4 weeks), the report of that initial service may constitute adequate acknowledgment of the referral. When a longer period will elapse, however, a separate referral acknowledgment is usually in order.

Such acknowledgments serve several purposes. They recognize that the referral has been received, express appreciation for the efforts of the referral source, assure the referral source that the requested service will be provided, and offer an estimate as to when it will be available. If, for some reason, the client fails to complete the referral, it will be on record that the referral was not lost.

In most instances, form letters can be used to acknowledge referrals. Word-processing or other computerized systems can, when available, generate appropriate acknowledgments economically and effectively. Such letters need contain only a few lines, acknowledging receipt of the referral, stating the approximate date when the service will be available, and promising a fuller report when initial services are complete and recommendations can be made.

Referral acknowledgments are also appropriate in comprehensive services centers where referrals come from other staff members and communication is via notes in client records. Again, when delays will occur before referrals can be completed, it is good practice to enter an acknowledgment in the record. Particularly in inpatient centers, where services must be delivered within the shortest possible time, it may be wise to enter acknowledgments even when a delay will extend for only a few days.

Reports of Initial Evaluations

In typical clinical practice, initial contact with any client involves completion of an evaluation. Conventionally, such evaluations occupy one or more sessions that include administration of some formal testing together with informal observations of the client's communicative behaviors. This "diagnosis precedes treatment" model is obviously rooted in the traditions of medical practice, which have strongly influenced the delivery of all human services. When sufficient information has been gathered, most clinicians prepare initial evaluation reports. Whether entered into a client record or prepared separately, an initial evaluation report should always contain at least four of the following five elements: reason(s) for conducting the evaluation, description of the client's communication, conclusions regarding the basis of the client's communicative disorders, description of previous intervention, and recommendations.

1. *Reason(s) for conducting the evaluation.* Every report should specify at the outset the essential reason or reasons for conducting the evaluation. For example, "Gloria came to our clinic for a complete hearing evaluation as a follow-up procedure to the screening program at her school," or "George's parents brought him to the clinic because of their concern about his slow speech and language development," or "Mrs. Dixon came for evaluation of her voice problem on referral of Dr. Steven Grimaldi, the otolaryngologist she consulted at the suggestion of her internist, Dr. Marshall Weiner." The approach taken within the evaluation, the extent of the evaluation, and the recommendations formulated may all depend upon the reasons for conducting it. Consequently, those reasons should be stated clearly at the outset.
2. *Description of the client's communication.* The extent and specificity of this description will depend on the purpose of the evaluation and of the report. Such a description in the report to a physician following a hearing evaluation on a child with recurrent otitis media may be brief and specific. In contrast, the report on a client with a language disorder that is to serve as the basis for planning intervention may be extensive and detailed. Also depending on the nature and purpose of the evaluation, the report may comprise test data and interpretations, or more general descriptions of communicative behaviors, or combinations of both.
3. *Conclusions regarding the basis of the client's communicative disorders.* Although many clinicians believe that evaluations should always reach conclusions about possible causes of observed communicative disorders, I believe that this is the one optional element of such a report. In fact, I believe that overreaching the limit of available data to draw conclusions about etiology is one of our profession's most frequent transgressions. In my opinion, such conclusions are important in evaluation reports only when the basis of the communicative disorder can be confidently identified and when those conclusions will significantly influence management (e.g., implicating structural anomalies, motor deficits, or hearing impairments in cases of delayed speech and language acquisition; recognizing vocal abuse or hyperfunction in cases of dysphonia; or identifying noise exposure as a likely cause of hearing impairment). Some conclusions about etiology may have little influence on our own intervention but may have major implications for other professionals (e.g., symptoms of retrocochlear hearing impairment, motor speech disorders that typify degenerative neurologic diseases, or communicative disorders that may signal psychopathology).
4. *Description of previous intervention.* Every diagnostic report should summarize previous efforts to ameliorate the client's communicative disorder. This information may form the major basis for whatever recommendations are made. Furthermore, when financial support for further services is sought, it may be crucial in determining whether such support will be granted.
5. *Recommendations.* The professionals who refer our clients, and the clients themselves, usually expect more than a description of their communicative disorders when an evaluation is completed. In most instances, they expect recommendations for management. Every professional should make whatever recommendations emerge from the evaluations, regardless of the referral source's original reason for instituting the evaluation. (For example, a physician may refer for completion of an audiologic evaluation as a prerequisite to formulating a medical diagnosis. Regardless of that limited purpose, however, the audiologist should make whatever recommendations for rehabilitation are appropriate.) At the same time, the clinician must be certain that all of the questions that precipitated the referral are addressed, either by providing answers or by delimiting areas for further study before answers can be found.

School speech, language, and hearing services may require another document in conjunction with evaluations. Under the terms of PL 94-142, parents must consent, in writing, before an evaluation may be conducted. (At this writing, revised regulations have been proposed that eliminate this requirement.) In current practice, a preliminary report is rendered to the parents, stating the reason for conducting the evaluation, briefly characterizing the components of that evaluation, and requesting their consent. A copy of this documentation of informed consent must then be filed in the child's school record.

Therapy Plans

Therapy plans may form one section of evaluation reports, or they may constitute separate entries in client records or separate reports to referral sources, to other agencies, or to third-party payers. Customarily, therapy plans cover specified periods (a given number of therapy sessions or a time interval in weeks or months). Therapy plans usually suggest ultimate goals as well as short-term objectives that seem feasible for accomplishment by the end of the specified period.

Not only is it good professional practice to clarify therapy plans as specifically as possible, this clear delineation is an almost universal requirement in any setting where regulations of governmental agencies, accreditation agencies, or third-party payers apply—which is to say, virtually all settings in which speech-language pathology and audiology services are delivered.

The Joint Commission on Accreditation of Hospitals (JCAH), the agency that accredits most health services institutions employing members of our profession, considers speech-language pathology and audiology within the standards applied to rehabilitation services. JCAH specifies the following with respect to therapy plans:

> There shall be a current, written plan of care for each patient receiving rehabilitative services. It should state the treatment objectives for the patient, as well as the patient's short-term and long-term rehabilitation potential. The plan should be reviewed at stated, regular intervals and revised as indicated. The patient and his family shall be permitted to participate as much as possible in the development of the plan of care.

Speech-language pathologists and audiologists who provide services covered by third-party payers should be aware of these standards, even in agencies where JCAH accreditation does not apply, since third-party payers often use JCAH standards when they audit records of clients served under their auspices.

In many medical and rehabilitation facilities, therapy plans must be reviewed and approved by the physician responsible for case management. Such approval is virtually a universal requirement by third-party payers. In these instances, client records must always include duly approved therapy plans.

The standards for accreditation by ASHA's Professional Services Board (1983) also require written evidence of therapy plans. The following indicators signal that this standard is met:

A. Each client is assigned to a qualified speech-language pathologist or audiologist who assumes primary responsibility for the management of the client's program.

B. Long- and short-term treatment objectives are specified and based on the conclusions and recommendations of a diagnostic evaluation.

C. Treatment plans include statements of prognosis.

D. Treatment plans are reviewed and modified to reflect the changing needs of the client.

E. Treatment plans specify the type, frequency, and duration of speech-language pathology or audiology services.

F. Conferences are held with other service providers to review client progress, to develop further plans, and to maintain an integrated and coordinated program.

School clinicians must also adhere to stringent regulations with respect to setting down therapy plans. Under the terms of PL 94-142, the content of the Individualized Educational Program (IEP) must be specified for each child who receives either special education or related services or both. When a child is enrolled for special education, a single IEP is usually written covering both special education and related services (presumably with speech, language, and hearing specialists contributing within their areas of expertise). When related services are provided by speech-language pathologists or audiologists to children who are not enrolled in other special education programs, the IEP is usually written primarily by that single professional, with appropriate consultations with concerned administrators, teachers, and parents.

Clinicians in other settings must also be familiar with IEP requirements. When they see children who are being considered for special school services, they are often asked to contribute to the preparation of the IEP. Furthermore, under the provisions of PL 94-142, which permit local education agencies to purchase services from nonpublic programs, an IEP must be written, specifying the services to be provided by the out-of-school agency, including all information required in any IEP.

Section 121.a 346 of PL 94-142 regulations (see Dublinske, 1978) specifies the following content in the IEP:

(a) A statement of a child's present levels of educational performance.
(b) A statement of annual goals, including short-term and related services to be provided to the child and long-term instructional objectives.
(c) A statement of the specific special education and the extent to which the child will be able to participate in regular educational programs.
(d) The projected dates for initiation of services and the anticipated duration of the services.
(e) Appropriate objective criteria and evaluation procedures for determining, on at least an annual basis, whether the short-term instructional objectives are being achieved.

Progress Notes and Summaries

Progress notes serve at least three major functions: First, they serve as a ready reminder of the plan and course of the treatment program to the clinician providing the service, a particularly important function to clinicians serving many clients. Second, they should enable another clinician unexpectedly to assume responsibility for the client's care, either temporarily or permanently, with as little disruption as possible. Third, progress notes must provide evidence that each service has been provided, evidence to support claims for providing the service, and evidence which will answer questions about the nature and the outcome of the service. Progress notes covering therapy sessions usually begin with a one- or two-sentence statement of the goals of the session. Next comes a short description of the activities pursued toward the goals. Then follows a concise evaluation of the achievements of the sessions. Finally, there should be recommendations for future sessions or for other services (e.g., contacts with the family or school, or other testing).

When clients are enrolled in long-term therapy programs, progress notes may proliferate to the point that storage becomes unmanageable. Usually, lengthy therapy programs are associated with slow rates of client progress. Progress notes, then, tend to be similar from one session to the next. In these instances, progress notes may be entered at specified intervals (monthly, every 6 weeks, even every 3 months), although, as a rule, the date of each session is recorded in the progress notes with the statement "seen for therapy." Before instituting this procedure, one should be certain that it is not a breach of institutional policies or of the requirements of third-party payers.

When clients are enrolled in group therapy programs, multiple copies of progress notes may be prepared and distributed so that one copy is filed in the record of each participant. Occasional individual progress notes may be added to characterize a particular client's responses to treatment or to record special recommendations.

Progress notes are usually associated with clients enrolled in therapy. But these notes may also apply to clients involved in evaluation procedures requiring successive visits. For example, the completion of a hearing evaluation of a 2-year-old often requires a series of several sessions. The referral may be acknowledged following the first visit, but the evaluation summary is usually not prepared until some tenable conclusions can be drawn. Observations from the individual testing sessions may be entered as progress notes. The same procedure may be followed when an adult is seen for a series of visits in connection with the selection and fitting of a hearing aid.

As has already been noted, progress notes are important as a legal record of ongoing services. They may also be important as a legal record of untoward occurrences or other potentially litigious situations. The following suggest some instances that should be recorded.

1. *Accidents or other unusual occurrences.* Any misadventures which occur within the vicinity of the agency should be noted, whether or not any injuries are apparent. Such misadventures include falls, episodes of vertigo, seizures, abrasions sustained by children in activity programs, etc. Larger agencies, particularly hospitals and rehabilitation centers, usually have prescribed procedures to follow in connection with such occurrences and provide special reporting forms. If no procedures are defined, the misadventures should be noted briefly and factually in the narrative portion of the clinical record. The note should state any recommendations for medical consultation or other emergency procedures related to the incident.

   Clients have been known to ascribe later problems to certain audiologic procedures. It is wise, therefore, to record statements about extreme or lasting discomfort, such as reactions to loud sounds used in testing, markedly adverse reactions to impedance measurement, concerns about procedures involved in taking earmold impressions, and other complaints relative to hearing aid selection and fitting.
2. *Complaints.* Every clinical program occasionally receives client complaints. If these relate in any way to the services provided, they should be noted in the clinical record. Allegations that a staff member has been tardy, unsympathetic, rude, abrupt, overly familiar, or neglectful should be recorded. Usually the notation is best made by the staff member who is the subject of the allegation, once again with a brief, factual statement.

   Client complaints are an inevitable part of delivering clinical services. Although they need not be overemphasized, they are usually best recognized openly. If such complaints lead to any legal action, the clinician or agency is in a more favorable position when the matter is documented in the clinical record. The failure to note a complaint may be interpreted as an attempt to suppress it and thus may imply guilt. Although embarrassment may attend the incident and the record entry, much greater eventual embarrassment may be forestalled by a frank notation.
3. *Deteriorating performance.* Speech-language pathologists and audiologists may occasionally be the only professionals who are maintaining frequent contacts with clients. Therefore, they may be in a crucial position to monitor significant changes in performance. Speech-language pathologists may observe increasing hoarseness among clients in voice therapy. They may see steadily deteriorating performance among adults with aphasia or motor speech disorders. Audiologists may see clients with rapidly increasing hearing impairment.

   In these instances, two considerations are important. First, the record should document the observed changes. Second, it should show efforts, preferably letters, to alert whoever is responsible for medical management to these changes. As the only professional in regular contact with the client, the speech-language pathologist or audiologist could legitimately be charged with negligence if his or her attempts to intervene are not clearly documented.
4. *Advice and referrals.* Advice and referrals offered during evaluations and at discharge are usually noted in records, but clinicians frequently neglect to note this information when offered during the course of a therapy program. Clients and their families may frequently seek advice regarding all manner of problems from speech-language pathologists and audiologists who are concerned and helpful. When the advice sought extends beyond the clinician's expertise, he or she need only suggest sources of assistance and, perhaps, suggest how the assistance can be obtained. All such recommendations should be noted in the record. Once again, any subsequent charges of negligence or other professional malfeasance can be dealt with more easily when the record shows how such inquiries were handled.

When continuing services are provided to clients, it may be necessary, from time to time, to summarize the outcome of those services. Progress summaries are required in most school programs, usually being prepared for the normal reporting periods of the school year. Such summaries are virtually mandated by PL 94-142 to enable conclusions as to "whether the short term instructional objectives are being achieved," and they frequently comprise the first step in the preparation of supplementary or continuing IEP's. In other clinical settings, third-party payers may require progress summaries of previously authorized services as requisites to authorization of further services.

Speech-language pathologists and audiologists who are substantially dependent upon referrals may be well advised to send routine progress summaries to referral sources. Many clinicians establish no contacts between the initial evaluation report and the discharge summary. But in the interest of continuity of care, referral sources should be apprised of progress at regular intervals, particularly when they are responsible for coordinating multiple clinical services. Furthermore, routine progress summaries are among the most effective devices for educating referral sources and encouraging further referrals, because they offer regular reminders of the services the speech-language pathologist or audiologist can provide.

Discharge and Transfer Summaries

Another routine of good clinical practice involves the preparation of summaries at the time any program of services terminates. Such summaries should be prepared regardless of the basis of termination: because no further services are needed, because the client is to continue services in another program, or because the client has discontinued the program through disinterest or dissatisfaction.

Discharge summaries should usually be sent to original referral sources in the hope of stimulating a review of the client's total program so that the need for any further services can be determined. Rehabilitation programs often involve a sequence of services, with some awaiting completion of others. For example, vocational counseling may be staged to begin after completion of the selection and fitting of a hearing aid with attendant aural rehabilitation services. Or decisions as to whether a surgeon will carry out additional procedures in treating a child with cleft palate may depend upon the relative success of a speech therapy program. In these instances, continuity of care can be seriously impaired when a speech-language pathologist or audiologist terminates services without apprising whoever is coordinating the client's care of the outcome of those services.

Many of the clients we discharge are likely to be considered for speech-language pathology or audiology services again in the future, often by clinicians in other programs. At that time, it may be extremely important to know the results of previous services. This may be particularly true for clients who are always eager to establish contacts with new agencies but who rapidly lose interest in pursuing whatever recommendations result.

It is customary for third-party payers to require that summaries of all previous therapy programs accompany requests for authorization of additional services. Concise discharge summaries are invaluable for this purpose.

Summaries similar in content to discharge summaries are also mandatory when a client's care is transferred from one clinician to another. This obtains whether services are to be delivered within the same agency or in another agency. Once again, transfer summaries are an essential ingredient of continuity of care.

Discharge and transfer summaries briefly recount the entire history of efforts to evaluate and treat a client's communicative disorder. They should begin with a concise summary of relevant services prior to the initiation of current services. Next, there should be a brief description of all services provided since admission to the current program, specifying the nature, goals, and extent of those services and summarizing their apparent results. Finally, there should be recommendations for whatever continued services and follow-up are needed.

Although preparing discharge and transfer summaries may seem an odious, time-consuming burden, ultimately they may effect significant economies in effort. Whenever it is necessary to retrieve information from a client record—particularly from a voluminous client record—well prepared summaries can provide ready guides to the character and extent of the client's problems and to the nature and outcome of whatever services have been provided in the client's behalf.

ORGANIZING CLINICAL REPORTS

Should each clinical report follow a formally established pattern of organization?

There are many clear advantages to prescribed outlines. Clinicians may provide more consistent services when reports must be prepared according to specified categories, since there is an implied protocol for all procedures. Consistently organized reports may also assist readers, who will always know the approximate scope of material covered and the location of specific information.

On the other hand, rigidly organized reporting systems have distinct disadvantages. It is virtually impossible to construct an outline that will cover all requirements. For example, no single format is equally suited to reporting on a prelingual 3-year-old, a 25-year-old stutterer, and a 70-year-old laryngectomee. When a set outline requires coverage of specific areas, clinicians may slavishly include information that is irrelevant to the case at hand, making reports overlong and misleading. The opposite may occur when conventional report structures do not include unusual but occasionally relevant factors and clinicians are led to overlook salient details.

Some facilities prepare specific forms to be completed by clinicians for reporting evaluations, therapy plans, progress summaries, etc. These forms may have at least two advantages. First, it may require less time to fill out the form than to prepare a narrative report. Second, it may standardize reporting so that all staff members include similar information. (This may be particularly helpful when students and inexperienced staff members are involved.) Furthermore, this standardization may facilitate the retrieval of information, since a reader will know immediately where to look for particular data.

Forms are especially suitable for certain types of reports. They are obviously the most efficient approach to reporting routine hearing evaluations., in which test results can be summarized graphically and numerically and other important information and recommendations can be summarized briefly. Forms may be less suited to reporting other speech, language, and hearing services. Again, when designed for use with most clients, they may be difficult to apply to any single client.

While all-purpose forms may be problematic when prepared for exclusive use in speech-language pathology and audiology programs, they become infinitely more problematic when intended to serve an array of clinical and educational services. The standard IEP forms developed by many school districts and the treatment planning and reporting forms used by hospitals, rehabilitation centers, and third-party carriers are frequent examples of all-purpose forms that are ill adapted for our use.

Some problems in report writing are caused by confusing protocols for clinical procedures with organizational structures for reports. This problem is best illustrated by traditional outlines used by physicians in reporting their primary physical examinations. They proceed through a routinized protocol, commenting on each item in turn (general appearance; head, face, and neck; eyes; ears, nose, and throat; thorax and lungs; cardiovascular system; abdomen; genitalia; extremities; nervous system; musculoskeletal system; etc.) without regard to any conceivable relationship of that item to the presenting complaint. Although this procedure may serve medical practice well, it serves as a poor model for the practices of other human services professions. Some cursory notation in the client's record to show that each aspect of communicative processes was considered may be helpful when future questions arise. But when clinicians compulsively comment on each aspect of their evaluation protocols in their reports, these reports become inefficient for both writers and readers.

Other models have been emulated in developing standard organizational systems for reporting speech-language pathology and audiology. Prominent among these are systems used by clinical psychologists. Huber's (1961, p. 37) recommended outline is typical:

Report of Psychological Examination

Name of Patient: Date of Examination:
Date of Birth: Tests Administered:
Referred by:

Referral Statement

(A brief statement of why the patient was referred for testing.)

Test Behavior

(Usually brief descriptions of appearance of test behavior pertinent to purposes of the report.)

Test Results

(The formulation of the case resulting from the analysis of test results.)

Summary and Recommendations

(Summary should be brief. Recommendations should be as detailed as is appropriate to the clinic for which it is written.)

This type of outline may serve speech-language pathology and audiology reports when the major focus is on the test results, as, for example, with many reports of audiologic evaluations. It provides little leeway, however, for the kinds of informal observations that most speech-language pathologists report, especially as questions increasingly arise as to the validity of speech and language tests. Even in audiologic practice, such emphasis on test results offers little room for the observations of real-life communicative behaviors that may actually be the most important areas for assessment.

Several standard outlines have been proposed specifically for speech-language pathology and audiology. For example, Johnson et al. (1963) recommended the following outline for reporting examinations by speech-language pathologists (these items are preceded by the usual items for client identification):

Problem

(A brief and clear indication of the type of communication problem, preferably stated specifically in the informant's own words.)

Referral

(Including the name, relationship, title, etc. of the individual or agency making the referral.)

History

(Organized under these headings: History of Problem, Developmental History, Social History, Medical History, School History, Family History, and Comments on the Interview.)

Examinations

(Detailing test results and other observations under three section headings: Speech, Voice and Language Examinations; Examination of Oral Speech Mechanism; and Audiological Examination.)

Psychological Evaluation

(This section includes a summary of a psychologist's report, abstracting data from that report and including major findings quoted in the psychologist's words.)

Impression

(A brief statement of the conclusions about the nature of the communication problem, its probable etiology, and the degree of its severity.)

Recommendations

(Summarizing decisions based on the findings of the examination and describing any counseling conducted with the client regarding those decisions.)

This outline is more generally applicable than are outlines based on either medical or psychological evaluation models. Nevertheless, even this outline should be adapted to accommodate the particular purposes of each report—adapted by deleting irrelevant sections or subsections or by adding other sections or subsections as needed. If doggedly applied in unalterable form to each and every evaluation report, any outline can be ineffective and uneconomical.

The outline should also be adapted to reflect the setting in which it is applied and the person to whom the report is directed. For example, if clients are routinely seen by other professionals in a particular setting and all significant history is covered in one or more of their reports, there is no need for a speech-language pathologist to reiterate the history in his or her report. Similarly, if the history is well known by the professional who has referred the client, there is no need to reiterate the history in the report sent to that referral source.

The organization of clinical reports may also be prescribed by the records system adopted by a clinical program. For example, the adoption of the problem-oriented record system entails a specifically described approach to report writing. Furthermore, newer methods for information storage and retrieval, utilizing modern computer technology, may also prescribe structures for preparing clinical reports. These considerations are discussed in Chapter 6.

Moore's (1969) comments about organizing reports are eminently sensible:

> The blueprint for a report may be supplied by a more experienced artchitect.... Hopefully it will be adapted for the information that must be transmitted, for the audience who will read the report, and for the peculiarities of the writer. The structure of the report should be flexible, complete, and logical. The design must serve the writer—it is the means to the end rather than the end itself.

SOME CHARACTERISTICS OF GOOD CLINICAL REPORTING

One hallmark of a profession is the capacity for distinctive contributions that can be made by no other profession. If speech-language pathology and audiology is a definable profession, it must then follow that we can make singular contributions to the delivery of human services. That singularity should be reflected in our clinical reports. This, then, is the first assumption that underlies definitions of good clinical reporting: reports should reflect the uniqueness of the discipline of their writers. Nevertheless, some characteristics of good reporting apply equally to all clinical reports, regardless of the writer's profession. To some extent, these characteristics arise from simple common sense, but other characteristics derive from efforts to reduce the growing complexities of human services delivery systems and to decelerate the escalation of costs within those systems. The characteristics cited below may apply to all clinical reports, but they focus on reports in speech-language pathology and audiology. Writers of clinical reports should: *be concise; focus on communication processes and behavior; emphasize new information; avoid overquantification; emphasize conclusions and recommendations rather than raw data; draw reasonable conclusions from available data; offer recommendations, not prescriptions;* and *write for a specific readership*. The illustrations come from reports I have received in connection with clients I have served. They have been altered only to prevent identification of the client, the writer of the report, and the agency or agencies involved.

Be Concise

Earlier enumeration of the various types of essential clinical reports might lead experienced clinicians to foresee schedules devoted primarily to report writing. This need not be the case, however, if the first, and most salient, principle of good reporting is respected. In fact, that principle may be restated: the best clinical reports are often the briefest reports.

Clinical reports are too seldom considered from the viewpoint of cost effectiveness. Yet costs can be substantial if one reckons the clinician time spent in preparing reports, the clerical time devoted to typing them, the time spent by professionals who read them, the cost of entering and storing them in clinical files and of retrieving them for future use, and, finally, the cost of time expended by professionals at some future date when they must locate specific information. Ultimately, clients must pay these costs, or someone else must pay them in the client's behalf. Therefore, responsible clinicians must continually inquire whether the expensive words they set down in their reports are justified in terms of their contribution to the client's care.

Cost factors are not the only consideration, however. Overlong and complex reports can actually interfere with client care. Relevant material which is written obscurely or buried in a morass of reiterations and irrelevancies is often overlooked by busy professionals. Conciseness is particularly important in reporting to physicians. Most physicians will not devote precious time to reading long reports; each paragraph beyond the first three or four is less likely to be read carefully.

Our profession's proclivity for overlong reports may originate during our student days. Student reports are usually designed to reveal mastery of all material relevant to a particular client's problems. The writer is eager to prove that no factors were overlooked in evaluations or therapy planning. It becomes the primary purpose of the report to impress an instructor, rather than to communicate efficiently with other professionals. This approach may carry over after graduation. Reports may still be the primary tool for clinicians to impress supervisors and other professionals with their enlightenment and acumen. It is quite true that a clinician's reports offer clues to his or her proficiency. But clinical proficiency is best demonstrated by clear and cogent reporting, specifically focused on whatever questions are in the minds of readers.

The following is a fairly typical report of an initial evaluation. It was written by an experienced speech-language pathologist employed in a large comprehensive medical center.

Evaluation Report

Ricky C., age 3 years 9 months, was referred to our clinic by Dr. Carleton H., because he does not talk and he drools excessively.

History

Ricky is the second born of two children. His birth and medical history are reportedly unremarkable, although his mother could not recall specific landmarks or details. He has had chronic colds and ear infections with associated high fevers. He is presently being treated for an "infection" in the right ear by Dr. H.

His motor development was reportedly within normal limits since he walked at 13 months. However, he is reportedly somewhat awkward and still not bladder trained. His speech development has been quite slow since he has only two or three clear words in his expressive vocabulary. He expresses his needs by pointing and vocalizing and does not imitate speech. His mother feels his comprehension is adequate and does not suspect a hearing loss.

Ricky was described as difficult to handle and frequently frustrated. He has frequent temper tantrums, but always for a reason. He reportedly gets along fairly well with his 7-year-old sister, but does not attend play school and has no peers to play with. It should be noted that his mother is divorced, being seen by Dr. Eugene Y., a psychiatrist, and openly admits that her household is chaotic. She also stated that she easily loses her temper and patience with her children and frequently yells at them.

Findings

Ricky readily came with the examiner and was cooperative throughout the evaluation. However, his attention span and concentration were inconsistent, and his response to speech was minimal. He was generally quiet and vocalized only to express his needs. He also needed continual help focusing his attention and, without structure, would randomly walk around the room. He was motivated to try and was pleased with his few successes, but he did not have the skills to complete most tasks presented.

No formal test results were obtained because of Ricky's inability to point, match, or imitate verbal speech. His receptive language appears limited to his name and a few contextual commands with visual gestural cues provided. He showed no response to verbal speech on a purely auditory level or to gross environmental noises. He was able to match colors and objects, but only after many demonstrations and repetitions. His responses even then were inconsistent and slow.

Expressive language was characterized by grunting noises when he was pointing to toys he wanted to play with. No words or word approximations were observed. As previously mentioned, he was generally quiet and did not babble or vocalize to himself or in an attempt to relate to the examiner. No verbal imitation could be elicited due to his inconsistent attention and withdrawal from direct interaction. Some gross motor imitation was elicited, but inconsistently and indirectly. It should also be noted that he drooled excessively throughout the evaluation.

Visual-motor and perceptual skills were significantly below age levels. He was unable to manipulate simple puzzles, string beads, to stack blocks without considerable help and direction from the examiner. He was able to draw straight lines, but only after repeated demonstration and help. His response to a circle consisted of circular scribbles. His gross motor skills were also observed to be quite awkward and uncoordinated. He walked on his toes and frequently lost his balance.

An oral peripheral examination was not possible because of his refusal to cooperate. Audiometric screening showed inconsistent responses to pure-tone stimuli. Consequently, he will be referred for a complete audiometric examination.

In summary, this youngster is functioning well below his chronologic age level in language and in visual-motor and perceptual skills. His language skills are severely limited, and he is generally showing no response to speech. He is, however, quite responsive provided he receives a structured teaching situation with immediate feedback and reinforcement.

Recommendations

It is recommended that Ricky receive a complete hearing evaluation to rule out the possibility of a hearing loss. This appointment has already been scheduled for March 2. It is also recommended that he receive speech and language therapy to further delineate his deficits and begin remediation of his existing problems. Regular parent counseling is also suggested in view of his mother's frustration over his behavior problems and her difficulty understanding his language deficits. He will be scheduled in our clinic at our earliest opening.

What this report does or does not illustrate about good clinical practices with respect to the approaches taken and recommendations made is not under consideration here. The point is that the clinician could have provided the same information clearly in half as many words:

Ricky C., 3 years 9 months, was referred by Dr. Carleton H. for evaluation because of failure to talk and excessive drooling.

History

As reported by his mother, Ricky's history reveals several potentially important factors:

1. Despite an apparently unremarkable medical history and grossly normal early motor development, he now seems awkward and has not yet acquired bladder control.
2. He has frequent colds and ear infections and is currently being treated for a right ear infection by Dr. H.
3. Although his mother believes Ricky's comprehension to be unimpaired, he uses only two or three words and does not imitate speech. He communicates by pointing.
4. Mrs. C., a divorced single parent, describes herself as impatient and volatile and her household as chaotic. She is currently seeing Dr. Eugene Y., a psychiatrist.
5. Ricky has little contact with other children but gets along well with his one sibling, a 7-year-old sister. However, his mother finds him difficult to manage, since he is easily frustrated and reacts with temper tantrums.

Findings

I administered no formal tests because Ricky was unable to point, match, or imitate speech. His attention was variable. Unless directly engaged, he walked aimlessly around the room. His responses on audiometric screening were also inconsistent.

Despite willing attempts, he failed at most tasks. He matched colors and objects only after many demonstrations and repetitions, and then slowly and inconsistently. He seemed pleased with his occasional successes.

He was quiet, except for grunting noises when pointing to toys he wanted. I heard no words or word approximations, nor could I elicit verbal imitations. His minimal responses to speech included responses only to his name and to a few commands reinforced by visual and gestural cues.

He would not cooperate for an oral peripheral examination. He drooled continuously throughout the time I observed him.

Ricky imitated some gross motor activities inconsistently, but his movements were awkward and uncoordinated. He walked on his toes, frequently losing balance. Visual-motor and perceptual deficiencies were apparent: he was unable independently to manipulate simple puzzles, string beads, or stack blocks. With assistance, he drew straight lines, but his circle consisted of circular scribbles.

In summary, Ricky is functioning well below age level in many respects. His hearing levels remain undefined. His speech is fragmentary and he shows little response to speech. Nevertheless, he seems amenable to structured teaching with immediate feedback reinforcement.

Recommendations

1. Hearing evaluation to be conducted on March 2.
2. Speech and language therapy to delineate deficits and begin remediation, scheduled when an opening is available.
3. Parent counseling to assist his mother with behavior management and to increase her understanding of Ricky's deficits.

The goal of conciseness underlies most characteristics of good reporting, which will be discussed in the remaining sections of this chapter, but two particular enemies of conciseness deserve special mention: *rituals* and *redundancies*. Already mentioned is the ritualistic behavior evident in too-rigid adherence to organizational protocols which leads to slavishly covering points that have no conceivable relevance to the case at hand. Another form of ritualism appears in consistent use of pat forms that add no useful information. The following are familiar to all clinical report readers:

Johnny was a sturdy, handsome, red-haired and freckle-faced little fellow.

Betsy came willingly into the test room with the examiner.

George was the product of a normal pregnancy and uncomplicated delivery. At his birth, his mother was 26 and his father 28.

There are instances when statements such as these provide essential support to conclusions about communicative disorders (although the conceivable relevance of red hair and freckles may be hard to hypothecate), but when they become stereotypical in all reports they contribute only verbiage.

Redundancies may result from clinical overkill where observation after observation is cited to establish a conclusion. This approach suggests an attorney laboriously eliciting the same point in repeated testimony to establish guilt or innocence. There may be times when reiterations are necessary, as, for example, when a clinician is questioning previous diagnoses or establishing information that may figure in a medicolegal proceeding. Usually, however, it is sufficient to cite conclusions with some brief recognition of the basis for those conclusions. If readers distrust the conclusions they will likely also distrust reports of the observations from which the conclusions derived. The number recounted is not likely to add to their credibility.

Redundancies may also result from overexplanation—amplifying what is already obvious. These statements came from the report of a language evaluation of an 8-year-old boy:

> David's ability to name opposites was tested using the Verbal Opposites subtest.
>
> The Manual Expression Test tests manual expression of ideas and concepts.

These came from a report on 6-year-old Sarah:

> In a spontaneous language sample of 50 sentences, Sarah showed development at the level of 3 years 8 months in her language development.
>
> The Grammatic Closure score shows that she has considerable difficulty in dealing with the grammar necessary for speech.

And this paragraph appeared in a report on 7½-year-old Dillard:

> The Northwestern Syntax Screening Test (NSST) is a measure of syntactic development based on standard American dialect groups. It may also be used to determine how well children of other dialect groups use standard American dialect, but it should never be used to judge a bilingual child or a Black-dialect child as language delayed or language deficient. One must be aware of these limitations when considering a child's score on the NSST. Dillard's expressive receptive scores were both below the 10th percentile.

In each instance, the redundancies both add unnecessary words and impair the cogency of the report.

E. B. White, in his introduction to his revision of Strunk's *The Elements of Style* (1959, p. ix), quoted a "masterly Strunkian elaboration" of a "noble theme"

> Vigorous writing is concise. A sentence should contain no unnecessary words, a paragraph no unnecessary sentences, for the same reason that a drawing should have no unnecessary lines and a machine no unnecessary parts. This requires not that the writer make all his sentences short, or that he avoid all detail and treat his subjects only in outline, but that every word tell.

There may be no better guide to writers of clinical reports.

Focus on Communication Processes and Behaviors

This statement may seem so obvious that it should go without saying, but speech-language pathologists and audiologists are sometimes so aware of their participation in a broad human services delivery system that they forget their specific role within that system. In some instances we may offer comments in areas peripheral to our discipline to alert other professionals to symptoms requiring further exploration. For the most part, however, our reports should concentrate within the proper scope of our profession.

The following is a verbatim reproduction of a report on Steven, a kindergartner referred for speech and language evaluation by his teacher, because of her concern about his immaturity:

> *Background Information*
>
> Steven was referred to this specialist by his kindergarten teacher, Mrs. G., who described the child as displaying short attention span, being very distractible, and being unable to work independently. Steven also manifested difficulty manipulating colors and pencil. Mrs. G. further reports Steven becomes easily frustrated during motor planning tasks.
>
> Steven is a slim, attractive youngster who seems to have difficulty controlling body movements during activity and at rest.

During parent conference with Mrs. F., she reported the child has a past history of seizures and sometimes after the seizures, the child tends to lean toward the left side of his body while walking.

Testing

Motor assessment: Steven writes with his right hand and seems to cut with either hand. The right hand has a stronger grip. Steven preferred to hop with his right foot. Though he displays difficulty with balance while balancing, he seemed to prefer his left foot. However, he would wrap this left foot around the right leg for better stability during balance.

Steven is bombarded by auditory stimuli both indoors and outdoors.

Diadochokinetic rate p-t-k was produced as p-k-k.

Visual-motor tasks: Though all the geometric shapes were adequately formed, considerable pressure was applied to the pencil. Considerable waviness occurred in the straight lines and in forming geometric shapes.

Recommendations

Mrs. F. was urged to take Steven to the R.L. Center for a psychomotor evaluation.

Steven should be considered for a learning disability class placement in order to strengthen visual-motor tasks and improve attention span.

This report covers an evaluation by a speech-language pathologist of Peggy, a 9-year-old with retarded growth and development:

Behavioral Observations

Peggy came willingly with the examiner. She was pleasant during the evaluation but not completely interested in the materials presented to her. She appeared rather passive but was always cooperative. She initiated some spontaneous conversation and seemed to enjoy herself.

Test Administered:

McCarthy Scales of Children's Abilities

Chronological Age: 8–10

Mental Age Estimate: Below 4–5

	Composite Raw Score	Scale Index	Standard Deviation From Mean
Verbal	57	24	−2½
Perceptual-performance	48	Below 22	Below −3
Quantitative	24	23	−2½
Memory	35	28	−2
Motor	43	Below 22	Below −3
General cognitive	129	Below 50	Below −3

Verbal Skills

Peggy retained 2 of 6 pictures from memory. She recognized and named 9 of 9 common pictures and gave simple definitions for 3 common words. She retained 3 words from a series, and gave back 7 of 11 key ideas from a story. Peggy named 2 to 5 items in 4 different categories She gave 6 of 9 analogies.

Perceptual-Performance

Completed building a tower, chair, and building but had some difficulty with the house. Solved 2-piece puzzles and some cuts from the more difficult ones. Sequenced 3 tones. Knows right and left on self but not on pictures. Imitated and copied only the simplest designs. For Draw-a-Child, Peggy received partial credit for some items and omitted others. Knew size, shapes, and colors and was able to manipulate to two variables.

Quantitative

Knew number of body parts and could do one problem of simple addition. Retained 5 digits forward. Repeated 2 digits backward. Was able to do only the most simple counting and sorting tasks.

Memory

Retained 2 of 6 pictures. Sequenced 3 tones. Retained 3 words from a series and gave back 7 of 11 key ideas from a story. Retained 5 digits forward. Repeated 2 digits backward.

Motor

Leg coordination. Could do all tasks but was inconsistent with skipping. Others included walking backwards, on tiptoe, walking a straight line, standing on right and left foot.

Arm coordination. Could not bounce a ball using one hand. Caught 3 of 9 bean bag tosses using one hand. Threw bean bag through target 3 times, hit target board 3 times. Peggy did well on this task.

Imitative action. Could do all imitative tasks such as cross feet, fold hands, twiddle thumbs, and sight through cube.

Motor. Imitated and copied only the simplest designs. For Draw-a-Child received partial credit for some items and omitted others.

Results

Overall cognitive development gives a mental age estimate of below 4 years 5 months. All subtest areas scored significantly below mean. Relative strengths appear to be in repeating digits and bean bag toss. Lack of interest, passive personality, and lack of experience may be contributing factors in Peggy's performance.

Even though Steven and Peggy were evaluated by speech-language pathologists, after reading these reports one knows virtually nothing about either child's communication. However accurate and perspi-

cacious the reported observations of motor abilities, visual-motor integration, memory, or whatever, for all the reader knows, either child could be virtually mute, have unusual verbal proficiencies, or fall somewhere between these extremes.

Speech-language pathologists' and audiologists' reports occasionally stay solidly within the scope of their expertise but still neglect to describe the client's communication. This is most likely to occur in audiologists' reports when evaluations are conducted in connection with medical diagnostic studies.

The following report was sent to an otolaryngologist after an audiologic evaluation. The referral was precipitated by the client's complaint of three episodes of vertigo, gradually increasing tinnitus, and some problems in understanding conversational speech, particularly in noisy environments:

> Mr. Garwood S. was seen for audiologic evaluation on your referral. As shown on the enclosed audiogram, pure-tone audiometry revealed a moderate binaural sensorineural hearing loss which was somewhat greater on the left than the right. Speech reception thresholds were at 15 dB in the left ear and 25 dB in the right ear. Speech discrimination scores were 82% in the left ear and 36% in the right ear. Type A tympanograms were obtained bilaterally. Acoustic reflexes were present at normal levels and symmetrical. There was no reflex decay.
>
> Because of the inordinate reduction in speech discrimination in the left ear and the reported episodes of vertigo, Mr. S. was seen for supplementary testing, including auditory brainstem reponse studies. Results of tone decay, SISI, and Bekesy testing were all compatible with cochlear impairment. On the ABR studies, a comparison of suprathreshold Wave V latency values showed differences within normal limits. These findings are also incompatible with a retrocochlear impairment.
>
> We recommend re-evaluation of Mr. S.'s hearing in 1 year. Thank you for your referral.

This report may or may not reflect an adequate assessment of the probable site of lesion in this client's auditory system. Nevertheless, the audiologist became so involved with efforts to establish a medical diagnosis, he overlooked the client's communication impairment. While the client may be pleased to learn that an acoustic neuroma is unlikely, he may still be frustrated when he tries to carry on a conversation in a less than optimal environment. Insofar as can be determined from the report, the audiologist ignored one of the client's major complaints. Not only has the audiologist failed to provide any real assistance to the client in this respect, he has offered the otolaryngologist no expert advice regarding possible rehabilitation, presumably one of the audiologist's most important roles.

If the unique expertise of our profession lies in the evaluation and amelioration of communicative disorders, that expertise must always be immediately apparent in our reports. We may contribute information about other aspects of client behavior and provide important evidence to assist other professionals in formulating their diagnoses, but these roles are secondary—a proposition that should be apparent to readers of our reports.

Emphasize New Information

Readers of patient charts in teaching hospitals are immediately entangled in masses of reiterated information duly recorded by the succession of students, trainees, and staff physicians who have participated, however slightly, in the patient's care. Statements of chief complaints, histories, and results of physical examinations are reiterated meticulously, as though being set down for the first time anywhere. To retrieve information from these records, a reader must either invest an hour or so in deciphering all reports or choose one that seems most likely to be reliable. This situation has parallels in university speech and hearing clinics where a succession of supervisors, senior clinicians, student clinicians, and various assistants have each recorded their versions of evaluations, therapy plans, progress notes, and summaries.

Clinical reports often involve lengthy repetitions of material that is already known to their readers. In striving for completeness, many reports merely achieve repetitiousness.

The following paragraphs are extracted from the pediatrician's report that accompanied her referral for speech and language evaluation of Brent, a 7-year-old with language and learning disabilities:

> Brent was a planned child. The pregnancy was uneventful except for the mother's excessive weight gain. He was born at 42 weeks. At delivery the cord was wrapped around his neck and was cut intrauterine. Upon delivery his color was poor, and he was without spontaneous respiration. He was breast fed for 3 months and then weaned suddenly due to a hospitalization of his mother.
>
> Brent's mother is unaware of any problems in early development. He sat at 6 months, walked at 1 year, toilet trained at 27 months, and used two- or three-word sentences at 3 years.
>
> The parents are mildly concerned about Brent's gross motor skills. This stems from the fact that he only recently learned to ride his bike and, in fact, is still a bit shaky on it. Until very recently he showed no interest in sports. Brent sometimes feels left out of the games and activities of his older brothers, Tom, age 10, and Gordon, age 8½.

The speech-language pathologist who evaluated Brent began his report to the pediatrician with the following section labeled "Background":

> Brent is the youngest of three boys. His siblings are ages 10 and 8 years. The family recently moved from Memphis, Tennessee. Pregnancy was uncomfortable and long—3 weeks past due date. Mrs. C. gained 40 pounds and experienced muscle spasms during the end of pregnancy—received muscle relaxant for these. She reported that the umibilical cord was wrapped around Brent's neck and was cut in utero. He was born "very dark colored"—had breathing difficulties during the first 3 minutes of life. Birthweight was about 7 lbs. 10 oz. Mrs. C. characterized him as a demanding and irritable baby and as being a more demanding chiid than the older children.
>
> He was breast fed until 3 months old, when he was weaned suddenly. Mrs. C. became ill and required immediate hospitalization. Brent was placed on a bottle and would not feed for 12 hours. Health history is essentially negative.
>
> *Developmental milestones*: sat up at 6 months; walked at 1 year; engaged in some baby sounds but not like two older children; first words "mama" and "dada" at 18 months, a few additional words at 24 months, and some 2- to 3-word sentences at 4½ years.
>
> Mrs. C. feels that Brent's overall gross and fine motor development has been slow and that he is distractible with a short attention span.

Two problems are apparent in the speech-language pathologist's report. First, the reiteration of information already found in the pediatrician's referral letter was wasteful, particularly since no implications were cited for Brent's present communicative disorders. Second, the reported history of speech development differed in the two reports, yet the speech-language pathologist ignored this discrepancy. In these respects, then, the report is both superfluous and obfuscating.

It may be helpful to begin reports with a cogent summary of relevant information gleaned from other reports. But ritualistic reiteration of already reported information is unnecessary and profligate.

Avoid Overquantification

In proposing this characteristic my bias is shown with respect to the quantification of communicative behaviors. In our quest for scientific respectability we have stressed the application of quantitative methods in the study of communicative disorders. However meritorious the objective—and it has unequivocal merit—our present technology falls far short of its realization. At the present state of our art, we may mislead the readers of our reports when we overemphasize quantitative data. (I recently received a report on a 7-year-old that features an "estimated language age of 4.74 years," which presumably converts into 4 years, 270 days, 2 hours, and 24 minutes.)

Two interrelated distortions may be engendered by excessive quantification in reports. The first rests on implications that the components of communication behaviors can be parceled out so that measurements of these presumed ingredients effectively quantify the total behaviors. This has been referred to as the "beads on a string" approach, i.e., viewing speech as sequences of discrete events following one another like beads on a string. Rees (1978), in a broader discussion of the evaluation of communication processes, pointed to the fallacy of approaches that "attempt to separate communication into its component units in a sort of building-block fashion" and further observed, "The building-block type of model tends to overlook that adding together all the components does not produce the total behavior in question." These approaches are manifested in clinical reports when the writer constructs a sort of profile by quoting scores of tests of vocabulary, syntax, articulation, etc., and implies thereby that the report affords a composite characterization of the client's communication.

A second kind of distortion comes from the implication that the results of whatever tests we have administered offer an objective and accurate picture of a client's communicative proficiencies. This implication ignores the complexity of communicative behaviors. Concerns about overquantification have been expressed most frequently by writers in the literature on language disorders, particularly by Siegel and Broen (1976) and by Leonard et al. (1978).

In another discussion of overquantification in clinical practice, Siegel (1975, p. 797) wrote:

> Whenever we reduce behavior to numerical indices we trade a loss of richness in detail for the conveniences that accrue to manipulating, averaging, and storing numerical data. There are sometimes important patterns, however, that can be discovered only in the data—the behaviors—themselves, or as close to them as our observations will allow us to get. The fact that a behavior can be reduced to numbers in some system is not necessarily a reason for embracing the system. It depends on what has been lost in the reduction.

Because audiologists may presume that they are engaged in psychophysical measurement, their scores may be even more seductive than the scores accrued by speech-language pathologists. Several writers in the audiologic literature have emphasized the hazards of assuming that the scores derived in conventional audiologic test batteries summarize actual communication performances. Among other problems, as observed by Giolas et al. (1979), "such procedures fail to assess comprehensively and accurately the hearing-impaired listener's response to a variety of listening situations." Furthermore, no standard tests assess hearing-impaired clients as discourse partners, observing how they manage discourse to their advantage or disadvantage.

The risks of quantification relate directly to the potential readers of the report. Those written expressly for other speech-language pathologists and audiologists may contain quantitative data with only the supplementary information required to interpret those data. Readers can then draw on their own familiarity with the tests to give the data whatever weight they deserve. Furthermore, it may be helpful to compare current data with data reported from previous administrations of the same tests.

Overquantification is most hazardous in reports prepared for readers from other professions or for an unpredictable readership. Numbers are too readily grasped by readers who have little appreciation of the complexity of the communicative behaviors they presumably quantify and have little understanding of how the numbers were derived. Although elaborately qualified and cautiously interpreted, the mere presence of numbers in a report can lead to their extraction from context and their use far beyond the intention of the writer.

Physicians are particularly prone to excessive reliance on numeric simplifications of complex processes. They seek summary expressions in age equivalents, percentiles, or percentages of complex communicative behaviors. Once they become available, these numbers can acquire a life of their own, sometimes completely unrelated to the context in which the data were offered. An excellent, if extreme, example of this situation occurred in the case of a 12-year-old girl who had been injured in an automobile accident. In seeking evidence of behavioral changes following the accident, to serve as a basis for litigation, her mother asked a speech-language pathologist to assess the youngster's "difficulty explaining what she has read or what she is trying to say." The speech-language pathologist's report of the evaluation consisted primarily of scores from the Illinois Test of Psycholinguistic Abilities. (The use of the ITPA in the assessment of a 12-year-old, much less as an approach to elucidating the behaviors observed by the mother, would, of course, never be condoned by even the most enthusiastic proponents of that test.) Not surprisingly, with three exceptions, the subtest scores exceeded the ceilings tabled on the Psycholinguistic Age Norms in the Examiner's Manual. The age equivalents of these three subtests were duly reported, including a 9-year 2-month equivalent on Auditory Sequencing and an 8-year 4-month equivalent on Visual Sequencing. (In each instance, a mere 2 more points in the raw score would have reached the ceilings of tabled scores.)

The speech-language pathologist's report was subsequently reviewed by a neurologist who concluded:

> The results of the Illinois Psycholinguistic Ability Test show marked decreased auditory and visual sequencing. There is marked scatter in these scores from her other scores, and this suggests that she is suffering from organic brain damage of the type that can be seen after trauma. More highly suggestive of this is recently she is having difficulty with both visual and auditory sequential memory. If these had existed all of her life she would probably have marked reading difficulties since the acquisition of reading requires sequencing.

The neurologist's overinterpretation of dubious fragments of quantitative data to justify a diagnosis of traumatic organic brain damage casts serious doubts on his professional competence. On the other hand, the speech-language pathologist must assume some responsibility for providing the dubious fragments of quantitative data in the evaluation report and thus misleading a reader who is unfamiliar with a particular test.

The pressures for reporting quantitative data have increased in recent years with the growing emphasis on accountability. For example, the "objective criteria" required in IEP's by PL 94-142 regulations are often assumed to imply test scores. One often hears members of our profession protesting that overemphasis on quantification in reports is required by the institutions that employ them or by their referral sources. However, if the consequences of that overemphasis lead to misdiagnosis, mismanagement, or distortion of the outcomes of intervention, some careful reappraisal is clearly necessary. The delivery of the best possible services to clients is always our pre-eminent responsibility. Acceding to practices that are not in our clients' best interests is unprofessional.

Emphasize Conclusions and Recommendations Rather Than Raw Data

This characteristic relates closely to the one just discussed. We often see clinical reports that consist almost entirely of recounting the raw data accrued during an evaluation. For example, the following is the entire report on an almost-6-year-old girl with a language problem.

Language and Speech Evaluation

Elena is a petite kindergarten girl. The first 4 years of her life she heard Spanish spoken at home. According to her mother, she started being exposed to English when she attended a preschool 1 or 2 days a week.

In April and May of this year, she was evaluated at the G. Speech and Hearing Center. In June she started receiving therapy there.

Two months ago, Elena entered kindergarten at Lincoln Elementary.

Formal Test Results

Syntax and Morphology

Test	Results
Assessment of Children's Language Competence	Missed 3 items in vocabulary prepositions (on, over, behind); and 2 items of two critical elements; one of three critical elements; and three of four critical elements.
Northwestern Syntax Screening Test	Scored below 10% in Receptive and Expressive.

Illinois Test of Psycholinguistic Abilities (ITPA) Grammatic Closure	Age Score: 2–2
Language Samples	Elena's language samples show that she is inconsistent in her use of the English language. She shows utterances of 3–5 words, sometimes 6 words. She verbs ("I don't know what is it?"). Sometimes she leaves out prepositions ("playing the kite"). Again, she is not consistent in omitting or reversing. She has some very complete sentences. ("What's she doing?" "She is not touching the horsey.") She also answers questions with inappropriate answers ("Why do we have a table here?" "Is a round table.").

Semantics
(Receptive)

Test	Results
Peabody Picture Vocabulary Test	Received a mental age of 3–6 years. Percentile score: 3%ile.
Boehm Test of Basic Concepts	Raw Score: 15/50 concepts correct. Concept Categories missed: 14 Spatial 14 Quantitative 2 Time 4 Miscellaneous
ITPA-Auditory Reception	Age Score: 3–5
(Expressive)	
ITPA-Verbal Expression	Age Score: 2–0

Integration

Test	Results
ITPA-Auditory Closure	Age Score: 3–10
ITPA-Auditory Association	Age Score: 3–11

Auditory Memory

Test	Results
Utah Test for Language Development Memory Sentences	Below the 3-year level, could not repeat a 12-syllable sentence at 4–5-year level.
Utah-Digit Span	Can repeat 4 digits at 4–5-year level.
ITPA-Auditory Sequential Memory	Age Score: 2–10

Phonology
(Articulation)

Test	Results
Goldman-Fristoe Test of Articulation	Elena has multiple substitutions in her articulation: th/sh, t/ch, w/r, d/dz, t/th, th/s, th/z, d/th. She omits /s/ in blends /skw/ and /st/. She says thl/sl.
Language Sample	All of the above articulation errors are present in Elena's connected speech. They frequently contribute to difficulties in understanding what she is saying, Elena also talks with a relatively immature tonal quality and inflection.

This approach to reporting bespeaks the same kind of infatuation with quantification already deplored. Even more insidiously, perhaps, it implies an unwillingness to assume professional responsibility for interpreting those data, drawing conclusions, and committing oneself to specific recommendations. In this report the clinician simply places the data on exhibit and implies, "Make of them what you will."

Of equal concern, this is the approach of a technician, not of a professional. Particularly in health care settings, it is well established that technicians secure data and professionals interpret those data. Whatever the limitations of this approach when applied to clinical laboratory, electroencephalographic, and radiographic studies, it is intolerable when applied to the assessment procedures used by speech-language pathologists and audiologists. The issue is not exclusively one of professional status. Our optimal contributions to client care derive from our ability to view behavior and formulate plans within a total context, contributions which far exceed the mere generation and reporting of data.

Draw Reasonable Conclusions from Available Data

Good science is characterized by making prudent interpretations and drawing reasonable conclusions from whatever data have been derived. This characteristic obtains whether the data have been derived from observations of a single subject or from observations of a group of subjects. The same obtains for good clinical reporting.

Good clinical reporting requires recognition of the limitations of the procedures used to generate data. It also requires recognition that the samples of behavior we elicit may not necessarily characterize a client's usual behavior. It is deceitful to draw sweeping conclusions from fragmentary observations, as in these examples:

> Results of the Peabody Picture Vocabulary Test indicate that receptive vocabulary is slightly below chronologic age expectancy. Results of the receptive portion of the Northwestern Syntax Screening Test indicate good comprehension for varying grammatical inflections. This combined information would suggest that reading comprehension should not be a problem for Trevor.

> Patricia scored above the normative ceiling of 8-7 on the Sound-Blending Test of the Illinois Test of Psycholinguistic Abilities. The results suggest adequate skills for the assimilation of phonically attacked words in reading.

> Ted's area of difficulty is auditory closure, which requires that he produce the word when only some of the sounds are given. This would relate to his ability to use phonetics and sequence sounds in words. Based on this information, it appears that Ted's needs center around a particular area of sound sequencing. He should be enrolled in speech therapy for remediation of these problem areas.

> Tommy performed below age expectancy on labeling tasks. This behavior demonstrates a weakness in the area referred to as "central language." Central language can be developed through small group discussion in the classroom. At home, parents can ask questions which will lead the child into "discovering" relationships and expanding concepts.

> The Wepman Test of Auditory Discrimination checks a pupil's ability to perceive differences between spoken words. If a pupil has difficulty with discrimination, he may have word confusions when he hears spoken messages. Greg had no errors on this test, which indicates this early processing skill is intact for this pupil. His confusion over directions does not appear to stem from auditory discrimination difficulties.

Someone once said, "I can only tell you what I know." Clinicians are well advised to restrict their reports to what is actually known at the end of whatever procedure they are reporting.

Offer Recommendations, Not Prescriptions

One of the most serious misapplications of a medical model to have plagued the delivery of speech-language pathology and audiology services is the assumption that evaluations lead logically to drafting specific prescriptions for management. In most instances, whatever prescriptions are formulated are to be carried out by other clinicians.

However attractive the prescription-writing concept may be in theory, that concept is essentially incongruent with the evaluation methodologies we employ. For example, Leonard et al. (1978, p. 373) commented with respect to the relationship between evaluation and management of children with problems in language acquisition:

> . . . the very fact that standardized test results are in quantitative terms makes the progression from test to treatment problematic. A finding that a child performs below the tenth percentile on a given test does not provide an indication of the feature of language that should serve as the initial or subsequent focus of remediation. . . . It might seem appropriate to select target features for remediation by performing an item analysis of the child's standardized test performance. However, for most standardized language tests, such an analysis would be insufficient. For example, it might be found that a child performed poorly on the preposition items on the Test for Auditory Comprehension of Language. Each of the prepositions on this test is assessed by a single test item. Thus, even if a clinician felt comfortable in assuming that prepositions should be taught on the basis of a total of six prepositions, a rather risky assumption, it would be entirely unclear which prepositions should serve as the initial focus. This is true for the majority of standardized tests designed to assess linguistic performance. In short, while an item analysis of a standardized test might provide information regarding features of questionable status in a child's linguistic behavior, more detailed probing of this feature would be necessary before it could be determined that the feature warrants treatment.

Rees (1978, pp. 13–14) further amplifies the concept that the results of evaluations do not necessarily direct specific approaches to management:

> . . . whatever the value of collecting behavioral data during diagnostic sessions, the data do not necessarily determine the structure of the remedial program. According to this point of view, diagnostic data allow the clinician to assess the severity of the communication disorder and to determine the objectives of a remediation program for the subject in question. The behavioral data collected during the diagnostic sessions also provide a handy baseline for measuring change over time. The results of assessment do not, in this case, translate directly into a design for remediation.

The following examples of prescription-oriented statements come from reports I have received:

> Work in the area of increasing his discrimination in noise, improving his attention to speech in noise, as well as quiet, and expanding his ability to concentrate on auditory input would be of great benefit to Stanley.

> Melanie's teacher should be advised to use visual reinforcers for auditory stimuli.

> Neil is significantly below his general level in both auditory and visual activities, primarily in the memory area; consequently skills which are presented in one modality should consistently be presented in both modalities, i.e., visual and auditory. This is possible by using a Language Master.

> Give Emily oral instructions seven to eight syllables in length with not more than three critical elements.

> The teacher and parents should use Peabody Level I Kit activities with emphasis on auditory visual sequencing, expressive language, and auditory association tasks.

> Icing 5 minutes, two times daily of oral musculature to increase kinesthetic awareness of oral pathways (for dysarthria) and use of mirror for articulation placement of tongue and lips, and use of Westlake button for articulation muscle control.

The first three examples offer unusual combinations of overspecificity and ambiguity. In each instance they prescribe something about input modalities, whatever that means, but fail to give clues about how the prescription is to be carried out, beyond the third example's lame reference to "using a Language Master." The other examples are much more specific, but imagine Emily's teacher composing each instruction during a day so that it is "seven to eight syllables in length with not more than three elements." The Peabody Language Development Kits may well be praiseworthy, but how are parents and teachers to determine which activities serve which of the prescribed functions? The final mind-boggler is best passed without comment. In each of these examples, clinicians deluded themselves and the readers of their reports because the evaluative procedures they applied did not permit the specificity of interpretations they offered.

Good clinical reports offer specific recommendations. But those recommendations should identify areas for further assessment, delineate important considerations for planning management, offer baseline descriptions of communicative behaviors, and suggest possible points of departure in therapy programs. Our assessment tools may someday permit greater specificity in prescribing therapeutic intervention—assuming this to be a desirable objective. For the present, however, prescription writing may actually interfere with clients receiving whatever help they really need.

Write for a Specific Readership

If reports are fundamentally a vehicle for communication, that communication will be facilitated by knowing as much as possible about the receiver or receivers. The information covered, the focus taken, the recommendations made, and the language used can then be accommodated according to whether the report is intended for physicians, classroom teachers, speech-language pathologists and audiologists, or for some other audience.

All-purpose reports are hard to prepare, particularly when those reports are available to anyone with access to the client's file or can be sent out at any time to anyone who follows proper request procedures. When program policies demand the preparation of all-purpose reports, they are best written in fairly general terms. The summary can propose that seekers of more specific information or recommendations contact the writer directly. Although this approach may seem evasive, it may ultimately facilitate good client care since readers are more likely to get specifically helpful information—specific to their professional roles and to the circumstances leading to their securing the report.

When reports about the same client must be sent to members of different professions, it may be infeasible to prepare separate special reports to each professional. But reports can be drafted so that different sections are sent to different professionals. A section offering summary statements may suffice for a report to the primary care physician. A section detailing information about hearing might be added in a report for an otolaryngologist. A section offering information about speech-related motor coordination might be added in a report for a neurologist. Recommendations about educational placement and management might be sent to school personnel. The complete report would probably be sent to the referral source or to another speech-language pathologist or audiologist.

This kind of selective reporting is particularly feasible when modern computer-assisted word-processing systems are available. The entire report is entered, but specific reports can be generated and printed simply by designating the paragraphs to be included in that report.

LANGUAGE USAGE IN CLINICAL REPORTING

The language of good clinical report writing is like the language of all clear and direct communication: simple, plain, and terse. As Strunk and White (1959) put it, "Do not be tempted by a twenty-dollar word when there is a ten-center handy, ready and able."

It is difficult to comprehend why so many clinicians affect styles in writing reports that they would never employ in any other communication. Yet clinicians who are capable of writing simple declarative sentences lapse into obscure words, intricate syntax, and archaic forms when they write their reports. Perhaps they are guided by notions of the gravity of their responsibilities, notions which have led them to distrust the language used in normal discourse. Perhaps they have an image of the respected clinician as meting out profound truths in oracular prose. For whatever reasons, clinicians, and particularly younger clinicians, are easily led to stylistic extremes. Strunk and White (1959, p. 55) observed:

> Young writers often suppose that style is a garnish for the meat of prose, a sauce by which a dull dish is made palatable. Style has no such separate entity; it is non-detachable, unfilterable. The beginner should approach style warily, realizing that it is himself he is approaching, no other; and he should begin by turning resolutely away from all devices that are popularly believed to indicate style—all mannerisms, tricks, adornments. The

> approach to style is by way of plainness, simplicity, orderliness, sincerity.

Unquestionably, there is a prevalent attitude that some unwritten stylistic rules traditionally govern report writing—rules that require avoiding at all costs the active voice, that forbid use of the first person singular, that insist on use of jargon, etc. But contrary to these assumed traditions, the reports of some of history's most eminent clinicians follow none of these rules. For example, the following case report comes from the collected papers of Hughlings Jackson (1932, p. 326), the renowned 19th-century British neurologist:

> About 12:30 p.m. on December 30, 1872, John D., aged 22, a strongly built soldier, came into the receiving room of this hospital in a state of mental excitement. His face was much congested, the conjunctivae were suffused, and for the moment it seemed as if he were the subject of delirium from drink. He was complaining in an excited manner of a "buzzing" in the right ear, and of intense pain, the character of which he could not describe. He frequently repeated that "he would go mad" if not relieved. His head rested with his right ear on the palm of his left hand, and it was noted that he frequently walked round and round, and always from right to left. The house-surgeon had some difficulty in getting him to be quiet, and explain his sufferings. When asked how long he had the pain, he said since he got out of bed that morning; in fact, he awoke in great pain; "The pain woke me, but has got worse and worse." Whilst I was deliberating as to the diagnosis, the patient said, "It feels like a large insect in my ear." This leading observation at once suggested an examination of the ear. Nothing was seen by ordinary examination, but with an ear speculum and reflected light from a mirror all the tissues appeared healthy, but on more close examination a small black dot was seen at the anterior wall of the tympanum and its junction with the mucous membrane of the external ear, and moving about as if trying to scratch its way betwixt the membrana tympani and the wall of the meatus. One syringeful of water brought out the offender, which proved to be a louse of rather large size, and dark. The patient was at once relieved, though his ear still felt "queer." He left the hospital in a sense of intense gratitude.

Except for some anatomic terms that might require reference to a dictionary, this case report is immediately intelligible to any moderately literate reader. If the gifted Hughlings Jackson could be so lucid, why should we humbler clinicians court opacity?

Since the rules that govern good clinical report writing are identical to the rules that apply to any good writing, such standard guides as Strunk and White (1959) and Barzun (1966) are as useful to report writers as to any writers. There are, however, some pitfalls in clinical writing that merit special attention; hence the following aphorisms: *use standard American English instead of jargon; use the active voice; use the first person singular in referring to yourself; make positive statements and be willing to commit yourself; avoid overgeneralizations; use uncomplicated sentence constructions.*

Use Standard American English Instead of Jargon

Every guide to clinical writing inveighs against jargon, yet the jargon content of most clinical reporting continues unchecked. One more reiteration here is not likely to solve the problem. Nevertheless, clinicians' proclivity for jargon remains one of the most serious obstacles to communication.

The following are gleaned from actual clinical reports written by speech-language pathologists and audiologists to physicians, classroom teachers, or other professionals.

> An analysis of his errors revealed that he responded, but incorrectly, on Low-Pass Filtered Speech, and had several no responses on the Competing Messages where he did not register the stimulus at all.

> The nonfluency appears to be either the bounce or the prolongation type of blocking.

> The profile grid further details that Juan is unable to make use of the redundancies of oral language in acquiring automatic habits of handling syntax and grammatic inflection.

> Sound-blending skills were adequate, although he experienced some confusion when there was no pictured referent.

> The Willeford Test of Central Auditory Processing

was also administered. Roy scored at normal levels for his age on the filtered words (where only a portion of the full frequency responses is presented) and binaural fusion when the low pass segment of the word was presented to the left ear. When the low pass was presented to the right ear, however, Roy could not integrate the two portions of the word successfully.

Any reader who is familiar with what these clinicians were trying to say could probably decode the approximate meaning of these statements. But other readers remain bewildered. No idea is expressed in any of these excerpts that cannot be communicated intelligibly to any professional, regardless of background, merely by relying on standard American English instead of such egregious jargon.

Use the Active Voice

Although the passive voice serves a very useful purpose in many contexts, it is seldom appropriate in clinical report writing. Its frequent use in clinical reports seems to accomplish the objective of absolving people of responsibilities. For example, the following depersonalizes the referral source:

> The reason for the referral was his demonstrated difficulty expressing himself, reluctance to respond, and incorrect word order in sentences noted when responses were elicited.

In this instance, the client's apparent difficulties become the absolute reason for the referral when, in fact, the referral was precipitated when the anonymous source concluded that problems existed and became concerned about those problems.

Clinicians often absolve themselves of responsiblity for what they do by resorting to the passive voice. For example:

> Specific training is also in progress regarding the expressive language areas related to development of correct usage and understanding of those verb forms he is presently omitting or using incorrectly, as well as pronouns, subject/verb agreement within sentences, and formulating question forms and the appropriate use of questions.

Clinicians also use the passive voice to assign responsibility to whatever testing procedure was used, rather than to focus on themselves as the interpreters of the test performances, as in the following examples:

> Impedance audiometry secured normal type A tympanograms bilaterally.

> Present performance on tasks used to measure underlying processes for learning appears age appropriate.

> Of educational significance are areas associated with manual expression. A very high score was found here. Negative educationally significant factors center around poor auditory reception and visual association. These factors might be indicators of learning-handicapped areas in multiple ranges.

The passive voice not only perverts the meaning of most clinical reports, it also impairs clarity. Such active statements as "Mrs. Edith Best, Jeremy's classroom teacher, referred him for . . . ," or "In my work with Susan, I have emphasized . . . ," or "I concluded from my evaluation of Mr. Silvester's responses using several different hearing aids that . . . " are much clearer than would be comparable statements written in passive voice.

Use the First Person Singular in Referring to Yourself

Closely related to the use of passive voice is avoidance of first person singular pronouns, once again to diffuse responsibility for the contents of the report. Such forms as the following are familiar:

> This speech-language specialist (referring to the writer) worked with Amy and five other kindergarten children five times a week.

> Mr. Liebert is one of the severest stutterers this examiner has ever seen.

Clinicians also affect the plural form in referring to themselves:

> We saw Gordon for hearing evaluation on March 13, 1981.

> During our contacts with Mrs. Naylor, we have tried to encourage her to use devices other than shouting to gain her children's attention.

Avoidance of the first person singular can also contribute to lack of clarity in reports, since a reader is often confused as to whether the writer is the person designated.

Make Positive Statements and Be Willing to Commit Yourself

If the reader of a report were not interested in the writer's conclusions he or she probably would not read the report. Facts should always be differentiated from observations, impressions, and opinions, but good clinical reports are always written in a forthright style.

Speech-language pathologists and audiologists often report their conclusions timorously:

> Pat appears to present an articulatory disorder of moderate severity.

> It is believed that a speech therapy program should be instituted immediately for Mrs. Bates.

> The recommended hearing aid seems to offer satisfactory gain.

> Problems in speech and language acquisition are not unusual among children with very low birthweight.

Moore (1969) reiterated Strunk and White's (1959) rule, "Avoid the use of qualifiers. Rather, very, little, pretty—these are the leeches that infest the pond of prose, sucking the blood of words." She then added (p. 537):

> The clinician knows other leeches: *somewhat, probably, seems to be, appears, quite, sort of, kind of*. It may give the clinician courage to omit these if he remembers that the clinic report is not and does not purport to be a divine revelation of wisdom. It is not the "pure" truth. It is the truth according to a particular writer. Certainly it must not be overstated but neither should it be a timid collection of "maybes" authored by a milquetoast.

Avoid Overgeneralizations

Sweeping statements should also be avoided. Clinicians must strike a balance between timidity and such excessive generalizations as:

> Like most children with problems in speech and language development, Kevin is experiencing difficulties in learning to read.

> Analysis of the ITPA profile showed that Sean was able to receive and derive meaning from verbally and visually presented stimuli.

> Robbie was quite mature for his age in all areas except speech and language.

> Most people with similar histories of exposure to industrial noise develop the kind of hearing loss Mr. Giacometti shows.

These examples of immoderation in report writing are closely linked to the hazards of making unwarranted generalizations from limited data, as discussed in a previous section.

Use Uncomplicated Sentence Constructions

Good clinical reports are comprised of unpretentious, tersely constructed sentences. If a clinician cannot state formulations clearly, those formulations are likely to be so muddy that they should not be reported. Consider the following:

> Debby had difficulty on the word recall task where a series of 50 pictures is shown to the child and she is asked to name them as quickly as possible on five repetitions at the same rate. However, the child is told that the rate of presentation will be faster, implying that the child's responses will need to be faster (word recall problems frequently become more apparent in such circumstances).

> While Terry has gross deficits in language skills, it is suspected that this is symptomatic of other problems rather than his primary problem because throughout the testing sessions he engaged in a great deal of self-stimulation (vocal, verbal, and visual) and he often seemed oblivious to the examiner and indifferent to social reinforcement.

> Dean's area of difficulty is auditory closure which requires that he produce the word when only some of the sounds are given and probably explains his inability to use phonetics and sequence sounds in words.

Diligent and attentive readers can divine the meaning from these sentences if they have sufficient background to know what the clinician was driving at. Uninitiated readers, however, soon give up in hopeless confusion.

Wendell Johnson's (1946, p. 49) familiar formulation of the scientific method specifies four steps:

> . . . (a) asking clear answerable questions in order to direct one's (b) observations, which are made in a calm and unprejudiced manner, and which are then (c) reported as accurately as possible and

in such a way as to answer the questions that were asked to begin with, after which (d) any pertinent beliefs or assumptions that were held before the observations were made are revised in the light of the observations made and the answers obtained.

Good clinical practices involve a similar four-step process involving (1) developing clear formulations of a client's problems, leading to (2) precise definitions of steps toward amelioration of those problems, followed by (3) impartial assessment of the outcomes of whatever steps are taken, which in turn elicit (4) appropriate readjustments in original formulations and definitions based on the results of those reassessments. Johnson observed, "The language of science is the better part of science." In a very real sense the same can be said about clinical practice—the language of good clinical practice is the better part of good clinical practice. Although skilled clinicians may express themselves unclearly and clear reports may disguise inept clinicians, both of these situations are exceptional. The clarity of clinical reporting usually offers the best single clue to the quality of the clinical services being reported.

SUMMARY

Clear, accurate clinical reporting is essential to the delivery of acceptable speech-language pathology and audiology services. Clinical reports serve to communicate information to other professionals. Such reports record information for future use by the person providing the described service or services. Furthermore, they document all services to afford a legal record of whatever has transpired. The first of these three functions, however, signifies the most important criterion for clinical reporting: it should always represent concise, factual, and intelligible communication.

References

American Speech-Language-Hearing Association Professional Services Board: Standards for PSB accreditation. *ASHA* 25:51–58, 1983.

Barzun J: *Wilson Follett Modern American Usage.* New York, Warner Books, 1966.

Dublinske S: PL 94-142: developing the individualized education program (IEP). *ASHA* 20:380–397, 1978.

Giolas TG, Owens E, Lamb SH, et al: Hearing performance inventory. *J Speech Hear Disord* 44:169–195, 1979.

Huber JT: *Report Writing in Psychology and Psychiatry.* New York, Harper and Row, 1961.

Jackson JH: *Selected Writings.* London, Hodder and Stoughton, 1932, vol 2.

Johnson W: *People in Quandaries.* New York, Harper and Brothers, 1946.

Johnson W, Darley FL, Spriestersbach DC: *Diagnostic Methods in Speech Pathology.* New York, Harper and Row, 1963.

Leonard LB, Prutting CA, Perozzi JA, et al: Nonstandardized approaches to the assessment of language behaviors. *ASHA* 20:371–379, 1978.

Moore MW: Pathological writing. *ASHA* 11:535–538, 1969.

Rees NS: Art and science of diagnosis in hearing, language, and speech. In Singh S, Lynch J: *Diagnostic Procedures in Hearing, Language, and Speech.* Baltimore, University Park Press, 1978.

Siegel GM: The high cost of accountability. *ASHA* 17: 796–797, 1975.

Siegel GM, Broen PA: Language assessment. In Lloyd LL: *Communication Assessment and Intervention Strategies.* Baltimore, University Park Press, 1976.

Strunk W, White EB: *The Elements of Style.* New York, Macmillan, 1959.

Supplemental Readings

Billings BL, Schmitz HD: *Report Writing in Audiology.* Danville, IL, Interstate Printers, 1980.

English R, Lilywhite H: A semantic approach to clinical reporting in speech pathology. *ASHA* 5:647–650, 1963.

Fisher LI: Reporting: in the schools to the community. In Van Hattum RJ: *Clinical Speech in the Schools.* Springfield, IL, Charles C Thomas, 1969.

Klopfer WG: *The Psychological Report.* New York, Grune and Stratton, 1960.

Knepflar KJ: *Report Writing in the Field of Communication Disorders.* Danville, IL, Interstate Printers, 1976.

Pannbacker M: Diagnostic report writing. *J Speech Hear Disord* 40:367–379, 1975.

Peterson HA, Marquardt TP: *Appraisal and Diagnosis of Speech and Language Disorders.* Englewood Cliffs, NJ, Prentice-Hall, 1981.

CHAPTER SIX

Systematic Record Keeping

The range of approaches to storing clinical information is very broad indeed. At one extreme in that range is the image—probably mythical—of the small-town family physician whose memory is a limitless repository of bits and pieces about each member of the families under his omnipotent care. When the need arises, he can retrieve the essential details of the pedigree; prenatal, natal, and neonatal course; childhood diseases, accidents, and injuries; adolescent emotional and dermatologic problems; marital adjustment; parenting behavior; extramarital affairs; menopausal and midlife problems; senescence and ultimate demise of each of his patients. Although he scrawls occasional notes in a shabby little vest pocketbook, these notes are mostly for the bookkeeper who handles his billing.

At the other extreme are the records found in many comprehensive medical centers. Patient "charts" consist of variegated pages loosely bound in grubby, bedraggled manila folders. The chart for any single patient may consist of several volumes, with a volume defined by the amount of paper a single folder can hold. Within these folders are dozens, even hundreds, of ruled papers with reports of physical examinations, treatment records, and nursing notes—most written hastily in illegible penmanship. There are dim third or fourth copies of laboratory studies. There are operative notes filed pages away from the notes of the pre- and postoperative evaluations. There are social workers' notes in pristine condition because they are seldom read by anyone. There are consultant reports, neatly typed and elegantly worded, that neglect to mention the purpose of the consultation. There are small slips of paper with such trenchant bits of information as "Dr. Johnson, please call Dr. Taylor about Mrs. Green." And there are countless other oddments that someone—physician, nurse, dietition, laboratory technician, therapist, speech-language pathologist or audiologist—at some time considered important to the patient's care.

Fortunately, most record keeping falls somewhere between these extremes. Too seldom, however, do clinical services programs—and this includes programs in speech-language pathology and audiology—have efficient, well integrated records systems which have been carefully developed to serve the unique demands of the services they support.

The following story reveals some common problems in records systems. Although some aspects are unique, similar problems can be found in many speech, language, and hearing services programs in medical centers, in rehabilitation centers, and in school programs, as well as in the freestanding speech and hearing center it describes.

Fifteen years ago, a service club in a midwestern city discontinued its program for preschool blind children. The demand for services to these children had all but disappeared because of the marked reduction in the incidence of blindness in infancy and because of growth of public programs. Since sponsorship of a service program for children was an essential rallying point for the club, they began a search for a new project. One member had a grandchild born with cleft palate. Out of this experience he had discovered that the community provided no organized speech therapy services for preschoolers with this condition. Therefore, he proposed such a program to the club, and the proposal ultimately achieved their enthusiastic support.

The program began on a three ½-day per week basis. Ms. Jean Dillon was employed as the speech-language pathologist/coordinator. No other professional staff was employed, but a professional advisory committee was appointed to consult as needed. Ms. Dillon was well qualified for the position. She had worked for several years as a speech clinician in the public schools, where she had been assigned most recently to a school for orthopedically handicapped children. She had also spent two summers as a speech-language pathologist at a special camp for children with cleft palate and similar impairments.

In instituting the new program, Ms. Dillon recognized the need for an appropriate records system. In view of the special mission of the program, however, a relatively simple system seemed adequate. The ultimate size of the program seemed foreordained. Considering the likely prevalence of cleft palate in the population area to be served, about 10 or 15 new admissions each year seemed likely. The program might ultimately become full time, but the demand for services was not likely to justify more than one speech-language pathologist.

The first record to be instituted was a schedule book. Ms. Dillon did much of the scheduling herself, but when she was working with children, the telephone was covered by volunteers who also made appointments. The schedule book noted for each appointment the name and age of the client, the referral source, and the service to be provided (i.e., evaluation, re-evaluation, follow-up, or therapy).

Beginning with the first client scheduled, Ms. Dillon also began a case record file. Because of the assortment of materials to be filed, including medical and surgical reports, audiologic studies, case history data, test forms, speech/language evaluation reports, therapy notes, miscellaneous letters, and release forms, she purchased heavyweight 9½″ × 13″ envelopes to hold the materials. Each envelope carried the client's name, last name first, on the upper right-hand corner. These envelopes were filed alphabetically in a locked file cabinet.

Within the first 6 months of operation, it became apparent that an additional file must be maintained for the volunteers. To discharge their responsibilities, they often needed to determine whether a particular child was known to the program, to know whether he or she was enrolled in therapy, and to find client addresses and telephone numbers. In order to retrieve this information from the case record face sheet, all materials were removed from the envelope. Not only did this procedure increase the hazard of losing material, it also placed confidential information under the scrutiny of all volunteers. To solve these problems, Ms. Dillon instituted an additional card-file system that provided the name, parents' name, address, and telephone number for each client. Clients actively enrolled in therapy were filed separately from clients seen only for evaluation or otherwise not enrolled in an ongoing program.

During the second year of the program's operation, Ms. Dillon was contacted by a neighboring university speech-language pathology program. Because of its unique nature, the faculty considered the program for cleft palate children to be a worthwhile clinical practicum placement. The service club, the professional advisory committee, and Ms. Dillon were pleased by this recognition and agreed to cooperate.

With more than one person providing therapy, more detailed reporting now seemed necessary. Furthermore, since the students frequently conducted therapy sessions when Ms. Dillon was also seeing a client, she wished to have therapy reports to review. From a practical standpoint, Ms. Dillon believed these reports should be as succinct as possible. She designed a form, 8½″ × 5″ in size, which was subsequently printed and padded for convenient use. These forms called for the client's name, the date of the therapy session, the specific objectives of the therapy session, the activities pursued to accomplish these objectives, an evaluation of the success achieved, and recommendations for conduct of the next session. These sheets were to be completed by the end of each day and given to Ms. Dillon for review. She then filed the therapy report in the case file. Frequently, however, a student's schedule precluded immediate completion and he or she took the reports home to finish and then submitted the therapy report later.

Also during the second year of the program, the service club decided to increase its fund-raising efforts to support the program. An important part of these efforts involved an extensive publicity campaign. A member of the local Ad Club volunteered to manage the campaign. He began by interviewing Ms. Dillon, who discovered, with some embarrassment, that she could not immediately answer questions about the number of clients seen, number of evaluations provided, total therapy visits provided, average number of services provided to each client, etc.

Another member of the club contacted an old friend who was on the board of a local charitable foundation. The friend encouraged submission of a request for funds and offered to assist in preparation of the application. This resulted in another request for statistical data about the services provided.

By canceling all appointments for a week and working through two weekends, Ms. Dillon was able to go through the case records and the schedule book to retrieve the data requested. This experience convinced her that an additional record was needed. She instituted an attendance reporting system. Cards were printed with squares for each day the program was in operation for a 12-month period. Volunteers transferred attendance data from the schedule book by placing in the square for a given date the letter "E" for evaluation, "R" for re-evaluation, "T" for therapy, "C" for cancellation, and "NS" for "no show" when a client failed to keep an appointment. Monthly statistical summaries were prepared covering all services provided. These summaries were stored in a looseleaf notebook.

During the second and third years of operation, it became increasingly difficult to be rigid in defining client eligibility for the program. First, children with other types of craniofacial anomalies were seen. Later, often at the urging of members of the service club who had some personal relationship with a child or his parents, preschoolers with other types of speech and language problems were seen. Eventually, because the program was able to provide therapy on a more intensive basis, neighboring school districts asked the program to continue services to more seriously handicapped children even after they reached school age. By the beginning of the third year, then, Ms. Dillon was not only working full time, but a second speech-language pathologist (who had participated in the clinical practicum program as a student) was employed full time as a clinical fellow.

Each of these new developments required some modifications in the records system. The schedule book had to be revised to accommodate a second clinician. The admission of children other than those with cleft palate required substantial reorientation of case records. Virtually all physicians in the area first referred children with cleft palate to the Craniofacial Anomalies Center at the state university medical school. Therefore, referral procedures to the service club program had been fairly straightforward; that is, all of the children seen came from the Craniofacial Anomalies Center. The center simply sent a copy of their composite summary which was filed in the case record. As the caseload of the program diversified, however, it became necessary to obtain diagnostic reports and other information from a wide variety of professionals in the community. These reports were also inserted in the case files.

By the beginning of the program's fourth year, some problems in record storage were apparent. There were now over 700 individual case records. Furthermore, the records for children enrolled in long-term speech therapy could not be contained in a single envelope; some records extended to three or even four envelopes. It also became difficult to prepare summaries for children leaving the program or interim reports in response to requests from surgeons, dentists, or other specialists. With various diagnostic reports, evaluations, summaries, test forms, therapy session reports, and letters, there could be 200 to 300 separate pieces of paper distributed among the various envelopes covering a single client.

Further problems arose in locating information about a client. Frequently, different addresses and telephone numbers appeared on the index card than appeared on the case record face sheet. When it was necessary to determine whether a client had received a particular service, it was sometimes necessary to reconcile disparities between the schedule book and the attendance record.

Yet, the two professional staff members were accustomed to the records system and found the problems only mildly annoying. Furthermore, Ms. Dillon had an excellent memory and could often supply details that could not be found in the records.

The fifth year of the program saw tremendous changes. The man who had proposed the original program died unexpectedly. His commitment was such that he had bequeathed his large home to the project with $500,000 to remodel it and to expand the program. Therefore, by the end of that year, it became the Lassiter Children's Speech and Hearing Center (named for its benefactor) and began to offer considerably expanded services. Soon, the staff included three speech-language pathologists in addition to Ms. Dillon (who functioned as director), an audiologist, and a teacher of hearing-impaired preschoolers. The professional staff was supported by a secretary-receptionist and a clerk-typist.

The center was now receiving referrals from many different physicians, from several community agencies, and from school districts. Within the next 18 months it grew from an agency providing about 600 client visits a year to one providing 2,500 visits a year.

It also soon became apparent that a complete change in the center's financial base must occur. The service club had originally insisted that the program serve children at no cost to their families. The magnitude of the new center's program, however, far exceeded the club's fund-raising capacity. Furthermore, Mr. Lassiter's bequest was disappearing rapidly under new financial demands.

Within the next 2 years, the center accomplished several goals. First, a fee-for-services system was established, with fees adjusted according to family financial circumstances. Second, the center was approved to receive payment for services to certain children from the state Crippled Children Services program and from the Regional Center for Developmentally Disabled Children. Third, the center was admitted as an agency of the local United Fund. Fourth, contracts were written with three local school districts to provide audiologic services and educational services for hearing-handicapped preschoolers.

Although Ms. Dillon and the center staff were elated by these developments, they soon discovered that each brought a new set of records problems. The previous attendance-reporting system served to provide information about individual clients and to accrue data for public relations efforts. Although errors were frequent, their effect was insignificant. As it operated, however, the system could not support the financial accounting required for billing families and agencies for services rendered. Therefore, the center instituted a "charge tag" system. At the end of each day, each staff member submitted a charge tag for each client served. The tag identified the client and stipulated the service provided. All tags were accumulated for use by the part-time bookkeeper who kept the financial records and handled the billing. After the charge tags were posted, they were filed with the client records in case questions arose about bills that had been rendered.

Further problems arose with clients seen under the aegis of Crippled Children Services (CCS) and the Regional Center. In both instances, prior authorization was required before services could be provided;

these authorizations specified a maximum number of visits. Unless the authorization was renewed when the maximum was reached, further payment was denied. Initially, the responsibility for keeping track of authorizations was assigned to the clinician serving the client. This approach soon proved unsatisfactory. Instead, a new card file was established in the office. The file contained 52 compartments, labeled for each week of the year. A card was prepared for each CCS and Regional Center client and placed in the compartment corresponding to the week in which the authorization expired. Regularly the clerk would review the cards 2 or 3 weeks in advance of expiration and inform the client's clinician. If services were to continue, the clinician would request renewal of the authorization. When received, authorizations were filed in the case records.

The United Fund also presented some special problems. That agency required more extensive reporting of service statistics than was required previously. Furthermore, they required reporting of family counseling, contacts with other agencies, and participation in conferences regarding clients. These data had never been recorded. The United Fund also required reporting clients within narrow age categories as well as precise information as to whether clients were on a full fee, partial fee, served at no charge, or were funded by another agency. Finally, because of charges of discrimination by some of their participating agencies, they also required reporting service statistics by sex, ethnicity, and approximate family income.

Several records procedures were instituted to accommodate United Fund requirements. Because family counseling and agency contacts did not appear in the schedule book, they could not be entered on attendance record cards, the current source of all service statistics. Since fees were not charged for these services, no charge tags were filed. Therefore, a staff daily report system was initiated. On specially prepared forms, each member of the professional staff recorded all major professional activities: direct client services, family interviews, contacts with other professionals and agencies (including telephone contacts), and meetings attended. These reports were turned in to the office at the end of the day, and eventually all noted activities were tallied by the clerk. On the bookkeeper's recommendation, these reports were also filed. The center received frequent questions from families about bills, questions which often revealed disparities between the schedule book and the attendance record (for example, clients were sometimes noted as canceled on the schedule but shown as attending a therapy session on the attendance record). It seemed, therefore, that the daily report form should afford an additional record of services provided to clients.

The issue of ethnicity and family income data caused considerable consternation. The legality of recording ethnicity was questionable according to state law. Furthermore, the office still relied on volunteers, and all but case records were readily available to them. The staff was apprehensive, therefore, about recording confidential data about family finances on any of the reports that were used for tallying information for United Fund reports. The only feasible solution was to designate the daily report as a confidential record. Whenever a client's name appeared on that report a two digit code followed the name; the first digit indicated ethnicity, the second the range of the family income. These data were also tallied by the clerk.

The school district contracts also required records modifications. The school districts contended that the children served were attending special programs under their jurisdiction, even though the programs were not actually conducted by the districts. They required, therefore, that cumulative folders, adhering to the format for records of all children in their districts, be maintained. Furthermore, since they received reimbursement from the state based on average daily attendance, they required attendance reporting according to the system employed by all schools in their districts.

The requirement for maintenance of cumulative folders caused concern. By school district policy, in fact by state law, these folders were available at all times for parental review. They were also available to school district administrative personnel, to pupil services workers, and to all special education personnel. Since center records frequently contained confidential referral information, the center's professional staff was reluctant to incorporate client records into cumulative folders. They decided, instead, to maintain cumulative folders adhering to school district standards separately from client records.

The attendance records for school district children created another problem. The school contracts included all services within a monthly per-child payment. In other words, such services as a hearing reevaluation, hearing aid selection and maintenance, parent counseling, and speech-language evaluation were all provided with no charge beyond the single lump-sum payment. These services, which were always recorded on the center's attendance record, were not reported to the school district on a monthly basis. The monthly report covered only attendance in the educational/therapy programs. On the other hand, all additional services were reported to the districts in an annual summary and were incorporated with other service statistics for the United Fund. For school district children, therefore, the clerk was required to tally the attendance card data twice; once for the monthly school district reports showing only "therapy" visits, and once for various annual reports showing all services.

It was soon evident, however, that this procedure was inaccurate. By center policy, clients seen by the audiologist for hearing aid-related services other than hearing aid evaluations were recorded as receiving "therapy." Yet, since the school district did not regard these as primary educational services, they could not be reported on school district monthly attendance reports. Furthermore, the data required for annual reports of family counseling and consultations with school district personnel were recorded on the staff daily report forms and hence could not be retrieved by the clerk tallying attendance records. The only solution seemed to be a separate reporting procedure for children in school district-supported programs. The staff serving these children were required to submit a supplementary daily report, noting only services for these children. Although this procedure was relatively easy for the teacher of the hearing handicapped, whose primary responsibilities related to these educational services, it was difficult for the audiologists or speech-language pathologists who provided occasional services to remember to submit the supplemental report. Since the staff also saw hearing-handicapped children who were not enrolled in school district programs, they had to determine whether a particular child was or was not seen under school district auspices.

By the center's tenth anniversary, it had become a large agency. It now employed, in addition to Ms. Dillon (who continued as director), a professional staff of 17 including nine speech-language pathologists, four audiologists, two teachers of hearing-handicapped children, a clinical psychologist, and a social worker. The center not only fully occupied the Lassiter house, it also leased space in a nearby church where the programs for preschool hearing-handicapped children and a new program for children with language disorders were conducted. The office staff now included a business manager, a bookkeeper, a receptionist, two clerks, and a secretary for the director. Throughout the school year, there were also three or four university students engaged in clinical practicum.

In that tenth anniversary year, some serious problems came into focus. The growing dissatisfaction of the staff with their records responsibilities could no longer be ignored. Their comments included: "For every hour we spend with a client, it takes a half hour to complete the records." "I can never complete all my reports by the end of the day, and by the time I get back to them I usually forget to record something." "If we have to keep all these records, we must be allowed at least 1 more hour a day for records and reports." (They were already allowed an hour each day for this purpose.) One of the more outspoken staff members summarized the majority feeling: "If I wanted to be a bookkeeper, I wouldn't have gotten a Master's degree in speech-language pathology."

There was also increasing strife between the professional staff and the office staff, particularly the business manager. Since he was frequently responsible for ameliorating problems resulting from inaccurate reporting, recording, or transferring of data, his concerns were understandable. He often deplored the lack of "business sense" among the professional staff and commented that they would never survive in the "real world" of free enterprise. The clerical staff constantly complained that their responsibilities were too heavy and more clerks were needed. It became increasingly difficult to produce reports. Eventually, the otolaryngologist on the center's Board of Directors reported colleague complaints to the effect that if delays in reporting were not eliminated, they would refer patients elsewhere.

Ms. Dillon discussed the problem of inadequate clerical staff with the board. While they were sympathetic, they could not identify sources of additional financial support to cover increased overhead.

Complaints about the volume of client case records were heard daily. These records had accumulated since the beginning of the program and now filled eight five-drawer file cabinets. These files included records for many clients seen once for a single evaluation several years previously. They also contained records on clients who had received such extensive services that their records were distributed in five or six envelopes. Since office space was limited, the clerical staff was rebelling against the purchase of additional file cabinets to accommodate more records.

A further source of professional staff complaints was an odious job that all shared. Several times each week the center received requests for summaries of services to previous clients. Frequently, the staff member who had provided these services was no longer employed at the center. As a result, an individual with no direct knowledge of the client had to review referral information, evaluation reports, test results, and dozens of therapy visit reports in an attempt to prepare an adequate summary.

As the professional staff fell farther and farther behind in preparing reports on both current and previous clients, they accumulated more and more client records in their offices. Originally, a rule had been established that all records were to be returned to the file at the end of each day, but this rule became so impractical that it was generally ignored. The clerical staff was constantly searching for missing records. The bulletin board became covered with notes inquiring, "Who has the record for . . .?" Both professional and clerical staff were embarrassed by urgent telephone requests for information which could not be handled because the record was missing.

When new information arrived at the center about clients whose records were out of file, it accumulated in a "to be filed" basket. This resulted in delays in the receipt of important information by the professional staff and further embarrassment.

Operating programs in two different buildings further complicated the records problems. Not only were records out of the file, they were sometimes in another building.

What the staff dubbed "the great records crisis" was precipitated by two incidents. The first grew out of a change in the state Medicaid regulations that permitted payment for certain speech-language pathology services when those services were provided by licensed rehabilitation centers. Since most children from families receiving public assistance were now served without fees, the center's board was interested in this additional source of revenue. The center applied to the state health department for licensure as a rehabilitation center and was subsequently visited by an evaluation team. Although the team commended the center's facilities, staff, and scope and the apparent quality of services, they were dismayed at the records system, which failed to meet most of the criteria specified in their regulations. Consequently, licensure was denied.

The second incident was the serving of a subpoena for the records of a client who had received extensive services several years previously. The child had been involved in an automobile accident during the time he was receiving therapy at the center. The family had been advised by their attorney to accept no settlement until all possible complications might appear. They were now seeking a large settlement. Prominent among their claims was that the child's speech had deteriorated as a result of the accident and that he had subsequently experienced serious social, emotional, and educational problems because of his deviant speech.

The child's case record contained a report of an initial evaluation together with the forms from the tests administered during the initial evaluation. There were also 72 therapy session reports. There was no mention of the accident anywhere in the record, but the attendance record showed that therapy appointments had been canceled for 4 weeks following the date of the accident. Two different clinicians had worked with the client. Neither was still on the staff, and, in fact, both were now living in other states.

Since no record had ever been subpoenaed from the center, Ms. Dillon contacted the attorney who served on the center's board. Under the circumstances, he declined to review the record personally but was aghast when the contents were described. In his view it was inconceivable that when the child had presumably been in the care of speech-language professionals during the interval in question, no data, or even subjective impressions, could be retrieved to either support or contradict the family's allegations. He not only shared his dismay with the other members of the board, he also offered a stern analysis of other possible legal implications of the inadequate records system.

These two incidents, the licensure denial and the subpoena, climaxed the growing discontent and frustration with the center's records system. In an unusual incursion into an area that had previously been considered a professional matter, the board instructed Ms. Dillon to institute an immediate total revision of the records system, a task that she and the professional and clerical staff soon recognized was akin to one of the 12 labors of Hercules: cleaning the Augean stables.

Without moralizing about the fable of the Lassiter Center, the most striking problems it illustrates can be identified:

1. *Short-sightedness.* With rare exceptions, speech-language pathology and audiology programs either grow or expire. In instituting a records system for a new program, regardless of how modest the beginnings, one should always assume continued growth. Therefore, every new records system should be planned so that it can grow in all dimensions to accommodate increasing numbers of clients and an increasing variety of information about those clients, and to serve an ever-widening range of clinical and administrative demands. Revising a total records system is always an expensive undertaking. Every new records system should have a virtually limitless capacity for multidimensional growth.
2. *Absence of a total design in the records system.* As new needs arose, new records procedures or new records documents were introduced without consideration of their relationships to a total records system.
3. *Indiscriminate records storage.* Virtually every piece of paper referring to a particular client was stuffed into an envelope with little regard to its future significance. Material was simply collected. It was never summarized. Once placed in an envelope, every piece of paper became a permanent part of the records. Furthermore, the system lacked any provision for retiring inactive records.

4. *Cumbersome inefficiency.* As the system proliferated, it made increasingly unreasonable demands on both the professional and clerical staff when they were called upon to enter or retrieve data. Even routine procedures became complex when those procedures involved clinical records.
5. *Insularity.* In developing the records system, the staff assumed that their records need contain only the information required to carry out day-to-day clinical activities within the center. They neglected to recognize the need for coordinating their records system with the systems of the other agencies serving the same clients. Furthermore, they failed to recognize that various regulatory agencies impose standards that must be considered in developing clinical records systems.

Having regarded some common problems in clinical records systems, we will turn the discussion to more positive matters. Six fundamental characteristics can be proposed for any clinical records system:

1. It must immediately reveal whether a particular individual is or ever has been a client of the agency.
2. It must provide essential identifying and demographic information about each client.
3. It must offer a clear and concise record of all services provided to and on behalf of each client.
4. It must facilitate continuity of care for all clients.
5. It must facilitate follow-up of clients served previously.
6. It must permit efficient retrieval of statistical data about the total program, and, when needed, provide data for research.

The remaining sections of this chapter address various aspects of developing clinical records systems that encompass these characteristics.

ESSENTIAL COMPONENTS OF CLINICAL RECORDS SYSTEMS

Two principles should guide the development of any clinical records system: *functionalism* and *economy*. The system must store and provide immediate access to whatever information is required to plan and carry out effective clinical services. It must also provide a continuing record of the nature and outcomes of those services. Hence, it must be functional. But the system must also be economical in terms of the professional staff effort invested in entering and retrieving information and of support staff effort in transcribing data and filing and locating records. Not incidentally, it must also be economical in terms of space required for storage.

Like all guiding principles, these two are sometimes incompatible. When one serves clients with complex communicative disorders, it is frequently difficult to differentiate between relevant and irrelevant data. Clinicians usually err, therefore, in the direction of including a wide range of information in records. Yet, the more information recorded, the more time spent entering the information and, later, searching for information when it must be retrieved. Ultimately, therefore, the volume of information recorded will influence the cost of the services we provide. Clinicians should develop a kind of monitoring reflex that leads them to pause to evaluate the likely functional value of every piece of information before entering it in the clinical record. In terms of these two principles, one must always ask, "Does the functional value of the information justify the economic impact of entering and storing it in the records system?"

The story of the Lassiter Speech and Hearing Center illustrated the problems that can result from proliferating the components of a records system. Each time a new need arose, a new component was added without regard for its relationship to the other components of the system. This proliferation was uneconomical because it involved the duplication of the same information in several places. Proliferation is also inefficient since it becomes necessary to search through multiple documents to retrieve a specific bit of information. Furthermore, proliferation substantially increases the frequency of errors since the same information must be recorded on several records. Under these circumstances, a staff member may forget to make a required entry or, even more frequently, when a particular bit of information changes, an entry may be revised in one place but not in another.

At the opposite extreme, overcentralization of records can also create problems. When, for example, all information on a particular client is entered in a single record, grave consequences may attend losing or misfiling that record. In such instances, it may be impossible to determine that a particular client has ever been known to the agency. This situation has serious professional, ethical, and legal complications.

Furthermore, overcentralization may result in inordinate use of a single record. When that record must serve all functions it will be heavily utilized for purposes that require only small segments of the total record. For example, if the only source of identifying data of clients is the case record face sheet, the entire record must be retrieved to find such trivial details as the client's address and telephone number. Or, when the only documentation of services provided is in the case record, that record must also serve all accounting functions. Again, this is highly inefficient.

Except in instances where records storage is computerized, a topic that will be discussed in another chapter, an optimal clinical records system consists of three component records: a *client directory*, a *services accounting record*, and a *client clinical record.*

The Client Directory

The client directory holds concise identification data on all clients served by the program. Each program must define what constitutes "served"; however, it usually entails direct personal contact between the client and a member of the professional staff. Many agencies provide extensive information and referral services by telephone to individuals who are not actually seen. Although data regarding these services may be reported to funding agencies, programs typically do not keep any kind of client records on individuals who do not receive direct clinical services.

It is usually wise to enter into the records system all individuals who receive any direct service. This may even include clients seen for brief sessions leading to the agreement that no significant problem exists or that immediate referral to a more appropriate program is advisable.

As the name implies, the client directory is a ready source for determining that a particular individual has been served and for retrieving essential identifying and demographic data. The directory will also provide access to the complete client case record. Typically, the client directory is a card file, situated near the individual or individuals who are most likely to be contacted for information.

The essential data which usually appear on client directory cards include the full name, birthdate, address, telephone number, parents' names when clients are children, or spouse's name for adults. Although recording social security numbers can offer a valuable identifier (except for birthdate, all other suggested entries are subject to change), many programs and clients consider the use of these numbers to be depersonalizing. For efficient operation, however, it may be useful to record such identifying numbers as Medicare or Medicaid numbers and client numbers assigned by such agencies as Crippled Children Services and departments of rehabilitation. In some settings it may also be helpful to show the original referral source in the client directory.

Some agencies enter a brief indicator of the nature of the client's problem in the directory, for example, by using one of the diagnostic codes to be described later. This offers some advantages for rapid identification of particular clients, but the practice is hazardous. An admitting diagnosis is likely to change, leading to frequent inaccuracies in the directory. Furthermore, the client directory is so generally used that it is a poor place for entering confidential information.

The client directory also provides entry into the client clinical records. As will be discussed later, alphabetic filing is inadequate for any but the most limited clinical record files. Therefore, the directory, which is filed alphabetically, also shows the identifying number of the client clinical record.

Because the client directory is the prime source for identifying the clients served, no card should ever be removed for a longer interval than is required to update information. Furthermore, directory cards should probably be maintained permanently. If agency policy directs destruction of outdated client case records, the client directory cards should be maintained in an auxiliary or "dead" file. When questions arise, it is better to respond, "Although our records show that John Doe was registered for service by this agency in 1955, we can provide no further information because client files are destroyed after 10 years," than to respond, "John Doe has not been seen by this agency during the last 10 years. We have no way of determining whether he was seen prior to that time."

The Service Accounting Record

Virtually every clinical services program must keep careful records detailing the services provided. In school programs, these data are used for computing excess cost reimbursement, for recording attendance, and for recording any other data required for periodic reporting of services provided. In agencies receiving overall program support from governmental agencies, service clubs, united funds, or foundations, the service accounting record will provide the data required to support budget requests and other applications for financial assistance. When fees are to be paid either directly by the client or in his behalf by a third-party payer, the service accounting record will provide the data for rendering bills. The service accounting record, then, must hold all of the information required to document the services that have been provided and to retrieve the data required to characterize clients in whatever agency reports must be prepared.

The service accounting record contains enough demographic information to identify the client and to meet reporting requirements. It should hold the information required to establish financial responsibility, i.e., the names of participating third-party payers together with the identification number they have assigned to the client and the nature of the services they have authorized.

Third-party payers, particularly health insurance carriers, often require that all claims show the physician who has recommended the speech, language, and hearing services and the diagnosis of the condition which is being "treated." Furthermore, their authorizations for services are usually specific, i.e., for evaluation only, for a specific number of therapy sessions, etc. These data should also appear on the service accounting record.

In most comprehensive medical or rehabilitation facilities, service accounting records covering all departments are maintained by a central office. Occasionally, despite centralized accounting records, each department compiles its own service statistics. In these instances, at least limited service accounting records are kept by the department as well as in the central office.

The Client Clinical Record

The client clinical record comprises all information regarding the professional services provided by the clinical program. It includes case history material, records for all evaluation, treatment, rehabilitative, and educational services, and reports to and from other concerned professionals and agencies. As a determiner of the quality of clinical services, it is by far the most important component of the clinical records system.

CLIENT CLINICAL RECORDS SYSTEMS

When speech-language pathology and audiology programs are conducted within larger institutions, they may be required to conform to the client record-keeping system of the entire institution. Although they may be able to adapt the system to serve their unique requirements, these adaptations must be essentially consistent with the overall plan of the records system.

Sometimes, however, speech-language pathology and audiology programs may have complete autonomy in the development and maintenance of client records systems. This is most likely to occur in freestanding programs, but it may also occur in larger institutions where no single records system has been adopted.

The succeeding discussion will consider records systems that are designed for entire multiservice institutions and systems designed to serve only speech, language, and hearing services programs. Although many systems have been designed, four were selected for discussion here: The *unit record*, the *problem-oriented record*, the *practice-oriented record*, and the *CASE information system*.

The Unit Record

The concept of the unit record was developed early in this century for use in hospitals and outpatient clinics. Previously, separate records were kept for each period of care for each specific complaint. This led to poor coordination of the various types of care provided to a single individual. The unit record system emerged, therefore, to support what was at the time a new concept in medical care. Benjamin (1977, p. 5) defined the essential characteristics of this system:

> The unit system is based on the concept that the patient and not the disease is the unit for record compilation and has only one case record folder, into which all documents relating to past and present medical care are placed. This system has the advantage of making complete medical histories available to all practitioners involved in the care of the patient.

The unit record, then, collects all information regarding services provided to a single client within the same institution. That information is compiled according to a specific plan. There is some variability among institutions in the way unit records are compiled, but most resemble the format proposed by Kurtz (1943).

The first sheet in the unit record is called the "front unit sheet." It is headed by the client's name, his age on first admission, and his "unit number," a number used in all aspects of client identification. The sheet is divided into two columns. The left column is headed "service." Here each major service is recorded with the date on which it was provided. The right column is headed "diagnoses and operations." In this column diagnoses are entered, usually using one of the standard systems described later. Operations are also entered using a standard nomenclature or code.

Following the front unit sheet is the chronologic record. The optimism of Kurtz's description of the chronologic record will be apparent to anyone who has worked in institutions using unit records (p. 18):

> It proceeds from the first contact with the patient to the last, through both clinic and hospital care. It is the basic record, and as such contains a great variety of material. Probably the doctors' progress notes in both out- and inpatient departments are the main component. They are freely interlarded, however, with all kinds of special examinations, ranging from thorough workups to simple laboratory reports, with individual treatment reports, including operation records, with brief social notes, with pertinent correspondence, and with authorizations. Such an intermixing is not nearly as confusing as it might seem, for each of these various insertions has a distinctive form which renders it easy to find. At the same time, they all lend meaning to the doctor's notes among which they appear.

The chronologic record includes five sections: *application data, initial examination, progress notes, special examination and treatment records*, and *authorizations and correspondence*.

APPLICATION DATA

This section includes all pertinent identification data: name, address, parents or other next of kin, age and/or birthdate, sex, birthplace, marital status, occupation, etc. Usually, information regarding insurance or other third-party coverage is also recorded. At one time, hospitals and clinics offering reduced fees to individuals with limited resources recorded family financial data among the application data. However, current regulations frequently preclude entry of such sensitive information on a record that can be scrutinized by so many people.

INITIAL EXAMINATION

The clinical record usually begins with a summary of the information obtained during the initial examination. It covers the history and physical findings, presumably the "logical starting point for any course of treatments or special investigations" (Kurtz, 1943). An initial examination usually begins the entire record, and initial examinations also usually precede every subsequent admission to the hospital or return to the clinic for investigation of a new complaint or for the re-evaluation of a previously studied complaint. Teaching hospitals (e.g. university-affiliated hospitals) may record repeated initial examinations by different individuals—for example, by a resident, an intern, and one or more medical students. This practice can be confusing to someone unfamiliar with the practices of teaching hospitals, particularly when disparities exist among the several initial examinations that have been conducted on the same day.

The traditional form for reporting an initial evaluation in the unit record is as classical as a Milton sonnet or a Bach fugue. It begins with a statement of the *complaint* (sometimes abbreviated *CC* for "chief complaint") which consists of the client's statement of the problem or problems that have led him or her to seek assistance. There follows a *family history,* with the primary focus on hereditary factors which may bear on the client's problem. Next is recorded the *personal history,* emphasizing factors in the accustomed environment which may impair health; the client's habits with particular reference to sleep, exercise, nutrition, use of tobacco and alcohol, etc; and previous illnesses, infections, allergies, and other recurrent symptoms. The *present illness* section includes the client's account of his symptoms, reinforced with answers to questions about such symptoms as pain, changes in weight, and other alterations of body functions. The *physical examination* section reports the results of the physician's examination. That examination is comprehensive, rather than focused on the presenting complaint. This report is also traditionally written in a standard format with each system (e.g., cardiovascular system, respiratory system, genitourinary system, and central nervous system) considered in turn. The initial examination report concludes with the *provisional diagnosis* which states the examiner's opinion, based on the information available at that time, as to possible diagnoses. These diagnoses are usually inconclusive and may be simply the basis for planning further studies or experimental treatment.

PROGRESS NOTES

Progress notes are a running record of all observations, conclusions, and recommendations made during the course of completing the diagnostic evaluation or providing treatment. Some comprehensive medical centers using unit records specify that only physicians may enter progress notes. Nonphysician specialists, such as speech-language pathologists, enter their reports among the "special examinations and treatments." In other centers everyone participating in the client's care may record observations among the progress notes. Medical centers may also make sharp distinctions between the progress notes covering outpatient care and those covering inpatient care. In some instances, special records are instituted when an individual is admitted for inpatient care, even though he or she had been receiving outpatient care previously. Usually, the records compiled during the period of hospitalization are combined into the main unit record following discharge.

When a distinction is made between inpatient and outpatient records, subsections of the progress notes may be defined: *hos-*

pital notes versus *clinic notes*. As a general rule, the form of these notes is essentially similar. Other unit records use a special category of progress notes identified as *follow-up notes*. These notes refer to the outcomes of a specific procedure rather than to the total care of the client.

The concept of the follow-up note may be particularly useful to speech-language pathologists and audiologists. They may report brief postoperative evaluations (e.g., following cleft palate surgery, or following Teflon injection into a paralyzed vocal fold) or brief re-evaluations of clients seen previously for speech therapy. Audiologists also may use follow-up notes to report postoperative evaluations, re-evaluations of hearing aid fittings, or re-evaluations of hearing-impaired children to determine the suitability of a recommended educational placement. Labeling such entries as follow-up notes shows that only those procedures necessary to answer one or more specific questions were carried out in lieu of a complete re-evaluation.

Sometimes unit records specify two supplementary categories of progress notes: *nurses' notes* and *social service notes*. Nurses' notes are most often entered when the individual is hospitalized. Because nurses have more frequent patient contact than the attending physician, these notes are usually more detailed than physicians' progress notes.

Social service notes often begin with a detailed evaluation covering all aspects of the client's family situation, living conditions, financial security, and attitudes toward the current situation. From time to time these notes are updated to reflect significant changes. The social worker is often the individual responsible for developing plans for immediate care following discharge from a hospital. These plans are also summarized in the social service notes.

Nurses' notes and social service notes may frequently be as valuable to a speech-language pathologist or audiologist as physicians' notes. For example, nurses often make excellent observations about variations in a client's communication from one day to another or from one time of day to another. Similarly, social workers routinely acquire information that is essential to rehabilitation planning. In particular, when the client is hospitalized, these notes may contain the information required for planning continued speech-language pathology or audiology services after discharge.

SPECIAL EXAMINATION AND TREATMENT RECORDS

This section of the unit record includes two different kinds of material: *laboratory reports* and *specialists' examination and treatment records.*

Laboratory reports consist of data yielded by laboratory studies ordered by the physician. Usually, these studies are reported by entering raw data on forms designed for the purpose. In medical centers, laboratory reports are generally completed by technicians. Such reports can only present data; they do not offer an opinion or a conclusion.

The role of the speech-language pathologist and audiologist must always be clear with respect to the way findings are reported. *They should never be entered as laboratory notes.* Laboratory notes consist of raw data presented by technicians for interpretation by a professional; in medical centers that professional is usually a physician. Although speech-language pathologists and audiologists administer tests that yield quantitative data, it is their province and responsibility to interpret those data. Among other considerations, most results from the tests we administer must be amplified by qualitative evaluations of client performance if their full value is to be exploited. Entries related to the results of speech-language and audiologic evaluations, therefore, differ substantially from the kind of data normally reported in laboratory notes.

Specialists' examination and treatment records include reports of such specialized diagnostic services as are provided by radiologists and pathologists. They also include reports from consultations by medical specialists in such fields as otolaryngology, ophthalmology, neurology, cardiology, and physical medicine and rehabilitation. These records also include reports of specialized treatment, particularly when the treatment involves surgery. Extended medical treatment, as opposed to surgical treatment, is usually reported in the progress notes section.

Speech-language pathologists and audiologists usually enter their evaluations among the specialist examination and treatment reports. When clients are enrolled in speech, language, or hearing therapy programs, these records may be entered either among the progress notes or among the specialist treatment records, depending upon the policies of the particular institution.

Serial graphic charting probably has limited applicability in speech-language pathology (although it can be used in a behavior modification context or, conceivably, when such a measurement device as the Porch Index of Communicative Abilities is employed). Nevertheless, such charting can be useful to audiologists in conducting serial studies of clients treated with ototoxic drugs or under treatment for sudden acute inner ear pathology. When a series of audiometric evaluations is recorded on a single sheet, significant changes in hearing levels are readily observable.

AUTHORIZATIONS AND CORRESPONDENCE

Many unit record systems specify that the last section of the record contain authorizations (e.g., authorizations for care issued by third-party payers, consent forms for release of information, consents for surgery and anesthesia, consents to serve as experimental subjects, or consents to be photographed), and all correspondence sent and received regarding the client. As more and more clients are covered by third-party payers, and as more and more legal actions emerge around clients' rights of privacy, this section becomes increasingly important.

Despite the earlier-noted optimism from the proponent of the unit record system, i.e., that "Such an intermixing is not nearly as confusing as it might seem . . .," the most frequent criticism of the unit record system is that it can create formidable obstacles to the rapid retrieval of information. When a client has received multiple services in an institution, unit records may be voluminous. Busy clinicians often ignore the records of previous examinations and begin as though the client had never been seen before. Specialists may develop easily recognizable forms for recording their data and simply ignore all other material. Others may rely on copies of summary letters sent to referring physicians rather than attempting to discover more complete information.

Some helpful modifications of unit records have been introduced. In some comprehensive medical centers, the various types of entries (progress notes, laboratory reports, surgical summaries, etc.) are recorded on color-coded sheets (usually with a band of color along the outer margin) to permit immediate identification. When a relatively limited range of services is provided, reports from each specialty may be assigned a color. Larger centers, however, usually assign colors by general function so that progress notes are indicated by one color, laboratory notes by another, etc.

Even more helpful is the division of the record into specific sections. Some centers use a rudimentary two-part division with diagnostic reports attached to the left cover of the record and all other reports to the right cover, or reports of inpatient treatment to one cover and outpatient treatment to the other cover. Much more useful is the designation, by tabbed dividers, of separate sections (using, for example, the section designations from the unit record system). This procedure may disrupt the continuity of the record (for example, the laboratory results forming the basis for a diagnosis or the report of an operation may be filed in a separate section from the notes entered in connection with the hospital stay for the surgery). Nevertheless, an experienced records user can usually retrieve information more expeditiously when sections are clearly marked.

Adapting the Unit Record System for a Speech-Language-Hearing Services Program

The essential characteristic of the unit record is the collection within a single record of all information concerning the care of a single client within a multidisciplinary setting, regardless of which department or staff member provides the services. It is not possible, therefore, to apply the entire unit record system to records documenting only speech-language pathology and audiology services. It is, nevertheless, possible to apply many features of this system in designing records for such programs. Many speech, language, and hearing services actually use systems derived from unit records, often without knowing it. A unit record-based approach for client case records in a speech, language, and hearing services program might take the following form:

APPLICATION DATA

As with the traditional unit record, the application data section contains all essential identifying and demographic data. Four considerations guide the selection of the information to be noted. First, what information is required to identify accurately the subject of the record and to specify what should occur in the event of emergency? Second, what other professionals or agencies are participating in the client's care and should be kept informed of major developments? Third, what information is essential to identify the financial basis for providing care to the client? Fourth, what information about the client should be included in the preparation of statistical reports about the program? (The latter information may be transferred to the service accounting record.)

When well planned and scrupulously completed, the application data section can contribute substantially to economy of program operation. If the data that are most frequently needed, particularly by clerical and administrative staff, are recorded here, time savings can be substantial. If such information must be gleaned from other sections of the record, the responsibility usually falls to professional staff. This is a poor use of the time of both professional and administrative personnel.

INITIAL EVALUATIONS

The initial evaluation section holds the essential data compiled to form at least preliminary impressions of the nature and extent of the client's communicative disorder, to decide the next steps that should be recommended, and to plan whatever continued services are to be provided by the speech, language, and hearing services program. Two general types of information will be found: information reported by other professionals, which may provide important background data, and information acquired in the course of the program's own evaluation of the client.

Despite the designation of "initial evaluations," it is usually most efficient to enter summaries of re-evaluations in this section as well. This obtains whether the re-evaluations occur following an interval during which no care is provided or as a part of reassessment of a client who is in continuous care. Compiling initial evaluations and re-evaluations in a single section offers a ready overview of the outcomes of care. It is both useful and efficient to distinguish between periodic re-evaluations and the regular entries regarding therapy sessions in the progress notes section.

PROGRESS NOTES

The progress notes section contains entries covering each contact between a member of the professional staff and the client or family. It is also good practice to enter instances of canceled appointments and failures to appear for appointments, even though these are also noted in the service accounting record, since these entries give immediate information about continuity of care. It is advisable, too, to enter notes about telephone conversations with the client or family or with other individuals in the client's behalf.

In all but the most luxurious programs, progress notes are handwritten or typed by the staff member providing the service. Special forms should be prepared for these notes, usually consisting of sheets of lined paper with space for client identification on each sheet.

In smaller centralized programs, it may be possible for the speech-language pathologist or audiologist to have the complete client case record at hand at each visit. In larger programs, or in programs where the clinician provides services in different locations (e.g., clinicians serving several schools or nursing homes or those providing home care), progress notes may be kept separately and, at intervals, filed in the case record. This situation has inherent hazards, as do all situations when at any particular time a complete record is not available at one location. So long as the availability and location of progress notes is understood, however, the hazards need not be serious.

TEST RESULTS

The policies of programs differ, but it is usually advisable to incorporate completed test forms in the client case record. When the test forms are voluminous, only the summary sheet may be included. At least two purposes may be served by incorporating test forms. First, when all raw data are included in the record, it may be unnecessary to reiterate these data in evaluation summaries. Second, clinicians may wish to refer later to data that might not be included in the summary. A detail that may seem insignificant on the initial evaluation may become important in the future.

Transcripts of spontaneous language samples are increasingly employed in the evaluation of children with communicative disorders. Such transcripts should always be filed in their entirety rather than merely entering summaries of conclusions drawn from those transcripts. Once again, a future clinician may be interested in some pattern considered insignificant by the examiner. Furthermore, as new approaches to the analysis of transcripts are proposed, future clinicians may wish to reanalyze previous transcripts.

In urging entry of entire test forms and transcripts, we may seem to violate our previous urging of economy in client records. Although these materials may require additional space, there may be substantial time savings when all data need not be transferred. Furthermore, the practice may preclude the repetition of certain tests in the future and otherwise facilitate efficient re-evaluations.

AUTHORIZATIONS AND CORRESPONDENCE

The final section of this single-discipline service adaptation of the unit record system resembles the authorization and correspondence section of any unit record. If more than five or six documents are filed in this section, it should be preceded by a list or log of entries. That list is divided into three sections: authorizations, consent forms, and correspondence. The authorization listing should show the name of the agency providing the authorization, the service or services authorized, the date of issuance of authorization, and the date of its expiration (again, these data are usually also entered in the service accounting record). The consent form list shows the precise purpose of the consent (to have a report sent to a particular agency, to be photographed in connection with a news release, to participate in a particular research project, etc.) and the date on which the consent was given. The correspondence list records letters and reports received, noting the writer and, when appropriate, the agency represented (usually noting whether the correspondence represents a report or a request for information). The correspondence list also records letters sent by the program. Following this index list, the actual documents are filed in date order within each of the three subsections.

The Problem-oriented Record

Concepts underlying problem-oriented records evolved, at least to some extent, from dissatisfactions with systems typified by unit records. As we have already noted, unit records can easily become diffuse, unfocused, and piecemeal. Although ostensibly the subject of the record is the crux of the system, the record may become a collection of unrelated or ill related fragments. In the final analysis there is no single guiding principle underlying the unit record design beyond the obvious one that all information about the same individual should be kept together. Problem-oriented records, on the other hand, attempt to classify and focus information in such a way that quality care is expedited.

Weed (1970), the original proponent of the problem-oriented system, suggested that clinical case records should be based on a scientific problem-solving process and that basic to this process was the clear and concise identification of problems. Weed (1972, pp. 51–52) elaborated the system's goals as follows:

1. The implementation of total care for the individual by more effectively organizing the combined efforts of multiple physicians, nurses, and other medical personnel (the all-knowing, ever-present, totally competent single physician never existed for an individual patient and no program can be designed to create one).
2. The conversion of the physician from a memory machine and oracle to one of the principal components of a guidance system in medicine.
3. The establishment of a set of rules for medical practice—rules that would:
   a) make possible corrective feedback loops on medical action.
   b) make fair and meaningful audit possible.
   c) make available to all patients for all problems one of the most powerful diagnostic tools—the effective use of time in the analysis of multiple changing and interacting variables.
   d) make the goals of medical care sufficiently well-defined and clear to students so that their development will be molded by the needs of patients and not by the parochial interests of specialized teachers.

In the problem-oriented system, the client case record is divided into four major sections: The *data base*, the *problem list*, the *initial plan*, and the *progress notes*. These four elements emerge from Weed's definition of "four phases of medical activity: 1. Establishment of data base; 2. Formulation of a list of all problems; 3. The initial plans for each problem; 4. Progress notes on each problem."

DATA BASE

The data base is a compilation of information about an individual recorded at the point of admission for service. It consists of six basic elements.

First, the *chief complaint* presents a concise statement of the reason the client is seeking care; preferably the statement is in the client's own words.

Second is the *client profile*. This element presents general information about the client's personal characteristics; the life style, including diet, work habits, and recreation; family relationships; and housing and work environment.

The third element relates to *present illness or illnesses,* which may fall into two categories. In some instances the illness is undiagnosed and is merely noted in terms of descriptions of the symptoms. In other instances, the illness may have been diagnosed previously and the individual is now seeking further care. In either instance, the illness is presented in terms of *symptomatic* information, i.e., *subjective* details observed by the individual or by the examiner, and *objective* information which is available from previous studies conducted in connection with the illness. Weed insists that these two types of information be "recorded separately and not interwoven in a single chronological sequence." As will be seen later, the clear distinction between subjective and objective information is an important characteristic of the problem-oriented system.

Fourth is the *past history* and *systems review*. Each aspect of the history and review is considered according to current function (what is the current level of function of the particular system?), past function (what problems previously existed, related to that system, which have disappeared?), and future function (what possible future risks may be present with respect to that system, e.g., with respect to work, dietary and other habits, problems in one system which may ultimately affect others, etc?). Weed recommends that the past history and system review be presented in the following order: social profile; family history, infections, diseases, immunizations; eye, ear, nose and throat; dermatology-allergy; dental; gastrointestinal; respiratory, cardiovascular, musculoskeletal, endocrine; breast; genitourinary; neurologic; and psychiatric.

Fifth are the results of the *physical examination*. The format is essentially similar to all standard physical examination protocols, except that completeness is particularly emphasized. A notable difference is apparent in the insistence that merely noting that a particular system is "normal" is of little value unless the procedure used for reaching this conclusion is specified. (This observation is of particular interest to specialists in communicative disorders because physical examination reports commonly note normal speech or hearing with no indication of the procedures employed to determine normalcy.)

The sixth element comprises *baseline laboratory examinations*. Within the data base are included only those results that are routinely obtained on any individual of the same age and sex, regardless of the presenting complaints. Those studies pursued to describe particular problems are reported in a later section of the record.

Institutions employing problem-oriented records vary in their practice relative to updating the data base. In some instances, the data base remains as compiled on first admission. Changes in and additions to those data are recorded as progress notes. In other instances, the data base may be amended or a new data base may be compiled on specified occasions, as, for example, when a client is readmitted for services following a period of inactivity.

PROBLEM LIST

Since the underlying philosophy of the problem-oriented record is that scientific methodology of client care depends upon clear definition of problems, the problem list is the heart of the record. Weed describes this list as a "table of contents and index combined." In most problem-oriented records, this list is placed at the beginning of the record.

Problems are defined very simply as anything that concerns the client and/or the examiner. For example, the client may be exclusively concerned about low energy. The examiner may be concerned about the client's obesity. Even though the same concerns are not shared, both would be entered in the problem list.

Weed proposes a four-part classification of problems according to "field of interest." Although that classification may be functional in a hospital, it may seem simplistic to clinicians concerned with the more complex aspects of human behavior, such as communication. The classification comprises: *medical problems*, which may consist of a diagnosis, a symptom or a physical finding (e.g., shortness of breath, high blood pressure, hearing loss), or an abnormal laboratory finding (e.g., abnormal electroencephalogram, high urine protein level); *social problems*, such as family discord, economic problems, or loneliness; *demographic problems*, such as occupational health hazards and unsanitary or unsafe living conditions; and *psychiatric problems*, which may be stated in conventional psychiatric diagnoses or in lay descriptive terminology.

Problems are further classified into *active problems*, i.e., problems that are present at the time services are provided, and *inactive problems*, or problems that are no longer present but may be important to understanding the current problems. For example, although a child may now be essentially healthy, "failure to thrive" in infancy may be an important inactive problem in terms of understanding such current problems as hyperactivity, poor fine motor coordination, and dysarthria. Or if an individual had a single Ménière's attack 2 years previously, it remains a significant inactive problem because of the possibility of recurrence.

A typical format for problem lists is shown in Figure 6.1. Column 1 is the date on which the patient is seen. Problem lists always identify each problem by number (column 2). Next, each current or active problem is identified. The fourth column notes either the date of onset or, depending on the policies of the particular program, the date of identification of the problem. (With many of the problems encountered by speech-language pathologists or audiologists, e.g., delayed language acquisition or prelingual hearing loss of unknown etiology, the date of problem recognition is obviously the important identifier.) The fifth column lists the date of problem resolution. The sixth column lists significant past or inactive problems; these problems are interspersed in the same sequence as the active problems, according to the date of onset or date of recognition.

A fundamental concept in the problem-oriented system is that the problem list should not be restricted to established diagnoses. All major expressed concerns of the client and of the participating clinicians should be entered. When further investigation shows no factual basis for the expressed concerns, the problem is noted as resolved. Entries in the problem list may be redefined at any time as additional information emerges.

In some medical centers that ostensibly use this system, only physicians are permitted to make entries in the problem list. In these instances, the problem list can become indistinguishable from the front sheet of a unit record, particularly since physicians are noted for their selective listening to patient complaints. Occasionally, institutions require problems to be entered according to one of the standard diagnostic codes. Such practices are fundamentally inconsistent with the philosophy underlying problem-oriented records and are insupportable.

INITIAL PLAN

The next step is the development of plans for the amelioration of each active problem found on the problem list. These plans are keyed to the problem list using the problem number. Plans may call for one or more of the following: (1) procedures to obtain further information (e.g., medical diagnostic studies; further testing; interviews with family, school personnel, or other individuals with information about the client); (2) treatment (medical treatment, surgery, therapy, etc.); (3) counseling and education (which may solve the problem, prevent the problem from becoming more serious, or help the client live more successfully despite an insoluble problem).

To illustrate, the following note might appear in the initial plan section of a problem-oriented medical record for a 10-year-old following the initial visit to a pediatric clinic.

Problem 1	*Hoarse voice*
Diagnostic	Obtain ENT consult
	Obtain speech-language pathology consult
Therapeutic	Prescribed antihistamine
Patient education	Explained to patient and parents that hoarseness may result from several factors and that consultations by ENT and speech-language are necessary. Explained that antihistamine may provide symptomatic relief and aid in establishing diagnosis.

The initial plan section is used only to cover the plans formulated immediately following the definition of a problem. Subsequent information about further evaluation, therapy, or client education procedures is entered as progress notes. It is, nevertheless, essential in the problem-oriented system that each entry in the problem list be supported by an entry in the initial plan section.

PATIENT NAME ______________________________

PATIENT I.D. No. ______________________________

PATIENT PROBLEM INDEX

List all potential, current, or significant past problems that affect the patient. Include date of onset or identification and the date of resolution for each problem.

Page ______

DATE	PROB. NO.	PROBLEMS POTENTIAL/CURRENT–ACTIVE	DATE OF ONSET	DATE RESOLVED	PROBLEMS SIGNIFICANT PAST–INACTIVE

FORM 21-PPI DHHA/CHS CONTINUE ON OTHER SIDE

Figure 6.1. Form for problem list in problem-oriented record prepared by Council of Home Health Agencies and Community Health Services of the National League for Nursing. (Reproduced by permission of National League for Nursing.)

PROGRESS NOTES

In problem-oriented records, progress notes are also keyed to the problem list, by problem number and name. These notes may be of two types: *narrative notes* and *flow sheets*. The form for narrative notes is identified by the acronym SOAP, covering each of the four facets of these notes: (S) *Subjective data* include the client's reports of symptoms, usually best stated as direct quotations, and subjective observations by the clinician. (O) *Objective data* include specific clinical findings, test results, and laboratory findings. (A) *Assessment* involves reconciliation of the subjective and objective data. (When disparities exist, it may be necessary to redefine the problem, to explore subjective impressions in greater detail, or to repeat or supplement the procedures used for the objective evaluation.) According to Weed (1972), "Herein lies the feedback loop, without which the medical record as a system runs wild." (P) *Plan* delineates the course of action to be followed, which may simply involve continued pursuit of the initial plan or may involve modification or reorientation of that plan. (Again, the plan is recorded according to the three-part breakdown of evaluation, treatment, and client counseling and education.)

Figure 6.2 reproduces a typical narrative progress note section form. The fabricated narrative covers the visit to a speech and hearing clinic of an 8-year-old with a coincident conductive hearing impairment and articulation problem.

Flow sheets are used to record those aspects of client progress that are easily summarized by recording measurements (e.g., the blood pressure of an individual being treated for obesity) or by recording aspects of progress that lend themselves to some kind of scaling. Flow sheets are usually designed so that problems are listed in a column at the left, followed by a series of columns with dates of services heading each column. The value or code number which indicates the status of the problem is then noted for each problem on each date that service is provided.

Flow sheets can be helpful in recording progress with reference to physiologic problems that lend themselves to some sort of objective measurement. It is difficult to conceive, however, of widespread applications in the treatment of the complex problems confronted by speech-language pathologists and audiologists. Occasionally, rehabilitation centers using problem-oriented records become overly enthusiastic in developing flow charts for recording responses to rehabilitation services. In these instances, speech-language pathologists may be urged to develop scales to indicate communicative competence. Inevitably, these scales must be so arbitrary that they defy any semblance of objectivity. Furthermore, from a practical standpoint, the broad categories of these scales obscure modest but significant gains in communication. As a consequence, clients who are showing steady progress may appear to be at a standstill on the flow chart. Speech-language pathologists may be well advised, therefore, to resist integration of their progress reporting into a flow chart format. Although they may seem uncooperative, they are probably serving the client's best interests.

Some problem-oriented record systems call for another type of progress note: the discharge or interim summary. Discharge summaries are recorded when a client leaves an inpatient or residential facility or when a particular course of outpatient care is discontinued. Interim summaries may be recorded any time, although program policies may call for their completion at regular intervals (monthly, every 6 weeks, every 3 months, etc.). These summaries may be prepared separately by each individual serving a client, or they may be composite summaries prepared cooperatively by all of the individuals participating in the client's care.

Discharge and interim summaries should list all problems noted as active at the beginning of the interval being summa-

PATIENT NAME OLSON, Gary

PATIENT I.D. No. 82-4379

NARRATIVE/ PROGRESS NOTES

Begin entries pertaining to subjective findings (S), objective findings (O), assessment (A), and plans (P) in the column appropriately headed and write through remaining columns to the right margin. The signature and title of the recorder must appear after each entry.

Page ______

DATE	PROBLEM NO.	NARRATIVE/PROGRESS S O A P
5/27/83	1	Conductive Hearing Loss
		S Gary seemed more responsive today. At no time did he misunderstand directions or ask for them to be repeated.
		O Audiometric check showed A.C. thresholds of 20-25 dB bilaterally at 250-2000 Hz as compared with 35-45 dB one month ago. SRTs consistent with puretone thresholds
		A Gary's hearing seems to be improving under current treatment regimen
		P Report audiometric findings to Gary's physician. Urge family to return to physician as recommended. Repeat audio in one month
5/27/83	2	Misarticulation of /r/.
		S. There was little change in the /r/ productions in Gary's conversational speech.
		O Acceptable /r/ productions achieved by imitation of words beginning with /dr/ and /tr/. Inconsistent acceptable productions by imitation of CVC words with /r/ in initial position. Accurate /r/ productions in spontaneous naming of 16 of 20 pictures of words beginning with /tr/ and 5 of 20 pictures of CVCs with initial /r/.
		A Although some progress is apparent in structured speech activities, no carry-over as yet achieved
		P Continue with current therapy plan.

FORM 21-NPN DHHA/CHS CONTINUE ON OTHER SIDE

Figure 6.2. Form for narrative progress notes in problem-oriented record prepared by Council of Home Health Agencies and Community Health Services of the National League for Nursing, with hypothetical entries regarding a child with coincident conductive hearing impairment and articulation problems. (Reproduced by permission of National League for Nursing.)

rized. Current information about each of these problems is then summarized, usually in the SOAP format.

Problem-oriented records are widely used in a variety of settings. They were originally proposed for use in institutions providing acute medical care, but the system may have achieved greater popularity in more specialized programs, such as rehabilitation and psychiatric facilities and home health programs. This situation may relate to the greater willingness of these programs to be innovative. Furthermore, these programs may be more aware of all of a client's problems since they are less focused on the treatment of specific symptoms and disease entities.

Several discussions of adapting problem-oriented records for specific settings have been published, among them: Bjorn and Cross (1970) described adaptation for use by a physician in private practice; Corbus (1977) discussed adaptations for long-term care facilities; Dinsdale (1970) discussed adaptations for rehabilitation facilities; and Gilandes (1972), Grant and Maletsky (1972), and Hays-Roth (1972) have presented modifications for use in psychiatric facilities. We have already cited the publication of the National League for Nursing (1974) which focused on the use of problem-oriented records in home care programs.

The most frequently quoted critical evaluation of the problem-oriented system was written by Feinstein (1973). He conceded that Weed and other proponents of problem-oriented records have achieved "admirable success in calling attention to multiple deficits in contemporary medical care, education and records" and have, therefore, achieved "many salubrious effects." He contended, however, that several purported advantages of this system are illusory and not necessarily more characteristic of problem-oriented records than of more traditional records. He asserted that such objectives as continuity and quality of health care, ongoing patient care audit, and integration of professional personnel can be served equally well by "old style" records systems when well used.

Feinstein described deficits that are merely perpetuated by the problem-oriented system, including the "fragmentation of a patient into different specialty zones" (hence losing attention to the "entire patient") and the absence of any editing process in the preparation of the data base (so that the data base becomes "hypertrophied" and burdened with unnecessary, extraneous, or even misleading information). He further asserted that problem-oriented systems contribute some new difficulties to clinical records because of the inherent redundancy in recording data (i.e., all data must be related to specific problems; hence the same data may be reiterated in support of several different problems); because of the unstandardized taxonomy of "problems"; and because students may not be educated in the "subtleties of scientific clinical skills" when, instead, we teach the "library technology used for cataloging data, indexing problems, and automating the processes of storage and retrieval."

Many of the deficits cited by Feinstein obtain specifically in traditional medical care settings. Since his point of view is likely shared by many physicians, this may further explain the greater popularity of problem-oriented records in less traditional and more specialized health care delivery programs.

Adapting the Problem-oriented Records System for a Speech-Language-Hearing Services Program

Once again, although conceived as a system for multidisciplinary services programs, problem-oriented records can be adapted for use in speech, language, and hearing services. This application has been discussed by Bouchard and Shane (1977) and by Kent (1980).

DATA BASE

The preparation of a consistent data base for all clients is important even in single-discipline programs. The initial evaluation reports prepared on clients with speech, language, and hearing problems may focus so specifically on presenting complaints that important information is neglected. Later reviews of these records may reveal that essential factors have been overlooked. Did a child who was seen because of problems in language acquisition have normal hearing? Did a child with a hearing loss show distortions in speech? Did an adult with a voice problem characterized by frequent pitch breaks show any evidence of dysarthria? Such vital questions may be unanswerable when the examining clinician recorded only that information which elaborated the presenting complaint.

The data base recorded for exclusive use in a speech-language pathology and audiology program need not be voluminous. It should discretely consider the factors that may be helpful in understanding the client's communicative disorders and in determining what services are needed and how those services can be best provided. Weed's six categories of data base information can be used.

The *chief complaint* is recorded as stated by the client and family, specifying as clearly as possible the reasons for seeking care. It is important to note instances in which the client and the family have different complaints (e.g., a wife is concerned about her husband's hearing, but he denies any problem; a child's hoarse voice is disturbing to the family but regarded as no problem by the child; an adolescent boy may be distressed about his high-pitched voice, while his mother finds it to her liking). It is also important to note instances where neither client nor family are concerned but are merely following through on a referral.

A *client profile* prepared in the problem-oriented format can also be helpful. Included here is the information that will reveal the client's social, educational, vocational, and cultural milieu. Such factors are essential to assessing the impact of communicative disorders.

The statement of *present communicative disorder or disorders* capsulizes the client and family description of symptoms and previously established diagnoses. For example, the following note might be recorded about Greg, a 5-year-old seen because of a possible hearing loss:

> Greg's mother reports that she has been concerned on several occasions during the past 3 years about his inconsistent responses. His kindergarten teacher also reports that he has trouble hearing in school "sometimes." His pediatrician has treated him for frequent bouts of otitis media, particularly during the past 2 years. Last month the pediatrician referred Greg to an otolaryngologist, who diagnosed recurrent nonsuppurative otitis media and recommended a hearing evaluation with subsequent consideration of myringotomy and placement of ventilating tubes.

The next section of the data base is the *past history*. It is always difficult to determine the ideal contents of a case history, but the following factors should be considered:

1. *Factors relating to the onset of the communicative disorder.* Although the precise etiology of a communicative disorder—when such can be determined—may have little significance in planning therapy, these factors do merit attention. The speech-language or hearing evaluation may be part of a complete diagnostic work-up, hence the speech-language pathologist or audiologist may contribute to the definition of diagnoses. In other instances, identification of the etiology of the communicative disorder may determine whether further evaluation or treatment should precede the institution of a therapy program. Understanding the etiology may also be important to formulating a prognosis. Clients and their families frequently assign major importance to identifying the causes of communicative disorders; consequently this question must often be dealt with before they can devote their efforts to finding solutions.
2. *Associated disorders.* Even in records designed to serve speech, language, and hearing programs exclusively, the case history must also incorporate commonly associated disorders. Several examples come into mind: the motor coordination and perceptual deficits of children whose neurodevelopmental disorders include delayed language acquisition; the tinnitus and vertigo that accompany the hearing loss of clients with Ménière's disease; and the dysphagia which is often coincident with the speech disorders of clients who have undergone surgery for head and neck tumors. These disorders may be highly relevant

in planning therapy for communicative disorders.

3. *Previous evaluations and treatment.* A detailed summary of all previous evaluations and treatment experiences is extremely important. Such a summary may offer clues about the essential nature of the communicative disorder, serve as a basis for predicting the outcome of further treatment, and be a key to understanding the attitudes of the client and family. For example, this section of the history of a client with spastic dysphonia might reveal that he has at various times been evaluated by five different otolaryngologists, received detailed neurologic evaluations on three different occasions, completed 2 years of twice-weekly psychotherapy, and been enrolled in speech therapy on three different occasions for periods ranging from 3 to 18 months, all with no perceptible changes in vocal production. From these data one can surmise that further evaluations are not likely to offer much new information, that the spastic dysphonia is not likely to respond to either further psychotherapy or to further speech therapy, and that the client has every reason to be skeptical about what professionals can offer. Clearly these are important considerations when one is contemplating what is to be recommended following an evaluation.
4. *Social and economic factors.* Recommendations which cannot be implemented because of social and economic constraints are of little value. It is necessary, therefore, to detail the background against which all recommendations must be set. Examples abound. Clinicians sometimes recommend to parents who speak only Spanish that a child with problems in language acquisition be exposed only to English. They may recommend purchase of hearing aids to oldsters on bare subsistence incomes. They may recommend intensive daily speech therapy to children living in communities with no possible resources for such a program. Although speech-language pathologists and audiologists are not sociologists, unless they are sensitive to social and economic factors they are not likely to be particularly effective in their areas of expertise.

In designing a case history format for a problem-oriented record, it is important to recognize its different focus from conventional case histories. Conventional histories tend to be "fishing expeditions," covering such areas as developmental history, medical history, school and vocational history, social history, family history, etc. The problem-oriented record history, on the other hand, highlights the specific areas that are most likely to contribute to the understanding of identified problems and explores those areas in many ways that can be applied in planning solutions.

In the data base of problem-oriented records designed especially for speech, language, and hearing services, it is probably unnecessary to divide initial examinations and baseline laboratory data. A single section, *initial evaluation*, should suffice. This section should include all test results and observations which led to the formulation of the initial plan. This does not necessarily imply that the total evaluation has been completed, since further evaluation may be the most important feature of the initial plan. One important advantage of the problem-oriented approach is that it defies the myth that the total evaluation must be completed and a "diagnosis" formulated before any intervention can begin. All that is required at the outset is enough information to formulate reasonable plans. The best evaluations of clients' communicative disorders may derive from efforts to help them overcome these disorders. The results of these further observations are entered as progress notes. Remember that subjective observations, objective data, assessment, and plans (SOAP) are included in each progress note. Therefore, each progress note records a current evaluation.

PROBLEM LIST

As in any problem-oriented record problem list, this list should contain the communication-related problems identified by the client and his family, together with the problems identified by the professionals serving the client. Furthermore, these problems should be specified as clearly as possible. For example, for a particular client with a voice problem, it is inadequate simply to enter "hoarseness" on the problem list. Such related problems as vocal fatigue, discomfort, and inability to project the voice in noisy environments should also be specified. Although all of these problems may relate to hoarseness, each may require specific intervention. Or in the instance of a hearing-impaired adult, it is not enough to list "moderate sensorineural hearing loss." Such related problems as impaired job performance, withdrawal from social contacts, and previous unsuccessful hearing aid use should also be noted. Once again, each of these problems will require special attention in planning the client's care.

The required specific documentation of each problem, even though problems are interrelated, may be one of the greatest assets of problem-oriented records. The danger exists in all clinical services programs that the problems a client finds most troublesome may be completely ignored when clinicians identify the problems they consider most important and concentrate on solutions to those problems. Worse yet are situations in which exclusive attention is focused on problems specified by a referring physician, teacher, or other professional.

It may be difficult to define the scope of problems to appear on the list prepared for use in a speech, language, and hearing services program. Should "hyperactivity" be entered as a problem when it characterizes a child with delayed language acquisition? Should "reading problem" appear on the problem list of a child with an articulation disorder? Should "poor dental hygiene" appear on the problem list of an adult with cleft palate who is using a speech appliance? Should "seizure disorder" appear on the problem list of an adult with post-traumatic aphasia? In each instance the answer is probably "yes" because the specified problems may have implications for planning and carrying out speech-language therapy programs. Furthermore, a speech-language pathologist may be the only specialist in regular contact with these patients. The notation of the problem list will remind the clinician to inquire regularly as to whether other measures are underway to alleviate these problems.

INITIAL PLANS

In a problem-oriented record each entry on the problem list must be reflected in a corresponding initial plan. In the instance of a record serving a speech, language, and hearing program, each initial plan would specify recommended further evaluations (including speech, language, and hearing evaluations as well as evaluations by other specialists), the therapy recommended, and any needed client and family counseling.

For example, the following initial plan statements might be entered in the record of 4-year-old:

Problem 1	*Delayed Language Acquisition*
Diagnostic	Continue observation to assess level of language performance. Refer to psychologist for developmental evaluation.
Therapeutic	Enroll in preschool language therapy program.
Family counseling/ education	Discuss current levels of language performance with family and suggest appropriate language stimulation strategies. Recommend participation in parent group of preschool language therapy program.
Problem 2	*Possible Mild Hearing Loss*
Diagnostic	Repeat hearing evaluations and impedance studies. Confer with pediatrician about ENT referral.
Therapeutic	None at present.
Family counseling/ education	Suggest approaches to observing responses to sound. Counsel regarding importance of obtaining further medical evaluations.
Problem 3	*Hyperactivity*
Diagnostic	Observe pattern of hyperactivity in preschool language program to determine consistency, precipitating factors, etc.
Therapeutic	Confer with pediatrician about trial of psychotropic medication. Pursue behavior modification program in the preschool language program directed at improving attention.
Family counseling/ education	Discuss with family approaches to managing the hyperactivity. Encourage continuing discussion of management in the parent group.

PROGRESS NOTES

The problem-oriented format is also useful in recording progress notes in speech, language, and hearing programs. The distinction between subjective observations and objective data may be particularly useful. Another advantage may lie in the required formulation of plans for next steps in the execution of each progress note. The following progress notes, written on a 70-year-old post-cerebrovascular accident client illustrate the format.

These illustrations of problem-oriented progress notes violate my earlier dictum about brevity. In part, this relates to making hypothetical notes comprehensible outside of the context of a complete record. Nevertheless, progress notes in this format must almost inevitably exceed the single paragraph limit specified earlier. It is important to remember, however, that in this system re-evaluation reports are integrated into progress notes. Therefore, summaries of re-evaluations may be unnecessary.

Problem 1 — *Word Retrieval Problems*

S: In informal conversation, Mr. Minelli seemed to be more fluent. Although his speech remains hesitant, with frequent instances of inability to retrieve appropriate words (usually he substitutes "You know"), his overall performance seems to be improving. Mrs. Minelli also notes improvement and insists that he is improving rapidly.

O: During today's session, Mr. Minelli named pictures of common household objects and pictures of woodworking tools with approximately 80% accuracy. He was able to recall correctly the first names of his four children and the names of seven of his nine grandchildren. Approximately half of the time he self-corrected initially incorrect responses. All errors were in-class errors. Although delays occurred with more than half of the correct responses, no delay exceeded 10 seconds.

A: Some disparities are evident between Mr. Minelli's performance in spontaneous conversation and on picture-naming tasks, where he has substantially less difficulty. Nevertheless, in comparison with his performance of 3 months ago, he shows substantial improvement in both spontaneous and structured responses. Mrs. Minelli, however, is overly optimistic in her evaluation of his rate of recovery.

P: Continue with similar therapy activities. Since playing cards was once a favorite recreational activity, begin with work on terms needed. Schedule session with Mrs. Minelli to review progress and prognosis. Repeat Porch Index of Communicative Abilities during next 2 weeks.

Problem 2 — *Language Comprehension Deficits*

S: Comprehension seems to be improving. Noted no inappropriate responses in therapy that seemed to result from failure to comprehend. He seems to have greater difficulty in following what his wife is saying, but she insists he understands everything.

O: Identified all named pictures with 100% accuracy. Made only one error in identification when use of pictured object was described; however, in this activity delays of 5 to 10 seconds were frequent.

A: The language comprehension deficits observed on initial evaluation seem to be subsiding. Some problems continue in his attempts to follow rapid conversation. He also shows some processing delays.

P: It does not seem likely that further structured work on language comprehension activities is indicated. Will begin discussions of processing delays and suggest ways in which he can make situations easier for himself. I will also counsel Mrs. Minelli about how she can make things easier for him.

Problem 3 — *Writing Deficits*

S: Still unable to hold pencil in right hand. Can print letters with left hand, but result is extremely crude.

O: No perceptible improvement in right hand use during last 4 months. Required 3 to 4 minutes to print barely legible name with left hand. Accurately spelled names of carpenter tools with movable letters.

A: Level of motor control probably precludes right-handed writing. Functional left-handed writing seems unlikely. Nevertheless, spelling proficiency does not seem to be severely impaired.

P: Work toward usable left-handed signature. No further work on writing seems important for the present. No further work on spelling is indicated.

Shortcuts are possible for recording notes on clients in continuing therapy programs. For example, it is quite feasible to refer to previous notes rather than reiterating information. Furthermore, complete progress notes need not be written at each visit. It may be sufficient simply to note that the client was seen for speech therapy on each date and to enter progress notes summarizing several visits at appropriate intervals.

To reiterate a previous statement, problem-oriented records emerge from a well defined philosophy that must be accepted if the system is to be adopted. Nevertheless, the system can tolerate many adaptations to serve the operational purposes of a particular program.

The Practice-oriented Record

The practice-oriented system is included in this discussion because it is the most fully realized of the systems that assume newer information technology. As presented by Lang and Dickie (1978), the system is designed strictly for use in medical care programs and, apparently, in programs using traditional single-physician-directed service models. Despite the traditionalism of the service model, however, the system is quite advanced in conception.

The basic philosophy of the practice-oriented system is that the record is not simply a medium for information storage. Rather, it is a communicative device and, as such, it should be developed from the basis of communications theory. Lang and Dickie (p. 33) elaborate this view:

> The basic function of the medical record is to communicate. This is true whether the data to be transmitted are stored on paper pages, or generated by a computer-assisted system on hard copy or appears on a volatile CRT system display. To serve this function well, the medical record must have two inherent characteristics: the ability to store an unabridged set of pertinent patient data and the ability readily to display these data in a form which can be quickly assimilated and acted upon.

The realization of these "inherent characteristics" requires that practice-oriented records be implemented through computer technology. Only a computer-assisted system can afford the immediate display of the essential and absolutely current information which this approach requires.

As described by Lang and Dickie, practice-oriented records are implemented through the Clinical Care Management System (CCMS). This system distinguishes between "archival data" and "operational management data." As they define it, archival data consist of the total body of information accumulated about the subject of the record. Operational management data, on the other hand, consist of only those data that are essential to planning and delivering the particular care that is immediately relevant.

The differences between these types of data can be illustrated with this example. Mr. Evans, age 73, became aphasic as the result of a cerebrovascular accident that occurred during hip replacement surgery 4 years ago. He has just been hospitalized on an emergency basis because of acute chest pain. While the archival information about the earlier surgery, its complications, and his aphasia are important, they are probably unrelated to his current symptoms. Consequently, while some reference would be made to the archival information in the record covering his hospitalization, the major emphasis would be assigned to the operational management data, i.e., the data related to the present condition, which will determine the course of immediate treatment.

This approach to data grows out of the authors' view that "the informational content does not have consistent value." A system, therefore, that affords easy and discrete access to immediately relevant information represents a significant step in clinical records technology.

Another of the authors' concepts is that "the informational value of data is variable and its worth is determined by the recipient." Individuals reviewing the same data may place different values on them. Information highly prized by one individual may be insignificant to others. This concept leads to the recognition that the operational management data may differ, depending upon which aspect of management is under consideration. Hence, in multidisciplinary settings, an ideal system would make immediately available different management data to different specialists yet still provide archival data and the total body of management data when needed. Such capacity is easily afforded by the CCMS.

The archival data essentially represents the data base of the record. In the practice-oriented approach the data base resembles the problem-oriented data base. It consists of three main categories: the *history section*, the *physical section*, and the *laboratory section*. The history section contains data about present and past illnesses; about the individual's family; about the occupational, social-cultural, and environmental background; and any other information that may be important to understanding the patient's problems. The physical section includes all data acquired from a complete physical examination. The laboratory section includes data yielded by all routine laboratory studies as well as those studies ordered to elucidate the particular problems the individual presents.

The system's uniqueness is evident in the storage of operational data through client profiles (called RECORDGRAMS in the CCMS). These profiles represent distillations of the information that is essential to current client management. The profiles may be generated on a regular basis (daily in acute hospitals; weekly, biweekly, or monthly in a long-term care facility) or irregularly, as needed (in conjunction with an outpatient visit or when some significant change occurs during the course of a rehabilitation program).

Client profiles are organized into six sections. The first section is the *client identifier* which contains the usual identifying information. Next is the *highlight section* that offers a therapy overview statement, that is, a brief summary of the objectives to be realized from the care provided (e.g., "long-term control for hypertension," "diagnosis and treatment of hearing loss," "increased independence in activities of daily living"). This is followed by the *problem listing section* which contains two types of listings: the established diagnoses (Dx list) and the functional problems (Fx list). Functional problems consist of those physical complaints for which no diagnosis has as yet been established, together with other problems that may be important in planning care (e.g., disorientation, apprehensiveness, limitations of language comprehension). Next is the *client services section* which contains summaries of the results of diagnostic studies, including abnormal laboratory findings and the findings of radiologic studies and function tests. Following this is the *physician order summary* which records the date, order number, service designation, and specific identification of each physician order. To illustrate, the following might appear in the physician order summary for a child with chronic otitis media:

Date	*#/S*	*SVC*	*Order*
800324	001	LB	CBC
800324	002	RD	Mastoid films
800324	003	AS	Hearing evaluation

On March 24, 1980, the physician recorded three orders: a complete blood count from the lab, mastoid films from radiology, and a hearing evaluation from audiology and speech pathology.

At the end of the patient profile is a *notes section*. Here are entered additions to and revisions of the profile. Some items that no longer obtain may be deleted (e.g., when a particular course of treatment is concluded, it will be deleted from the orders section), other entries will be revised (e.g., when a diagnosis is established, the functional problem may be deleted and the diagnosis inserted; for instance, if the diagnosis of Ménière's disease were established, that diagnosis would be entered and the functional problem, "vertigo," would be deleted). The results of all studies completed since the last profile was generated would also be entered. Finally, new orders would be added. All information in the notes section is subsequently entered into the computer so that the next profile to be generated will reflect these additions and deletions.

The virtues of such systems as CCMS are abundant. In providing care to a client, one has available at all times a completely current summary of his or her situation. This summary includes all currently relevant data, even though those data were recorded at a time long past. Past data which are not immediately relevant, however, have been deleted so that all information is current at the date the profile is generated. This is in notable contrast to other records systems, which often necessitate review of extensive notes to determine what is relevant currently.

In the CCMS system, if a review of the entire program of care that has been provided to a client is required, all previous profiles are available. Furthermore, when a specific program is completed, the relevant information may be added to the data base and become a part of the archival data.

As described by Lang and Dickie, the practice-oriented approach is primarily intended to record data covering hospitalization for acute care or covering outpatient care provided in a physician's office or a medical clinic. The system assumes a single case manager who reviews all incoming data and determines which data are to be entered into the data base and client profile. The prototype practice-oriented record is described as divided into three sections in a three-compartment folder. The left compartment is a plastic envelope in which incoming laboratory reports are filed. The middle compartment contains handwritten narrative notes entered by the various professionals participating in the client's care. The right compartment contains the computer-generated data base and the patient profiles (with the case manager's hand-written notes at the bottom of each profile).

As proposed, the practice-oriented system probably suffers from its assignment of omnipotence to a single case manager. When complex problems are present, no single individual can possibly be expert enough to judge the ultimate value of all data. These problems relate, however, to an application of the system and are not necessarily indigenous to the system. So long as they are trained in the system and willing to use a common language, there is no reason why different individuals could not add notes to client profiles which would then appear in the next generated profile. It would also be completely feasible to record separate client profiles for the use of each discipline (for example, in a rehabilitation center, each specialist in speech-language pathology, physical therapy, occupational therapy, and rehabilitation nursing might maintain a separate profile). At any time, however, a composite profile could be generated which would permit a complete overview of the client's situation.

Considerable adaptation of the practice-oriented system would be required for application to a freestanding speech, language, and hearing services program. Nevertheless, some features of the system could be applied. A computer-stored data base which could be updated at intervals would certainly be useful. Similarly, easily generated current profiles would also be helpful. One might, for example, enter regular progress notes in the conventional fashion and at specified intervals summarize these notes on the last client profile so that an updated profile could be generated. Any clinic supervisor would revel in the capability for immediate generation of concise client profiles on each client currently receiving services. It would also be helpful to be able to generate immediately the case-closure profile of inactive clients. Computer-assisted records storage will be discussed in Chapter 7. As the best realized of the various systems assuming computer technology, the practice-oriented record system merits careful study by anyone considering the development of a computerized system.

The CASE Information System

The most fully developed records system especially designed for speech-language pathology and audiology services is the CASE information system (ASHA, 1976). CASE is an acronym for "comprehensive assessment and service evaluation." The system was formulated through the NEEDS II Project of the School Services Department of the American Speech-Language-Hearing Association. While intended to support public school speech, language, and hearing services programs, many elements of the system are directly applicable in any program that serves children. With some expansion, elements of the system could also be employed by programs serving adults.

The authors characterize the system as follows (p. 7):

> It was designed to be evaluation oriented and to provide a broad data base that can be used for planning, increasing program efficiency, documenting program and staff practices, and analyzing the degree to which services provided were appropriate and effective.

It is also described as a "prototype" system, not designed automatically to supplant existing records systems. Elements of the system can be used without adoption of the entire system. Furthermore, these elements can be adopted and modified to serve the special requirements of an individual program.

The CASE system differs from those described previously in that it is more than a system for client clinical records. It inherently distinguishes two types of data: *case level data* and *program level data.* The case level data consist of information concerning individual clients: the data required to document screening, assessment, placement, and intervention services. The program level data involve information needed to summarize the nature and scope of all client services, to implement cost analysis, and to assist in the completion of reports to interested local, state, or federal agencies. Of the records systems that have been discussed, CASE is the only one that includes the storage and retrieval of overall programmatic information as an inherent feature. Since many speech, language, and hearing services must report such data, this feature makes CASE attractive.

Unlike the practice-oriented system, CASE does not assume the availability of computer technology. On the other hand, it is designed to afford an "automation potential." All segments of the system are designed to enable efficient adaptation to a computer mode.

The CASE system is process oriented. Its authors have studied the various processes involved in the delivery of clinical services in the schools and have devised the records needed to support these seven processes: *referral/screening, parent contact, assessment, planning and placement, intervention, case coordination,* and *program management.*

REFERRAL/SCREENING

The referral process is supported by records used to alert the case coordinator and the parent or guardian that a referral for speech-language pathology and audiology services has been effected. Records covering the screening process summarize the information obtained during speech, language, and hearing screening. The *Referral/Screening Form* has five sections. The first section contains identification information—demographic data regarding the primary language of the client and family. The second specifies the reason for the referral. The third section contains screening information, noting whether the client has passed screening, requires rescreening, or requires rescreening in one or more of the "communication areas": hearing, language, articulation, voice, and fluency. The fourth area notes the disposition—the clinician notes the types of assessment indicated (hearing, language, speech, educational testing, etc.). The fifth section consists of comments.

PARENT CONTACT

The parent contact record shows the maintenance of communication with the family throughout all phases of service delivery. It notes efforts to promote family understanding and cooperation and to ensure the basic rights of all concerned parties. The *Parent Contact Record* again begins with client identification information. The remainder of this record documents all parent contacts together with the outcomes of those contacts. These contacts may include communications relative to referral, screening, assessment, and the formulation and modification of plans for intervention or for termination of services, together with consents for release of information.

ASSESSMENT

The assessment records summarize those procedures employed to determine the presence or absence of communication problems, to obtain differential diagnoses of such problems, and to develop general recommendations for management. The assessment program is supported by seven different records forms: the *General Language-Speech-Hearing Case History Form*, the *Comprehensive Language-Speech-Hearing Case History Form*, the *Audiologic Assessment Form*, the *Language and Speech Assessment Form*, the *Local Education Agency (LEA) Record of Special Services*, the *Student Summary Record*, and the *Student Summary Record Information Update*.

The *General Speech-Language-Hearing Case History Form* is designed for completion by the parent or by the client prior to assessment. It affords spaces both for narrative answers to questions and for responding "yes," "no," or "do not know." These questions relate directly to the client's communication as well as to potentially related aspects of development, health, and behavior.

The *Comprehensive Case History* is completed by the examining speech-language pathologist or audiologist on the basis of interviews with the family and client. It contains a comprehensive review of demographic and family data, the educational history, the pregnancy/birth history, the behavioral/social history, the special services history (recording other services provided in connection with communicative and related problems), and communication skills information (i.e., auditory behavior, language behavior, vocal behavior, and fluency).

The *Audiologic Assessment Form* summarizes the components of conventional audiologic evaluations. It also summarizes hearing aid test results, including rechecks of the client's aid(s) and evaluations of new aids. Another section is devoted to "special tests," e.g., tests designed to identify sites of lesion in the auditory-neural system. A final section summarizes results and recommendations.

The *Language and Speech Assessment Form* is divided into nine sections. As usual, the first section contains identifying information. The second section contains general information about the client's perceptions of the communicative disorder and about any previous intervention, together with a summary of the clinician's general impressions. The third section summarizes the results of an examination of the oral peripheral mechanism. The fourth, fifth, sixth, and seventh sections, respectively, summarize the results of the articulation assessment, the language assessment, the voice assessment, and the fluency assessment. The eighth section, labeled "additional information," includes impressions of overall intelligibility and evaluations of communication-related behaviors and motor skills. The final section contains conclusions and recommendations, including diagnostic summary statements and severity ratings together with specification of recommendations for management, which may consist of intervention and referral for evaluation by other professionals.

The *LEA Record of Special Services* allows for listing all special services provided both by the education agency and by other agencies and individual practitioners outside the school program. The *Student Summary Record* and *Student Summary Record Information Update Form* provide for a cumulative record of the client's status in the speech, language, and hearing services program. These records identify the types of disorders present, summarize the "overall functional communication status," and stipulate the client's placement and requirements for further services.

PLACEMENT

Information regarding placement is recorded on the *Language-Speech-Hearing Individual Placement Plan.* This form is designed to satisfy the requirement for an "individually written educational plan," as specified in Public Law 94-142. Placement decisions are made following completion of the initial assessment process, on the basis of the deliberations of a placement team (with the client's parents serving as members of that team). The first section, with the usual identifying information, is followed by a second section summarizing the client's current status with respect to the nature and degree of the communicative disorders and the overall communication status. The third section contains general recommendations for the individual educational plan, specifying the type of services required and the frequency with which the services should be provided. The fourth section details the placement plan, identifying the annual goals and specifying the precise schedule for providing whatever services are required. That section concludes with summary totals of the number of sessions and hours of service provided during the particular reporting period.

INTERVENTION

Four different forms are devised for recording data relative to intervention: the *Response Data Form*, the *Master Response Data Form*, the *Session Summary Data Form*, and the *End-of-Period Progress Report.* Two alternatives are provided for reporting intervention services; the selected alternative may reflect the orientation of the clinician or the nature of the service provided. When activities can be summarized in terms of stimuli used and the correctness of the elicited responses, the *Response Data Forms* are used (one records data from individual sessions; the other records compiled data from a series of sessions). The second alternative involves use of the *Session Summary Form*, which also requires documentation of levels of success (usually expressed in percent) in the achievement of specified instructional objectives, but which can be used where precise response counting is not possible. The *End-of-Period Progress Report* summarizes services provided during a specified interval (in terms of the type of service provided, the number of sessions, and the amount of "intervention time"), the need for further services at the end of the period, and ratings of the severity of the communication disorders and the functional communication status at the beginning and end of the period. It also contains narrative summaries of terminal/target behaviors, instructional objectives and criteria, and results of services provided.

CASE COORDINATION

The case coordination process strives for the delivery of efficient speech, language, and hearing services and for cooperation with the providers of whatever additional services are being rendered to the same client. This process involves the continuing review and integration of data from all forms described thus far and does not require any documents devised especially for this process.

PROGRAM MANAGEMENT

The functions involved in program management entail two different categories of reports: student information reports and cost analysis reports. The various report forms included in the first category are essentially compilations of the data found on the forms completed for individual clients. These compilations provide composite summary data regarding the total speech, language, and hearing services program, including *Screening Results, Assessment Records, Placement Report, Summary of Communication Disorders/Differences Population* (which summarizes, by school and grade, unduplicated counts of clients assessed as having communication disorders or differences and the number of clients for whom special placements have been effected), an *LEA Summary of Communication Disorders/Differences Population* (which provides compilations of the above-noted data for the entire local education agency), an *End-of Period Service Status Report*, and a *Summary of Language-Speech-Hearing Student Services.*

The second category of program management records, the cost analysis reports, is discussed in Chapter 10.

The CASE system admirably realizes its announced intention of developing an information system to support a total clinical program. Among its many virtues is the data base afforded by the forms developed to support the assessment process. These forms make excellent models for the development of a data base for any system for recording speech, language, and hearing services.

Clinicians in smaller, self-contained programs may be overwhelmed by the system's inevitable emphasis on the efficient management of large amounts of quantified data. It is also inevitable that the system's approach to documenting intervention is restricted. The system emphasizes quantitative appraisals of change that can be used in generating programmatic data. One could not enter the detailed qualitative information found in the progress notes of other systems. As noted at the outset, however, one functional precept of the CASE system is that adoption need not be total. Adopting specific elements of the system implies no commitment to the total system. Therefore, in instances where more detailed documentation of intervention is necessary, other forms could be devised to serve that function.

ACCREDITATION AND LICENSURE STANDARDS FOR RECORD KEEPING

Client records are always appraised by accreditation agencies in reviewing clinical services programs. Accreditation standards stress the importance of records in planning treatment and in ensuring continuity of care. They specify that these records must provide official documentation of all services; must facilitate communication among the various professionals participating in the client's care; and must protect the legal interests of the clients, the clinicians, and the institution.

The Joint Commission on Accreditation of Hospitals (1983) sets forth this principle, relative to records: "The hospital shall maintain records that are documented accurately and in a timely manner, that are readily accessible, and that permit prompt retrieval of information including statistical data." JCAH further defined five standards for records (pp. 83–91):

I. An adequate medical record shall be maintained for every individual who is evaluated or treated as an inpatient, outpatient, or emergency patient, or who receives patient services in a hospital-based home care program.
II. The medical record shall contain sufficient information to identify the patient, to support the diagnosis, to justify the treatment, and to document the results accurately.
III. Medical records shall be confidential, secure, current, authenticated, legible, and complete.
IV. The medical record department shall be provided with adequate direction, staffing, and facilities to perform all required functions.
V. The role of medical record personnel in the hospital patient care evaluation programs and in committee functions shall be defined.

In interpreting Standard II, the following are specified as essential components in all records: identification data; medical history; report of relevant physical examination; diagnostic and therapeutic orders; evidence of appropriate informed consent; clinical observations, including the results of therapy; reports of procedures and tests, and their results; and conclusions at termination of hospitalization or of evaluation and treatment.

JCAH reviews most medical facility-based speech-language pathology and audiology services under their supplementary standards for rehabilitation programs/services. These standards particularize requirements for records even further (pp. 164–165):

> Records for each patient referred to a rehabilitation program/service shall include at least the following data:
>
> —The diagnosis, and problem list where appropriate, pertinent to the rehabilitation process;
> —Precautions necessitated by the patient's general medical condition or by other factors;
> —The short-term and long-term goals of the treatment program as appropriate; and
> —A statement regarding the frequency of review, when it is desired more often than monthly, of the patient's progress within each rehabilitation program/service providing treatment to the patient.
>
> There shall be a current, written plan of care for each patient receiving rehabilitation services. It should state the treatment objectives for the patient, as well as the patient's short-term and long-term rehabilitation potential. The plan should be reviewed at stated, regular intervals and revised as indicated. The patient and his family shall be permitted to participate as much as possible in the development of the plan of care.
>
> The medical record on admission shall document baseline assessment of the patient's medical condition, functional limitations, prognosis, any possible need for corrective surgery or use of prosthetic and/or orthotic devices, the attitude of the patient and/or the family toward the rehabilitation, and the existence of any sociopsychological problems affecting rehabilitation. The medical record should also document, at least on a monthly basis, an assessment of rehabilitative achievement and an estimate of further rehabilitative potential. Justification for continued rehabilitative care shall require either evidence of problems necessitating active treatment, or evidence of observed or expected improvement in functional ability.
>
> Individuals providing rehabilitative services to patients shall enter such information into the medical record as specified, and in the location determined, by those performing the medical review function. These determinations shall be made by the medical record committee where one exists.
>
> The medical record shall evidence a team approach, with participation of the professional and administrative staffs, the patient, and, as appropriate, the patient's family. The medical record shall document the written instructions given to the patient and/or the family concerning appropriate care after discharge from the hospital.

The Professional Services Board of the American Speech-Language-Hearing Association (1983) applies the following principle, relative to records: "Accurate, complete records shall be prepared and maintained for each client seen for any clinical service. Records shall be accessible and systematically organized to facilitate storage and retrieval." PSB standards further specify that case records contain at least the following information: (1) case identification data; (2) referral source; (3) pertinent information about the client (e.g., medical records, psychological reports, educational tests, and observations); (4) designation of the speech-language pathologist or audiologist responsible for the case; (5) diagnostic reports, treatment plans including specific objectives, and treatment reports; (6) chronologic log of all services; and (7) client release consent forms.

As discussed elsewhere, many states license facilities providing speech-language pathology and audiology services, primarily as a prerequisite to providing services under such public third-party payment programs as Medicaid. Such licensure standards may address records systems. Usually these requirements follow JCAH standards. In some instances, however, state licensure requirements are more specific. In California, for example, standards for licensure of rehabilitation facilities specify that client records show the principal and associated diagnoses; the prognosis; the onset date of the illness or injury; the extent of previous services and the benefits accrued from those services; the therapeutic goals; the anticipated time to achieve goals; the type, number, and frequency of services provided; and the results of those services. Records audits by state health department staff can lead to suspension of licensure when the records do not meet the established standards. More limited infractions may merely lead to denial of payment for inadequately documented services. All speech-language pathologists and audiologists who are responsible for planning and maintaining case records should explore the licensure regulations enacted in their state to be certain that their records systems and procedures conform to those regulations.

SUMMARY

No other facet of service delivery is more important than effective and economical clinical records keeping. An efficient records system provides immediate identification of every client served, offers clear and concise information about all services delivered, facilitates continuity of client care, encourages efficacious follow-up, and affords easy retrieval of statistical and research data.

In many instances speech-language pathology and audiology programs must employ the records systems of their parent organizations: school districts, medical centers, rehabilitation facilities, etc. Often these systems are not well suited for recording the kinds of information speech-language pathologists and audiologists consider essential. Yet, virtually all systems can be adapted or expanded to meet the special needs of programs serving clients with communicative disorders. Functional adaptations and expansions can be accomplished without undermining the integrity of the larger system.

In other instances, records systems serve only speech-language pathology and audiology programs and can be designed to serve their singular missions. Nevertheless, in all work settings, as providers of health, education, rehabilitation, and social services, we must always reckon with the mandates of the public and private institutions and agencies that establish the laws, regulations, and standards that govern the delivery of those services.

References

American Speech and Hearing Association: *Comprehensive Assessment and Service Evaluation Information System.* Rockville, MD, American Speech-Language-Hearing Association, 1976.

American Speech and Hearing Association Professional Services Board: Standards for PSB accreditation. *ASHA* 25:51–58, 1983.

Benjamin B: *Medical Records.* London, Heinemann Medical Books, 1977.

Bjorn JC, Cross HD: *The Problem Oriented Private Practice of Medicine.* Chicago, Modern Hospital Press, 1970.

Bouchard MM, Shane HC: Use of the problem-oriented medical record in the speech and language profession. *ASHA* 19:151–159, 1977.

Corbus H: Problem-oriented medical records in long-term care. *J Gerontol Nurs* 3:24–31, 1977.

Dinsdale S: The problem-oriented medical record in rehabilitation. *Arch Phys Med* 51:488–492, 1970.

Feinstein A: The problems of the "problem-oriented medical records." *Ann Intern Med* 78:751–762, 1973.

Gilandes A: The problem-oriented record in a psychiatric hospital. *Hosp Community Psychiatry* 23:336–339, 1972.

Grant R, Maletsky G: Application of the Weed system to psychiatric records. *Int J Psychiatry Med* 3:119–129, 1972.

Hays-Roth F: The problem-oriented medical record and psychiatry. *Br J Psychiatry* 121:27–34, 1972.

Joint Commission on Accreditation of Hospitals: *Accreditation Manual for Hospitals.* Chicago, Joint Commission on Accreditation of Hospitals, 1983.

Kent LR: Problem-oriented record in a university speech and hearing clinic. *ASHA* 22:151–158, 1980.

Kurtz DL: *Unit Medical Records in Hospital and Clinic.* New York, Columbia University Press, 1943.

Lang GS, Dickie KJ: *The Practice-oriented Medical Record.* Germantown, MD, Aspen Systems, 1978.

National League for Nursing, Department of Home Health Agencies and Community Health Services: *Problem-oriented Systems of Patient Care.* New York, National League for Nursing, 1974.

Weed LL: *Medical Records, Medical Education, and Patient Care.* Chicago, Year Book Medical Publishers, 1970.

Weed L: The problem oriented record. In Hurst JW, Walker HK: *The Problem Oriented System.* New York, Medcor, 1972.

CHAPTER SEVEN

Storing and Retrieving Clinical Records

Many professionals contend that such technical details as clinical records storage methods are not their concern. Consider, however, the plight of the speech-language pathologist who must describe the amount of progress a child has shown since the last evaluation when the record of the last evaluation cannot be located. Or what of the audiologist who answers a series of questions from a physician about Gerald Smith's hearing, only to discover that the record quoted concerned another Gerald Smith? Such incidents painfully illustrate the relationships between the efficiency and accuracy of records storage and the quality of professional services.

Eight criteria can be specified for an adequate records storage system:

1. It must provide immediate access to records.
2. It must minimize hazards of losing, misfiling, and other impediments to locating records.
3. It must afford the easy addition of materials.
4. It must make only reasonable demands on the total space available to the clinical services program.
5. It must be readily understandable to the professional and support staff who use it.
6. It must be sufficiently economical that it does not add inordinately to the overhead costs of the clinical program.
7. It must protect the rights of privacy of the clients whose records are stored.
8. It must provide for the efficient management of inactive records and for their easy identification.

These eight criteria apply whether the records system is a modest set of file folders kept by a single private practitioner or whether it is a most elaborate records system serving a huge comprehensive medical center. Furthermore, they apply both to conventional records storage systems and to systems employing the latest computer technology for information storage and retrieval.

CONVENTIONAL RECORDS STORAGE

Earlier, the optimal clinical records system was characterized as consisting of three components: the client directory, the service accounting record, and the client clinical record. Each component requires a different approach to storage.

Client Directory

The client directory was described as usually consisting of a set of file cards, which hold the information essential for identifying and locating clients and the numerically filed client case records. These cards must, therefore, be filed alphabetically. When few directory cards are required, a drawer file system is utilized, usually either the type of drawer files used for library card catalogs or the tray files that are found in vertical filing systems.

Service Accounting Record

Unlike the client directory and the client clinical record, the service accounting record has a comparatively short active life. Usually, these records need be immediately accessible only during periods of active service or until payment is received for any service that has been provided. Even when services are provided on a long-term basis, the service accounting record seldom covers longer than a 12-month interval. (Service statistics are tabulated at least annually, and financial records are "closed" at least once a year.) After summaries are prepared and accounting data posted, the service accounting record is usually placed in an inactive file, or even destroyed.

The storage system for active service accounting records, therefore, may hold far fewer records than either the client directory or the client case records file. Nevertheless, it is the most active component of the system, since an entry is always made at each client contact. Consequently, these records must be readily accessible to the individual responsible for keeping them current.

Virtually all programs serving large numbers of clients have adopted computer-assisted systems for service accounting records. Almost by definition, therefore, programs using conventional filing systems for these records serve a limited number of clients. Thus, alphabetic filing is usually most practical.

Client Clinical Records

The management of client clinical records entails a much different approach. These records usually hold substantial bodies of information that must be retained for a long time. Accordingly, they require a storage system that will provide ready access to voluminous records accruing for 8 or 10 years or even longer.

Drawer filing cabinets, whether vertical or horizontal, are suitable for storing client clinical records only so long as limited numbers are on hand. Such cabinets occupy excessive space in relationship to the number of records they hold. Furthermore, filing and retrieving records become unnecessarily complex when many records are stored. Shelf files, either open or closed, are much more functional, both from space usage and accessibility standpoints.

ALPHABETIC SYSTEMS

Client clinical records should be filed alphabetically only in those rare instances where few clients are seen and there is no likelihood that the number of clients will increase substantially during the next decade. Conversion of a filing system from alphabetic to numeric is always a cumbersome and expensive procedure. It is far better to establish a numeric system from the outset, even though the program is serving few clients.

The disadvantages of alphabetic filing are many. Filing errors are frequent. When a drawer or shelf is filled, all files must be moved to permit expansion. If the files must be expanded to other areas, a portion of the alphabet will be in one area, the remainder in another. In addition to the other shortcomings of alphabetic filing is the inescapable fact that some clients may change their names.

NUMERIC SYSTEMS

Numeric systems are virtually always better than alphabetic systems for filing client clinical records. Entry to the numeric system is provided by the client directory. For systems serving single-discipline services programs or moderate-sized multidiscipline services programs, simple but functional numeric identification can be achieved with six-digit numbers. The first two digits indicate the year the client was first admitted for service, the next four denote his place in the sequence of patients registered. For example, the first client registered during 1980 would be identified as 80-0001, the next 80-0002, the next 80-0003, and so on. Once assigned, the number remains the same regardless of future readmissions. For example, a child with delayed language acquisition was seen for evaluation in 1976 at age 3 years and given the number 76-2315. No therapy was recommended. Three years later the child was seen for re-evaluation and entered in the therapy program. The case record continued to be identified by the number originally assigned.

Obviously, this relatively simple numeric system assumes that a program is likely to register at least 1,000 new clients each year and will not register more than 9999. When there is no chance that more than 999 new clients will be registered annually, either presently or during the forseeable future, the system can use a five-digit number (e.g., 80-327). When more than 9999 new clients are registered, the agency probably represents a large multidisciplinary program that uses a system designed for terminal digit or middle digit filing.

Terminal digit and middle digit systems were developed to serve institutions where large numbers of case records must be stored and retrieved. When records are stored sequentially, as in the system proposed above, the major activity is focused in a small section of the files. Particularly in medical centers, records are most heavily used during the first 3 months following admission. Therefore, when filed sequentially by date of registration, the greatest activity in the records storage area occurs within limited segments of the files. In terminal and middle digit filing, new files are distributed throughout 10,000 predesignated sections.

Both terminal and middle digit filing involve six-digit numbers, divided into three two-digit groups; for example, record 317582 is identified as 31-75-82. For terminal digit filing, the storage shelves are divided into 100 equal sections numbered from 00 to 99. Each of these sections is subdivided with guide cards in 100 subsections. Through this division and subdivision, then, the filing system has 10,000 compartments.

In terminal digit filing, the numbers are read in two-digit groups, beginning with the third group. In the example of 31-75-82, 82 is the primary number, 75 the secondary number, and 31 the tertiary number. To file this record, one would first identify section 82, then subsection 75, where it would be filed as the 31st record in that subsection.

The dispersal of new records throughout the system can be illustrated by filing three successive new records 31-75-82, 31-75-83, and 31-75-84. As has been shown, the first record would be filed in section 82, the second in section 83, and the third in section 84. Or, illustrating the system in another way, when filing record 31-75-82, one would find that the two preceding records would be numbers 30-75-82 and 29-75-82, respectively. In other words, 10,000 records have been opened during the interval between each successive record in the file.

Middle digit filing resembles terminal digit filing. In this system, using the same illustration of record 31-75-82, 75 is the primary number, 31 the secondary number, and 82 the tertiary number. (The record would be filed in section 75, subsection 31, the 82nd record in that subsection.) Middle digit filing, while achieving some dispersion, groups records more nearly in temporal sequence than does terminal digit filing. For example, the records following 31-75-82 would be 31-75-83 and 31-75-84, hence these records are actually in temporal sequence. However, the record following 31-75-99 would be 31-76-00, to be filed in section 76, subsection 31, the first record in the next 100-record sequence. The next record to be filed in section 75 would be record 32-75-00, a record that occurs 10,000 records later in sequence.

The advantages of middle digit filing result from keeping 100 sequential records together, but at the same time dispersing these sequences throughout the entire system. Again, from the sample, the 100-record sequence of 31-75-00 through 31-75-99 will be found together in section 75, but the next 100-record sequence of 31-76-00 through 31-76-99 will be found in section 76. Assuming that the most recently opened records are also the most active records, these most active records will be focused in specific areas, but those areas will be distributed throughout the filing system.

IDENTIFICATION OF INACTIVE OR OBSOLETE RECORDS

One of the criteria for records systems stipulated that it must provide for easy identification of inactive or obsolete records. This is another important determiner of the method used for records identification. Assume that a program places in dead storage the records of all clients not seen for the previous 7 years. If alphabetic filing is used, every record must be checked to determine whether the client has been seen during the interval. If a system uses the year of registration as the first two digits of the identifying number, only records with first two-digit numbers denoting registration 7 or more years previously need be examined. In other numeric filing systems, the first and last number assigned each year are logged so that earlier records can be identified. For example, if in 1980 all records of clients not seen since the beginning of 1973 were to be retired, one would consult the log to discover the first client registered in 1973 was given the number 17-26-54. Therefore, all records in the active file with numbers of 17-26-53 and below would be reviewed to ascertain whether the clients had been seen since January 1, 1973.

COLOR CODES

Sometimes client clinical records filing systems are reinforced with color. When the records of several different programs are kept in a single filing system, different colored file folders may be used to denote the program serving the client. In other instances, filing numbers are reinforced by colored stripes, representing each digit, in the interest of rapid identification of a particular record on a shelf. Individual pages for client clinical records may also be color coded (with each color representing the section of the record in which the page should be filed). This expedites the entry of new material into records.

OUT-OF-FILE RECORDS

Another of the designated criteria for filing was related to the ease of location of records that are out of file. Two considerations are important. First, procedures should be instituted which reduce the number of times the record is removed from the file and the length of time it is withdrawn. Generally, a record should be removed from the file only when it is necessary to refer to the information it holds. When new information is to be added, it is usually best to record the information on appropriate sheets or forms for subsequent filing in the record by a clerk. As already noted, progress notes may be recorded separately and at intervals filed in the clinical record.

When files must be removed, it is essential that some consistent procedure be instituted. Usually, the position in the file the record normally occupies is marked with a tracer card which shows the whereabouts of the record. The problem of missing records can also be reduced by restricting the number of people permitted direct access to the files.

CENTRALIZED VERSUS DECENTRALIZED STORAGE

Large multidisciplinary programs must often weigh the merits of centralized versus decentralized records storage. On the one hand, there are substantial advantages to keeping all records on the same client together, so that all specialists are at all times aware of the services provided and of the results of those services. On the other hand, centralized records soon become ponderous and may be in such demand that they are often unavailable. A practical solution may lie in a centralized client clinical record holding only the data base and short summaries of evaluations and treatment, with supplementary departmental records that hold detailed data of primary interest to that department. When records are decentralized, a central client directory should be maintained which identifies the existence and location of clinical records. Furthermore, a common identification system, usually a client number, should be used for all records.

COMPUTER-ASSISTED RECORDS STORAGE

Technology is now available to computerize all components of most clinical records systems. Computers can easily store numeric data, narrative descriptions, and even graphic representations such as test profiles and audiograms. The stored information can be retrieved immediately, either in segments or in its entirety, and displayed on a screen or printed out. Computer-stored records can even be transmitted immediately to any other facility that has the necessary hardware.

Computer technology antiquates all conventional systems of records storage. That technology readily satisfies most of the criteria we established for records storage.

Computers can immediately access substantial bodies of information. Except in the hands of inexperienced users, there are minimal hazards for loss of records or problems in locating records. Current hardware makes modest demands for space in comparison to the magnitude of information stored. Although entering information into computerized systems may require more training than can be offered to all staff, most can be readily trained to access whatever information they need. Because of the amount of information that can be stored in miniscule segments of discs and tapes, records can be maintained indefinitely, precluding the problem of dealing with inactive and obsolete records.

The two less easily met criteria relate to economy and clients' rights to privacy. In the long range, computerized systems may well be more economical than conventional systems. Nevertheless, costs of initial installation are substantially greater in computerized systems and are thus beyond the reach of many programs. But the transition to computerized systems can be gradual, so that costs may be spread over several years. In considering the economics of computer systems, it is also important to recognize a unique situation. In contrast to virtually every other technology, equipment costs have declined steadily and sharply in recent years. If this trend continues, as seems likely, automated information systems will become increasingly feasible for more and more clinical programs.

One of the most widely discussed of all topics about computerized information storage is the protection of the privacy of the subjects of that information. This same issue has concerned critics of such federal agencies as the Internal Revenue Service and the Federal Bureau of Investigation, as well as consumer advocates investigating the practices of such institutions as banks and credit bureaus. The issue has received the careful attention of people who are concerned about uncontrolled access to the computerized records kept by educational and medical programs. When records consist of papers bound in manila folders, access can be controlled with locked files and restricted release to authorized individuals. When records are computerized, however, they can become available to any person with a compatible terminal who knows the codes required to access the system. Nevertheless, although no system is perfect, reasonable safeguards have been designed. These safeguards must be integral to the planning of any computerized clinical records system.

Levels of Automation

As noted earlier, the computerization of clinical records systems need not be total. Based on our characterization of an optimal system, four levels of automation can be defined: *computerized client directories, computerized service accounting records, computerized client clinical services summaries,* and *computerized client case records.*

COMPUTERIZED CLIENT DIRECTORIES

Here, only the essential identifying information is stored for each client. This level affords immediate determination of whether a particular client is known to the program and provides whatever information is required to locate other records about the client.

COMPUTERIZED SERVICE ACCOUNTING RECORDS

At this level, ongoing data about services provided are also automated. These data are merely quantitative, specifying the services provided, the dates of the services, and, when appropriate, the fees assigned to the services. In a variant of this system, many comprehensive medical centers, particularly inpatient facilities, use computer-assisted scheduling so that all recommended services are entered in advance to ensure that all are carried out. When service accounting records are computerized, we can easily document services provided to individual clients and also easily compile summaries of all services provided by the entire program.

COMPUTERIZED CLIENT CLINICAL SERVICES SUMMARIES

At this level, some aspects of the client clinical record are automated. These might include a data base (containing succinct demographic, case history, and diagnostic data), together with periodic summaries of the services provided and of the outcomes of those services. The client profiles of the practice-oriented system described earlier illustrate this level of automation.

COMPUTERIZED CLIENT CASE RECORDS

At this level, essentially the entire clinical record is automated. Copies of letters and reports sent and received, and original copies of completed test forms and authorizations, may be filed in the conventional manner, but the primary case record containing all the data we have attributed to these records is automated.

At the present time, many programs providing speech, language, and hearing services employ some level of automation. Most medical and rehabilitation centers use computerized systems for service accounting; many also employ computerized client directories. Many school districts automate identifying information about their pupils, often including attendance data and data about special services provided. Even small clinical services centers and individual private practitioners may use automated accounting procedures, either directly or on contract with computer services companies. Programs using complete computerized records systems are rare; however, this situation is likely to change during the next decade.

Data Input

Regardless of the level of automation, whatever data are to be stored must first be entered into the system. This procedure may be accomplished either off-line or on-line.

Two different off-line input procedures are possible. The first procedure consists of recording data in a form that is subsequently coded and digitized for keypunching on cards or tape for eventual entry into the computer. This has been the most widely used of all approaches to data input.

The second off-line procedure involves recording data in such a way that they can be read automatically and then entered into storage. The most familiar examples of this approach are machine-stored multiple-choice tests in which specially designed answer sheets are marked by the examinee and subsequently read and scored automatically. Similar procedures have been employed in preparing patient-completed health history forms.

On-line input involves direct data input, usually by means of a typewriter terminal. This procedure is used by most newer clinical records systems. Again, two approaches are possible. In the first, the data are entered immediately by the individual accruing the data. For example, the person responsible for initial registration of clients may enter the identifying information for the client directory and the service accounting record as that information is collected during the registration procedure. Presumably, a member of the professional staff could record the results of the initial interview directly on a terminal as he or she conducts that interview. For many practical reasons, however, this practice is seldom used.

The second on-line procedure involves entering data at some time following acquisition of the data. For example, the results of an evaluation or of a therapy visit are summarized and subsequently entered into the computer. Again, entries may be made directly by the clinician who rendered the service or, secondarily, by a clerk working from the clinician's written summary. In both instances, the clinician or clerk enters the information directly into a terminal.

Regardless of whether entry is off-line or on-line, and regardless of the procedure used to enter the data, automated systems require careful consideration of the language used to represent the information to be stored. Unless newer technology with substantial memory is available, closed information systems are employed. In these systems a finite number of options are available for the language used to encode the data. All numeric data are entered directly, but other data must be expressed in a standard vocabulary in which each term has a standard numeric designation (for example, by using one of the standardized diagnostic codes); by choosing from a closed set of options (for example, by placing family income within one of 10 different ranges or characterizing educational placement within a set of specified categories); or by making binary choices (yes or no, present or absent, left or right, etc.). Closed information systems must always be used for off-line entry involving punch cards or scanner sheets. Many on-line entry systems also employ closed systems.

Other on-line systems use semi-free language. Here, data are entered, using normal vocabulary, directly into the computer. The data may be entered by listing, in paragraph form, or in outline. They may be entered using standard English sentences or in telegraphic form. Words may be abbreviated or entered in their entirety. Few language restrictions are any longer imposed by available technology; there are only practical constraints related to the particular application.

Despite the absence of technologic constraints, some cautions are advisable in considering the language used for computerized records. Most systems are enhanced by some standardization of language. Records will be more functional when all users agree on the terminology for diagnoses, for identifying procedures, and for documenting the outcomes of services. Without this standardization, some of the most valuable features of computerized records are lost. An important advantage of automated systems is their potential for multiple modes of access. For example, one can access all clients with a particular diagnosis in a particular age range, or all clients tested with a particular instrument, or all clients subjected to a particular intervention strategy. Such access is only possible when a standard vocabulary is used in the initial entry of information.

One further consideration is important with respect to vocabulary. For a variety of practical reasons, professionals themselves seldom enter their data into computers. An intervening clerical step is almost always involved. The likelihood of erroneous entries increases substantially when no standard vocabulary is employed. Even more hazardous is the practice of expecting the clerk to translate a professional's idiosyncratic vocabulary into a standard vocabulary. This practice is frequently employed in medical centers where random physician notes are edited and entered into the computer by clerks. The results can be disastrous. As a general rule, therefore, any system involving the entry of professionals' notes by clerical personnel should entail a reasonable amount of vocabulary standardization.

Data Output

Current technology also provides several options for data output. The general options relate to a visual display of data (essentially on a television screen) or the generation of hard copy via an automatic typewriter or printer. Several systems permit review of records through visual display, with immediate productions of hard copies whenever they are required.

Frequently, it is not necessary to review an entire record but, rather, to consult only one segment: a particular medical report, a section of the case history, the results of a particular test, etc. It is possible to "thumb through" a conventional client clinical record to locate such specific information, but computer-stored information cannot be scanned in the same way. It is essential, therefore, to devise a standard code for identifying record entries so that individual segments can be accessed easily. In this way data output need not be an all-or-none procedure.

PERMANENCE AND RETENTION OF CLINICAL RECORDS

Clinical information should be recorded in such a way that it will survive throughout any period that is likely to be needed. When a client is first seen during childhood, this period may be 20 years or longer. Permanence, then, requires consideration of the medium used for recording the information as well as of the material on which it is recorded. Obviously, handwritten notes should always be in ink. Typed text should be either the original or the first copy. Photocopy processes vary widely in longevity; therefore, the estimated life of copies must be considered in selecting equipment used to duplicate clinical records. The paper on which information is recorded must be of sufficient weight to survive years of storage and use. Onionskin copies, certain lightweight photocopies, and most pressure-sensitive copy papers deteriorate too rapidly. The choice of recording processes and materials must also consider their amenability to producing legible photocopies, both immediately and in the future. Records should be bound in such a way as to provide adequate protection.

Although usually not included in the clinical record, speech-language pathologists should recognize the value, from a legal standpoint, of retaining audiotaped speech samples from certain clients. Among these are pre- and postoperative samples of the speech of patients undergoing palatal or laryngeal surgery (e.g., removal of growths, Teflon injection, recurrent laryngeal nerve sectioning, or pharyngeal flap procedures); samples of the speech of patients seen because of surgically induced speech problems (e.g., following glossectomy or surgery for cancer of the hard and soft palate, or instances of recurrent laryngeal nerve impairment following thyroidectomy); and patients with trauma-induced speech problems (e.g., automobile accidents, industrial accidents, gunshot wounds). These situations can lead to litigation in which speech-language pathologists are called as expert witnesses. The availability of high-quality tape recordings can make the clinician's task considerably easier by providing a means of illustrating the condition of the client's speech rather than offering subjective descriptions.

Decisions about the retention of clinical records can also be thorny. Since many speech, language, and hearing problems are permanent, some data may seem relevant for a very long time. On the other hand, few clinical programs have sufficient space to continue endlessly the retention of all records.

The Joint Commission on Accreditation of Hospitals (1983, p. 86) made nonspecific recommendations in their interpretation of records standards:

> The length of time that records are to be kept is dependent upon the length of time that they may be needed for continuing patient care and for legal, research, or educational purposes.

ASHA's Professional Services Board (1983, p. 57) is more specific:

> Clinical records are retained for a period of time in accordance with state or federal statutes.

As noted in the Professional Services Board standards, many states have laws governing the retention of client records, particularly when they are considered "medical records." These laws vary widely, ranging from 7 years in California to 25 years in Nebraska, Kansas, and South Carolina. Special provisions may govern the retention of records concerning children. Some states require that children's records must be kept for a period of years after the subject has reached the age of 21.

Many speech-language pathology and audiology programs merely adhere to the retention policies of whatever agency or institution provides their administration. However, freestanding programs must define their own policies based on state laws, accreditation standards, prevailing community practices, and practical considerations as to storage facilities and characteristics of the population served. (A program exclusively serving a geriatric population obviously can adopt different retention policies than programs serving preschoolers.) This is but one other area in which no absolute standards should be proposed.

SUMMARY

Many professionals consider problems related to storing and retrieving clinical records to be technical matters unworthy of their concern. These problems can, however, significantly influence the quality of professional services. When conventional storage and retrieval systems are used, they must afford efficient and immediate access to active records, provide adequate methods for retiring inactive records, and ensure security and confidentiality. The computerized records systems that are now achieving widespread application in human services agencies offer ideal solutions to some of the problems that characterize conventional systems, but they also introduce some new and unique problems. Computerized systems may complement conventional systems or replace them entirely.

External factors also influence the procedures agencies adopt for records storage and retrieval. Among these factors are state laws and regulations and the standards imposed by accrediting agencies.

References

American Speech-Language-Hearing Association Professional Services Board: Standards for PSB accreditation. *ASHA* 25:51–58, 1983.

Joint Commission on Accreditation of Hospitals: *Accreditation Manual for Hospitals.* Chicago, Joint Commission on Accreditation of Hospitals, 1983.

Supplementary Readings

Benjamin B: *Medical Records.* London, Heinemann Medical Books, 1977.

Elliot LL, Vegely AB, Falvey NJ: Description of a computer-oriented record-keeping system. *ASHA* 13:435–443, 1971.

Elliot, LL, Vegely AB: Notes on clinical record-keeping systems. *ASHA* 13:444–446, 1971.

Peterson HA: More about computer-assisted record keeping. *ASHA* 19:617–618, 1977.

Weed LL: *Automation of the Problem-oriented Medical Record.* Burlington, VT, University of Vermont Promis Laboratory, 1977.

CHAPTER EIGHT

Coding Systems for Clinical Information

One curious characteristic of our profession is that despite our presumed dedication to solving problems of human communication, we have never been able to adopt a common vocabulary to facilitate intra- and interprofessional communication. We have no universally accepted nomenclature for either the disorders that concern us or the services we provide.

In earlier days our semantic arguments were fairly harmless diversions. Does a child have an articulation problem or a phonologic disorder? Should it be functional hearing loss, psychogenic hearing impairment, or pseudohypacusis? Is speech denasalized or characterized by rhinolalia clausa? Is a particular client's voice quality rough, hoarse, or characterized by aperiodicity? Can a child with a congenital or developmental problem be enrolled in a rehabilitation program, or must it be a habilitation program? For at least three important reasons, these word games are no longer innocuous. First, our growing involvement with other professions precludes such idiosyncratic language usage. Second, the increasing definition of our services—particularly of the conditions under which those services may and may not be provided—in laws and regulations and in the policies of third-party payers, demands consistency in terminology. Third, the growing use of automatic data-processing technology in record keeping and administration procedures requires a common language.

Regrettably, our profession assumed little initiative in developing standard nomenclatures to meet these exigencies. Consequently, we have been presented with, and are increasingly required to adopt, terminology that serves us badly. Until we can agree among ourselves, however, we have little choice but to use these systems as best we can, adapting them as much as they allow to serve our special needs.

Nomenclature systems are considered here as they are applied in codes used in various applications for recording, storing, and reporting clinical data. Two general areas are discussed: *diagnostic coding* and *procedure coding.*

DIAGNOSTIC CODES

Health care was the first field of human services to recognize the need for consistent terminology. Initially, that concern grew out of efforts to standardize, at national and international levels, approaches to reporting epidemiologic and mortality data. Unless common terminology was used, it was obviously impossible to gather reliable data. The first taxonomies, therefore, were devised to serve this kind of data gathering.

Gradually, however, as other needs for consistent reporting grew, the taxonomies were adopted for other uses. Individual institutions use such systems for compiling data about the clients they serve and the services they provide. The taxonomies are used to access records as a basis for identifying possible research subjects. Third-party payers frequently define covered conditions and services according to these nomenclatures. Each year sees new and expanded applications.

These taxonomies are commonly referred to as "diagnostic codes." Of the many systems proposed, six will be discussed here. The *Standard Nomenclature of Diseases and Operations* and the *International Classification of Diseases* (ICD) are the two major systems employed by health care institutions and programs. The *Diagnostic and Statistical Manual of Mental Disorders* (DSM) is widely used by mental health programs. Two approaches to the development of specific taxonomies for speech, langauge, and hearing services are the *Iowa Quality Assurance Program System for Disorder Classification* and the *CASE Classification Schema*. Finally, although incomplete, *The Rehabilitation Codes* offer an alternative approach to taxonomy that may have important implications for developing more useful diagnostic codes in speech-language pathology and audiology.

Standard Nomenclature of Diseases and Operations

The Standard Nomenclature represented the first major effort to establish a system of medical terminology for universal application. It was initially published in 1933 by the National Conference on Nomenclature, a group sponsored by the Commonwealth Fund. Four years later, however, the responsibility for periodic revisions and republications was assumed by the American Medical Association.

The system specifies the classification of each disease according to two parameters: topographically, in terms of the organ or tissue principally affected, and etiologically, by the causative factor. For example, vocal fold paralysis is coded 336-569. The first set of three digits (336) designates the topography. The second set of three digits (569) specifies the etiology.

The topographic classification is based on the following 10-part breakdown:

0 Body as a whole (including psyche and body generally), not a particular system exclusively
1 Integumentary system (including subcutaneous areolar tissue, mucous membranes of orifices, and the breasts)
2 Neuroskeletal system
3 Respiratory system
4 Cardiovascular system
5 Hemic and lymphatic systems
6 Digestive system
7 Urogenital system
8 Endocrine system
9 Nervous system
X Organs of special sense

The second digit in the topographic code locates the disease further within the system. For example, within the respiratory system:

31 Nose
32 Accessory sinuses
33 Larynx
34 Trachea
35 Bronchi and bronchioles
36 Lung
37 Pleura

Or, within the special sense system:

X1 Structures concerned in vision
X2 Structures concerned in vision
X3 Structures concerned in vision
X4 Structures concerned in vision
X5 Structures auxiliary to the eye
X6 Structures auxilary to the eye
X7 Acoustic sense
X8 Acoustic sense
X9 Vestibular equilibratory sense

The third digit in the topographic code locates the disease even more precisely. For example, the following topographic specifications are available for laryngeal diseases:

330 Larynx generally
331 Epiglottis
332 Arytenoid cartilages
333 Thyroid cartilage
334 Cricoid cartilage
335 Perichondrium
336 Vocal cords
337 Laryngeal ventricle
338 Articulations
  3381 Cricoarytenoid articulation
  3382 Cricothyroid articulation
339 Intrinsic muscles
33X Intrinsic vessels

Or diseases of the ear may be located topographically with greater specificity as follows:

X70 Acoustic sense, generally
X71 Ear, generally
X72 Auricle
X74 Cartilage of auricle
X75 External acoustic meatus
X76 Osseous meatus
X77 Tympanic membrane
X78 Lobule
X79 Cartilaginous meatus
X80 Middle ear, generally
X81 Auditory ossicles
X82 Muscles of tympanum

X83 Auditory tube (Eustachian tube)
X84 Mastoid antrum and mastoid air cells
X85 Internal ear
X86 Osseous labyrinth
X87 Cochlea
X88 Organ of Corti
X89 Perilabyrinthine tissues
X8X Petrous portion

The etiologic classification, denoted by the second set of three digits, is based on a 13-part breakdown:

0 Diseases due to prenatal influence
1 Diseases due to a lower plant or animal parasite
2 Diseases due to a higher plant or animal parasite
3 Diseases due to intoxication
4 Diseases due to trauma or physical agent
50 Diseases secondary to circulatory disturbance
55 Diseases secondary to disturbance of innervation or of psychic control
6 Diseases due to or consisting of static mechanical abnormality (obstruction, calculus, displacement, or gross change in form) due to unknown cause
7 Diseases due to disorders of metabolism, growth, or nutrition
8 New growths
9 Diseases due to unknown or uncertain cause with the structural reaction (degenerative, infiltrative, inflammatory, proliferative, sclerotic, or reparative) manifest; hereditary and familial diseases of this nature
X Diseases due to unknown or uncertain cause with the functional reaction alone manifest; hereditary and familial diseases of this nature
Y Diseases of undetermined cause

The etiologic classification is elaborated further by the second and third digits. For example, in category 0 (diseases due to prenatal influence), 5 as a second digit indicates "diseases due to infection, intoxication, or trauma before or during birth; abnormalities of pregnancy and labor." These are elaborated by a third digit as follows:

050 Injury during birth
052 Due to maternal infection
053 Due to maternal intoxication
054 Injury prior to birth
057 Due to maternal metabolic disturbances
059 Due to genetic disturbances prior to birth

Another example of the three-digit refinement of an etiologic classification can be drawn from category 50 (50 to 54, diseases secondary to circulatory disturbance). The subcategory 51 refers to "diseases due to diminished blood supply," with the subcategory elaborated as follows:

510 Generally or unspecified
511 Due to thrombosis of nutritional artery
512 Due to embolism of nutritional artery
513 Due to spasm of nutritional artery
514 Due to section, ligation, compression, or constriction of nutritional artery
515 Due to arteritis or endarteritis
516 Due to sclerosis of the nutritional artery
517 Due to sclerosis of the intrinsic arterioles
518 Due to reflex or other disturbance of vasomotor control
519 Due to disorders of heart beat
51X Due to phlebitis

The use of the Standard Nomenclature system can be illustrated by deriving some common conditions in speech-language pathology and audiology:

Vocal Fold Paralysis

3	Disease of respiratory system
3	Disease of larynx
6	Disease of vocal fold
−56	Due to disturbance of efferent innervation
9	With paralysis due to pressure on or lesion of nerve
336−569	Vocal Fold Paralysis

Cleft Palate

6	Digestive system
1	Mouth
6	Palate
−0	Disease due to genetic and prenatal influence
3	Supernumerary part; duplication, division, bifurcation; diverticulation
7	Nonfusion
616−037	Cleft Palate

Serous Otitis Media

X	Organs of special sense
8	Acoustic sense
0	Middle ear generally
−1	Diseases or infections due to lower plant (bacteria or viruses) or animal parasite (bacteria or viruses)
90	Unknown or unclassified organism generally (nonsuppurative infection unspecified)
X80−190	Serous Otitis Media

It must be remembered that the Standard Nomenclature system was developed for use in recording classical medical diagnoses. The system is woefully inadequate in dealing with many of the behavior disorders that concern speech-language pathologists and audiologists. Many of the diagnostic terms that apply to these disorders are found in the catch-all designation, "supplementary terms," terms which are exclusively topographic. It is noted that these terms are to be used as supplements to any of the diagnoses listed in the nomenclature of diseases. In other words, they are presumably used in addition to designations of the underlying disease. Among these terms are the following:

271	Ataxia
322	Aphonia
320	Change in voice
321	Hoarseness
992	Acalculia
984	Agnosia, acoustic
9551	Agrammatism aphasia (jargon aphasia)
955	Agraphia, developmental
951	Agraphia
952	Alexia
967	Alexia, developmental
957	Anarthria
9550	Aphasia
9552	Aphasia, amnesic
976	Aphasia, developmental
95X	Aphasia, dysarthric
9553	Aphasia, expressive (motor)
9554	Aphasia, global
9557	Aphasia, nominal
955X	Aphasia, receptive
9561	Aphasia, semantic
9562	Aphasia, syntactic
9563	Aphasia, verbal
9564	Aphasia, visual
990	Aphonia, developmental
9630	Apraxia
991	Apraxia, developmental
9632	Apraxia, ideational
9633	Apraxia, ideomotor
9634	Apraxia, motor
9301	Delayed speech with mental deficiency
9303	Delayed speech without mental deficiency
958	Dyslexia
953	Dysphasia
959	Dyspraxia
928	Echolalia
994	Special spelling disability
9305	Speech disorder due to habit (after repair of cleft palate)
9302	Stammering
X09	Conduction deafness
X08	Deaf mutism, symptomatic
X59	Deafness, neural, cause unknown
X47	Deafness, neural, due to vascular lesion of higher centers
X56	Deafness, sensory, cause unknown
X58	Deafness, sensory-neural, cause unknown
X06	Deafness, unspecified
X071	Diplacusis
X00	Ménière's syndrome
X01	Middle ear deafness
X02	Nerve deafness
X04	Tinnitus
0124	Word blindness
X03	Word deafness

In reviewing these terms, the shortcomings of the Standard Nomenclature for use in speech-language pathology and audiology become readily apparent. When the precisely designed system did not accommodate essential diagnoses they were simply added on. Furthermore, they were added piecemeal with little regard to their relationship to the total system. No guidance is offered for their use. When, for example, should X02 Nerve deafness be used and when should X58 Deafness, sensorineural be used? Or when should 0124 Word blindness be used in preference to 952 Alexia or 958 Dyslexia? Moreover, the distinguishing characteristics of the 11 different notations for aphasia are elusive and seem to rely on no consistent system of terminology.

If a speech-language pathologist or audiologist works in a facility using Standard Nomenclature, he or she would be well advised to select a set of terms from those available and to prepare a glossary of how those terms are to be used. The number of terms used should be sharply reduced; for example, 9550 Aphasia as a generic classification for all aphasic disorders and 9630 Apraxia for all clients with apraxic disorders should be used, rather than attempting to classify clients in more discrete categories. If a more refined system is needed for the purposes of the speech-language pathology and audiology department alone (for example, for the identification of possible research samples), an in-house elaboration of the system can be developed.

In some medical centers, only physicians may record diagnoses. Particularly in these instances, the use of a simplified system for noting communicative disorders should be encouraged. Since most physicians have only rudimentary knowledge of speech, language, and hearing problems, all kinds of difficulties result when they are expected to use the complex, yet inadequate, supplementary terminology of the Standard Nomenclature.

International Classification of Diseases (ICD)

The *International Classification of Diseases* has become the most widely used diagnostic coding system. More specifically, the system used by most American health care programs is the ICD-9-CM, i.e., the ninth revision of the ICD in its "clinical modification."

The antecedents of the ICD originated in a resolution adopted at a meeting of the International Statistical Congress in 1853, ultimately presented for approval 30 years later as the *International Classification of Causes of Death.* This classification system was expanded and revised and ultimately adopted as the official system of the Health Organization of the League of Nations for the tabulation of morbidity statistics. With the advent of the United Nations and the subsequent founding of the World Health organization (WHO), there began wider concern for achieving consistent reporting of all aspects of health maintenance and care. No longer did the mere collection of morbidity statistics suffice. Consequently, in 1948 the sixth revision of the system that had begun as the *International Classification of Causes of Death* was substantially expanded to become the *International Statistical Classification of Diseases, Injuries, and Causes of Death.* The succeeding 30 years saw three further revisions; the most recent, the ninth revision, was published in 1976.

The ICD-9-CM, published in 1978, is a clinical modification of the WHO *International Classification of Diseases*, ninth revision. The purpose of the modification is stated in the introduction (p. xxiii):

> The term "clinical" is used to emphasize the modification's intent; to serve as a useful tool in the area of classification of morbidity data for indexing medical records, medical care review, and ambulatory and other medical care programs, as well as for basic health statistics. To describe the clinical picture of the patient, the codes must be more precise than those needed only for statistical groupings and trend analysis.

The basis for the classification of diseases and injuries is essentially etiologic, although some catch-all categories are provided. The primary classification is divided into 17 categories. The number range assigned to each category is noted:

1. Infectious and parasitic diseases (001–139)
2. Neoplasms (140–239)
3. Endocrine, nutritional, and metabolic diseases and immunity diseases (240–279)
4. Diseases of the blood and blood-forming organs (280–289)
5. Mental disorders (290–319)
6. Diseases of the nervous system and sense organs (320–389)
7. Diseases of the circulatory system (390–459)
8. Diseases of the respiratory system (460–519)
9. Diseases of the digestive system (520–579)
10. Diseases of the genitourinary system (580–629)
11. Complications of pregnancy, childbirth, and the puerperium (630–679)
12. Diseases of the skin and subcutaneous tissue (680–709)
13. Diseases of the musculoskeletal system (710–739)
14. Congenital anomalies (740–759)
15. Certain conditions originating in the prenatal period (760–779)
16. Symptoms, signs, and ill-defined conditions (780–799)
17. Injury and poisoning (800–999)

The following items from the basic ICD index illustrate entries that are of particular interest to speech-language pathologists and audiologists:

161.0 Malignant neoplasm of the vocal cord
307.0 Stammering and stuttering
315.0 Specific reading disability
315.3 Developmental speech or language disorder
381.0 Acute nonsuppurative otitis media

381.1 Chronic serous otitis media
381.2 Chronic mucoid otitis media
384.2 Perforation of tympanic membrane
385.1 Adhesive middle ear disease
385.3 Cholesteatoma of middle ear and mastoid
386.0 Ménière's disease
386.3 Labyrinthitis
387 Otosclerosis
388.1 Noise effects on inner ear
388.3 Tinnitus
389.0 Conductive hearing loss
389.1 Sensorineural hearing loss
389.2 Mixed conductive and sensorineural hearing loss
478.3 Paralysis of vocal cords or larynx
478.4 Polyp of vocal cord or larynx
478.5 Other diseases of vocal cords
744.0 Congenital anomalies of ear causing impairment of hearing
749.0 Cleft palate
784.3 Aphasia
784.4 Voice disturbance
784.5 Other speech disturbance (including dysarthria and slurred speech)

The ICD also provides for further elaboration of some of these diagnoses through additional decimal coding. For example, 749.0 Cleft palate, can be refined as follows:

749.00 Cleft palate, unspecified
749.01 Unilateral, complete
749.02 Unilateral, incomplete
749.03 Bilateral, complete
749.04 Bilateral, incomplete

In addition to the basic classification system, the ICD-9 provides a "Supplementary Classification of Factors Influencing Health Status and Contact with Health Services," designated as the "V Code." The V Code may be particularly useful to speech-language pathologists and audiologists since it permits the coding of client reports and presenting complaints, rather than requiring completed diagnoses. These V Codes are also useful in situations involving physicians who are sensitive to the use, by other professionals, of diagnoses which, they believe, should be reserved for their use.

The V Codes are intended for use under two different sets of circumstances:

> When a person who is not currently sick encounters the health services for some specific purpose, such as . . . to discuss a problem which is in itself not a disease or injury.
>
> When some circumstance or problem is present which influences the person's health but is not in itself a current illness or injury.

Several features of the V Codes are particularly relevant to speech-language pathologists and audiologists. These codes enable the identification of clients who are evaluated despite no immediate evidence of pathology (e.g., V19.2 Family history of hearing loss, V40.0 Problems with learning, or V20.2 Routine infant or child health check). They also permit broad entries that may be employed in instances where the diagnosis is delayed or for other reasons is unavailable (e.g., V40.1 Problems with communication, including speech, V41.2 Problems with hearing, and V41.4 Problems with voice production). Another feature of the V Codes allows speech-language pathologists and audiologists to record the procedure they have carried out (e.g., V53.2 Fitting and adjustment of hearing aid, V57.3 Speech therapy, V67.0 Follow-up examination following surgery, V71.3 Observation following accident at work, V72.1 Examination of ears and hearing, V79.3 Special screening for developmental handicaps in early childhood, and V80.3 Special screening for ear diseases). V Code listings may also be useful when third-party payers require entry of ICD diagnoses on claim forms, since these codes often cover speech-language pathology and audiology evaluations that cannot be specified using the pathology-based listings from the primary ICD codes.

Although not without problems, the ICD-9-CM is substantially easier to apply to speech-language pathology and audiology services than is the Standard Nomenclature. Nevertheless, some quandaries are inherent. For example, in coding a general entry for hearing impairment, should one use 389.9 Unspecified hearing loss or V41.2 Problems with hearing? Should a general entry about a voice disorder be 784.4 Voice disturbance or V41.4 Problems with voice production? Furthermore, many ICD categories permit little precision in entering speech, language, and hearing problems. Everything from grossly delayed acquisition of language to a mild phonologic problem is included under 315.3 Developmental speech or language disorder. Contact ulcers of the vocal folds, nodules, and leukoplakia are all coded 478.5 Other diseases of the vocal cords. There is also little provision for coding degrees of impairment. For example, a 30 dB sensorineural hearing loss with good speech discrimination and an 80 dB impairment with grossly impaired discrimination would both be coded 389.1.

Some of the limitations of ICD can be offset by local policies. A staff may agree on the use of a particular entry when two or more seem apt. Additionally, the ICD listings can be elaborated locally by further decimal coding. Using a previous example, a particular clinic could employ 478.52 to identify contact ulcers, 478.53 to identify nodules, 478.54 to identify leukoplakia, etc. When data are fed into some larger network, only the usual ICD listing is used, but the local refinement of the system can be used for all in-house functions.

The virtual universal adoption of the ICD makes it an important tool for any speech-language pathologist or audiologist working in health care agencies. The system is revised and expanded at least once each decade. Each succeeding revision has shown substantial improvements in the sections most likely to be used by our profession. Inevitably, with increasing emphasis on national health care planning and programs, greater standardization of data will be required. Every professional working in health care programs is well advised, therefore, to become versed in the use of the most likely medium for reporting such data, i.e., the ICD.

Diagnostic and Statistical Manual of Mental Disorders (DSM)

The American Psychiatric Association published the first DSM in 1952. Two subsequent revisions have appeared; the third revision, DSM III, was published in 1980. DSM was originally developed in the belief that the ICD provided an inadequate means for the classification of mental health problems. Nevertheless, each edition has been developed to maintain compatibility with the latest edition of ICD. Therefore, DSM III is designed to relate to ICD-9.

DSM III represents a substantial departure from the two previous editions. Among the innovations is the use of a "multiaxial" system for evaluation, with five axes, the first three of which constitute "an official diagnostic evaluation." Axes I and II contain listings of various diagnoses of mental disorders. Two classes of these disorders, Personality Disorders and Specific Developmental Disorders, are assigned to Axis II; all others are assigned to Axis I. The stated rationale for this division is that "This separation insures that consideration is given to the possible presence of disorders that are frequently overlooked when attention is directed to the usually more florid Axis I disorders." A single individual, then, may present disorders which are recorded in either or both Axis I and Axis II. Thus, in recording diagnostic information about a specific case, entries may occur for both Axis I and Axis II, or "no diagnosis" may be recorded in one of these axes when no entry is appropriate.

Axis I categories and subcategories are as follows (for the purpose of this overview, code numbers are omitted):

Disorders usually first evident in infancy, childhood, or adolescence:

- Mental retardation (subclassified mild, moderate, severe, profound, and unspecified)
- Attention deficit disorder (subclassified with hyperactivity and without hyperactivity)
- Conduct disorder
- Anxiety disorders of childhood and adolescence
- Other disorders of infancy, childhood, or adolescence (schizoid behavior, elective mutism, identity disorder, etc.)
- Eating disorder
- Stereotyped movement disorders
- Other disorders with physical manifestations (stuttering, functional enuresis and encopresis, sleepwalking, etc.)
- Pervasive developmental disorders (including infantile autism)

Organic mental disorders:

Section 1. Organic mental disorders whose etiology is a pathological process, taken from the mental disorders section of the ICD-9-CM. (This section includes dementias arising from the senium and presenium, as for example, degenerative dementias, and substance-induced dementias from such agents as alcohol and hallucinogenics.)

Section 2. Organic brain syndromes whose etiology or pathophysiological process is either noted as an additional diagnosis from outside the mental disorders section of ICD-9-CM or is unknown (e.g., delirium, amnesic syndrome, organic personality syndrome, etc.).

Substance use disorders (alcohol abuse, barbiturate abuse, tobacco dependence, etc.)
Schizophrenic disorders
Paranoid disorders
Psychotic disorders not elsewhere classified
Neurotic disorders
Affective disorders
Anxiety disorders
Somatoform disorders (conversion disorder, psychogenic pain disorder, hypochondriasis, etc.)
Psychosexual disorders
Disorders of impulse control
Psychogenic factors affecting physical condition
V Codes of conditions not attributable to a mental disorder that are a focus of attention or treatment (e.g., malingering, borderline intellectual functioning, antisocial behavior, academic problem, marital problem, parent-child problem, etc.)

Axis II categories include:

Specific developmental disorders:

Developmental reading disorder
Developmental arithmetic disorder
Developmental language disorder
Developmental articulation disorder
Mixed specific developmental disorder
Atypical specific developmental disorder

Personality disorders:

Paranoid
Schizoid
Schizotypal
Histrionic
Narcissistic
Antisocial
Borderline
Avoidant
Dependent
Compulsive
Passive-Aggressive
Atypical, mixed or other personality disorder

DSM III offers an important improvement over other diagnostic codes in that it provides statements of diagnostic criteria. The following are typical of these criteria:

Diagnostic Criteria for Mental Retardation

A. Significantly subaverage general intellectual functioning: an IQ of 70 or below on an individually administered IQ test (for infants, since intelligence tests do not yield numerical values, a clinical judgment of significant subaverage intellectual functioning).
B. Concurrent deficits or impairments in adaptive behavior, taking the person's age into consideration.
C. Onset before the age of 8.

Diagnostic Criteria for Stuttering

Frequent repetition or prolongation of sounds, syllables, or words or frequent unusual hesitations and pauses that disrupt the rhythmic flow of speech.

Diagnostic Criteria for Developmental Reading Disorder

Performance on standardized, individually administered tests of reading skill is significantly below the expected level given the individual's schooling, chronological age, and mental age (as determined by an individually administered IQ test). In addition, in school, the child's performance on tasks requiring reading skills is significantly below his or her intellectual capacity.

Diagnostic Criteria for Developmental Language Disorder, Expressive Type

A. Failure to develop vocal expression (encoding) of language despite relatively intact comprehension of language.
B. Presence of inner language (the presence of age-appropriate concepts, such as understanding the purpose and use of a particular household object).
C. Not due to mental retardation, childhood onset pervasive developmental disorder, hearing impairment or trauma.

Diagnostic Criteria for Developmental Language Disorder, Receptive Type

A. Failure to develop comprehension (decoding) and vocal expression (encoding) of language.
B. Not due to hearing impairment, trauma, mental retardation, or childhood onset pervasive developmental disorder.

Diagnostic Criteria for Developmental Articulation Disorder

A. Failure to develop consistent articulations of the later-acquired speech sounds such as r, sh, th, f, z, l, or ch.
B. Not due to developmental language disorder, mental retardation, childhood onset pervasive developmental disorder, or physical disorders.

Axis III provides the repository for entries regarding "any current physical disorder or condition that is potentially relevant to the understanding or management of the individual." Diagnostic codes from the ICD-9-CM are employed for these entries.

Axis IV contains an entry which estimates the "severity of psychosocial stressor." Here the clinician estimates the "overall severity of a stressor judged to have been a significant contributor to the development or exacerbation of the current disorder." Ratings are to be based "on the clinician's assessment of the stress an 'average' person in similar circumstances and with similar sociocultural values would experience from the particular psychosocial stressors." Among the types of stressors to be considered are conjugal (marital and nonmarital), parenting, occupational, legal, developmental, and physical illness and injury. For Axis IV entries, clinicians employ a seven-level severity rating scale from 1, to indicate "none," to 7, to indicate "catastrophic."

Axis V contains an estimate of the highest level of adaptive functioning during the past year. Adaptive functioning is defined as a composite of three major areas: social relations, occupational functioning, and use of leisure time. Again, a seven-level rating system is employed, with level 1 indicating superior functioning (usually effective functioning in social relations, occupational functioning, and use of leisure time), and 7 indicating grossly impaired functioning (gross impairment in virtually all areas of functioning).

Two hypothetical examples of recording the results of a DSM III multiaxial diagnosis follow (although omitted above, the appropriate code numbers are included):

Example 1: A 4-year-old child with hyperactivity, delayed language acquisition, and neuromuscular problems.

Axis I:	314.01 Attention deficit disorder with hyperactivity
Axis II:	315.31 Developmental language disorder
Axis III:	781.3 Motor incoordination
Axis IV:	Psychosocial stressors: inconsistent parental management Severity: 4 Moderate
Axis V:	Highest level of adaptive functioning last year: 4 Fair

Example 2: An adult stutterer who has bouts of alcohol abuse.

Axis 1:	307.00 Stuttering 305.02 Alcohol abuse (episodic)
Axis II:	V71.09 No diagnosis on Axis II
Axis III:	None
Axis IV:	Psychosocial stressors: 0 No information
Axis V:	Highest level of adaptive functioning past year: 5 Poor

Since its basic purpose is the coding of behavioral diagnoses rather than physical ailments and deficits, the DSM III may be more readily used by speech-language pathologists than either the Standard Nomenclature or the ICD. However, because of its conservative view of what constitutes "mental disorders," the DSM III does not offer several categories required to document speech and language disorders. Furthermore, the system offers little that would be useful to audiologists. Although diagnoses relative to hearing levels can be coded on Axis III, there are no Axis I or II categories that can appropriately denote several of the most common behavioral components of hearing impairment.

Few speech-language pathologists or audiologists would choose the DSM III for their own practices; nevertheless, an increasing number are finding employment in psychiatric hospitals, in other mental health facilities, and in programs for the developmentally disabled which use DSM III. These clinicians may be required to use the system.

The essential naïveté of the listings relative to speech and language disorders represents a troublesome cultural lag, particularly in the statements of diagnostic criteria. The state of our art had long since surpassed such simplistic formulations at the time DSM III was being prepared. Yet, the diagnostic criteria can be refined for use in a particular facility and more discrete diagnostic categories added, again by the addition of further decimal codes.

Sophisticated clinicians may also be troubled by the simplistic categories recorded in Axes IV and V. Inevitably, the Axis V rating can be interpreted as a severity rating and used as a basis for documenting progress in treatment as revealed by evaluations. Substantial gains might be achieved which were nevertheless insufficient to produce a one-digit change in the estimate of "highest level of adaptive functioning" (for example, the mastery of two or three functional communication signs by a severely autistic child). In these instances, services can be discontinued because the rating system employed seems to show no progress.

DSM III represents substantial advances over DSM I and DSM II. Although it lags far behind the state of the art in areas of our major professional concerns, it can probably be modified sufficiently within its essential structure to be used by speech-language pathologists serving programs that use this system.

The Rehabilitation Codes

The Rehabilitation Codes grew out of projects that were initiated by the Association for the Aid of Crippled Children and further developed by an independent agency supported by grants from the United States Public Health Service. Regrettably, the project did not win the level of general support needed to carry it to completion. In my view, this approach represented the ultimate answer to developing a completely utilitarian system for diagnostic coding in speech-language pathology and audiology programs.

Speech-language pathologists have long recognized the precariousness of medical or disease-oriented diagnostic systems for classifying speech and language disorders. Yet the codes discussed thus far are clearly based on such diagnostic systems; consequently, they intermingle essential pathologies with descriptions of communication behaviors. For example, when a client with articulatory problems and excessive nasal resonance resulting from cleft palate is seen, what ICD code should be applied? Should the fundamental physical condition of cleft palate be coded (709) or should the speech disorders, the actual basis for the involvement of the speech-language pathologist, be coded (784.49 and 784.5)? Or should all three codes be entered? The same quandary is faced by all rehabilitation services. If a child with cerebral palsy has difficulty walking, should the essential condition of cerebral palsy be coded (343) or should the gait problem be coded (781.2)?

In recognition of these problems, *The Rehabilitation Codes* make a fundamental distinction between the *cause* of the impairment (i.e., the essential pathology) and the impairment itself, defining the impairment in terms of its functional manifestations. To record the cause, therefore, one enters the appropriate ICD listing. The impairment is recorded using entries from an Impairment Code, a code that identifies the nature of the impairment and, when appropriate, the degree of limitation in one or more aspects of function. For example, in the instance of the client with cleft palate, the ICD entry for "cleft palate" would be recorded as the cause, and the functional manifestations in communication, e.g., impairment of articulation, excessive nasal resonance, etc., are recorded using the Impairment Codes.

The section of the Impairment Code of particular relevance to speech-language pathologists and audiologists includes four major sections for coding communicative disorders: Impairment of Hearing Function, Impairment of Voice Function, Impairment of Language Function, and Impairment of Speech Function. The entries for impaired hearing function cover impaired hearing sensitivity (expressed in degrees of impaired hearing sensitivity for speech), dysfunction of hearing affecting intelligibility, and other dysfunctions such as lowered tolerance for sound, inability to localize sound, and intermittent hearing impairment. The section covering impaired voice function includes absence of phonation, impairment of pitch level, impairment of loudness level, impairment of control, impairment of intonation, impairment of quality associated with phonation (breathy quality, rough quality, etc.), and impairment of quality associated with resonance. The section covering impaired language function is divided into two subsections: Impairment of Language Comprehension and Impairment of Language Use. Each of these is further subdivided as to aspects of symbolic functioning where problems are manifest, i.e., nonverbal symbols, verbal symbols (spoken and graphic), and numeric symbols. The section covering impaired speech function has entries for impairment of articulation, impairment of fluency, impairment of stress, and impairment of rate.

The structure and terminology used in *The Rehabilitation Codes* may reflect some superannuated notions about human communication processes; they were, after all, written almost 20 years ago. Nevertheless, the fundamental differentiation between functional manifestations and inherent pathology deserves serious consideration from anyone involved in designing coding systems for programs in speech-language pathology and audiology.

Iowa Quality Assurance Program System for Disorder Classifications

With the advent in the early 1970's of emphasis on peer review of all phases of health care, the Iowa Speech and Hearing Association instituted a Quality Assurance Board. The first charge to the Board was to develop procedures for "a statewide system of data retrieval, analysis, and joint problem solving." One essential facet of this effort was the adoption of a standard set of disorder classifications which could be used by all cooperating individuals and agencies in reporting service data. The Board described these efforts as "an attempt to fit traditional speech, language, and hearing terminology into a medical classification system used and understood by Medical Records persons and third-party carriers."

This system offers three types of classifications. The first involves a general heading "designed to include medical and communicative disorder terminology in one category which is concise and yet explanatory." Second, is the communicative disorders classification which offers "the specific disorders to be evaluated or treated by speech, language, and hearing pathologists." The third classification consists of the ICD code or codes which are included among the specified communication disorders.

The most recent published version of the Iowa Quality Assurance Program *Manual* (1977) predates the ICD-9-CM. As a consequence, the third classification is based on an earlier ICD system. In presenting the system, therefore, we will not attempt complete presentation of the third level of classification, but will simply note illustrative diagnoses. The system is organized into 11 major disorder categories:

1. Articulation disorder
   Communication Disorder: Articulation disorders with unknown etiology
   ICD codes: Presumably drawn from section covering specific delays in development
2. Cerebral palsy
   Communication disorder: Dysarthria and/or language deficits
   ICD codes: Cerebral palsy
3. Cerebrovascular disease, trauma, and other CNS disorders
   Communication disorder: Aphasia, apraxia, dysarthria, confused language, and/or disorientation
   ICD codes: Includes such diagnoses as cerebral hemorrhage, cerebral thrombosis, cerebral embolism, malignant neoplasm of the brain, multiple sclerosis, myasthenia gravis, etc.
4. Cleft palate and/or lip, miscellaneous craniofacial anomalies
   Communication disorder: Articulation disorder, language disorder, and/or voice disorder
   ICD codes: Includes cleft palate, cleft lip, dentofacial anomalies, anomalies of skull and face bones, etc.
5. Developmental language disorder
   Communication disorder: Deficits of receptive and/or expressive language skills
   ICD codes: Presumably drawn from section covering specific delays in development
6. Hearing loss
   Communication disorder: Receptive language

disorder, expressive language disorder, hearing disorder, speech disorder, and/or voice disorder

ICD codes: Includes entries drawn from hearing loss section as well as various entries covering specific ear diseases

7. Laryngeal disorders or disease (excluding malignant neoplasm of larynx leading to total laryngectomy)

   Communication disorder: Voice disorder

   ICD codes: Includes such entries as benign neoplasm of larynx, chronic laryngitis, polyp of vocal cord or larynx, hoarseness, etc.

8. Laryngectomy

   Communication disorder: Aphonia due to total laryngectomy

   ICD codes: Malignant neoplasm of the larynx

9. Mental retardation

   Communication disorder: Articulation disorder, language disorder, voice disorder, and/or dysfluency

   ICD codes: Mental retardation and subcategories

10. Minimal cerebral dysfunction

   Communication disorder: Language disorder, articulation disorder, voice disorder, and/or dysfluency

   ICD codes: Presumably drawn from sections covering specific delays in development

11. Stuttering

   Communication disorder: Stuttering dysfluency

   ICD codes: Stuttering and stammering

A notable contribution of the Iowa Quality Assurance classification system is that it presents a system specifically designed for use in speech-language pathology and audiology programs which is also cross-referenced with ICD. This concept may be useful when such programs are components of large centers that use ICD, because they may use terminology that is specific to their services which, nevertheless, articulates with the generally employed diagnostic code system. It is even relatively simple to program computerized information systems so that the diagnoses used in speech, language, and hearing programs can automatically be translated into ICD codes when needed.

Some theoretical questions can be raised about the Iowa Quality Assurance system. One might, for example, question the appropriateness of parallel categories which handle such general descriptions of communication problems as "articulation disorder" and such medical diagnostic classifications as "cerebrovascular disease, trauma, and other CNS disorders." Furthermore, problems seem inherent in separating clients into such categories as "developmental language disorder" and "minimal cerebral dysfunction." Nevertheless, the system seems functional, and whatever confusions exist can be resolved on the basis of common agreement among the clinicians using the system.

The CASE Classification Schema

The *CASE Information System* (1976) has already been described in some detail. The system employs a classification schema throughout which is highly economical but which, nevertheless, can be extremely useful when relatively broad categories of communicative disorders suffice. The schema differentiates between "communication disorders" and "communication differences." The latter are defined as "maturational or cultural/ethnic linguistic variations that are not considered communication disorders." This is the only system of those discussed that makes such a differentiation, a provision that may make it particularly useful in some service settings.

The communication disorders are subclassified as follows (pp. 26–28)

A. *Articulation disorder* is defined as the abnormal production of one or more phonemes (speech sounds). There are four basic types of abnormal productions: Omission of phonemes, substitution of one phoneme for another, phonemic distortions, and the inappropriate addition of a phoneme.

B. *Language disorder* is defined as the abnormal acquisition, comprehension, or use (including all receptive and expressive language skills) of spoken or written language. The disorder may involve all, one, or some combination of the phonologic, morphologic, semantic, or syntactic components of the linguistic system. Individuals with a language disorder frequently have problems in sentence processing or in abstracting information meaningfully for storage and retrieval from short- and long-term memory. For the purposes of this classification system, the following definitions are operational:

—Phonologic disorder involves the sound system of a language: the particular sounds that comprise the sound system and the ways in which the rules of a language permit them to be combined to form larger units of a language such as words.

—Morphologic disorder involves the structure of words and the construction of word forms from the basic elements of meaning: morphemes. Inflectional suffixes indicating plurality and tense are examples of morphologic units.

—Semantic disorder involves the meaning of individual words and the combination of word meanings to form the meaning of a sentence.

—Syntactic disorder involves the rules governing the order and combination of morphemes in the formation of sentences and the relationships among the elements within a sentence or between two or more sentences.

C. *Voice disorder* is defined as the absence or abnormal production of voice characterized by defective vocal quality, pitch, and/or loudness.

D. *Fluency disorder* is defined as the abnormal flow of verbal expression, including rate and rhythm.

E. *Hearing impairment* is defined as abnormal hearing sensitivity and/or damage to the integrity of the physiological auditory system. An individual with a hearing impairment has a communication disorder when the abnormality in the physiological auditory system prevents or impedes normal development, comprehension, use, or maintenance of effective communication behaviors.

Although the simplest system discussed thus far, the CASE classification schema offers many advantages, not the least of which is its essential simplicity. It also is exclusively based on data accrued by speech-language pathologists and audiologists, since no medical diagnoses are required to classify a client's problem. The schema is, therefore, most applicable in programs where relatively broad categorizations of disorders suffice and where clinicians must rely primarily on information accrued by speech-language pathologists and audiologists.

There are, nevertheless, no inherent restrictions on expanding the system, with specific refinements within the broader classifications. Individual programs could effect whatever refinements they consider useful. Furthermore, as with the Iowa Quality Assurance system, a program could articulate the CASE schema with a more comprehensive system like ICD, so that each category could translate automatically into a comparable ICD code. The schema could also serve the approach proposed by *The Rehabilitation Codes*. ICD entries could be used to record underlying pathologies and the CASE schema used to enter the manifest communicative disorders.

PROCEDURE CODING

Two factors have spurred speech-language pathology and audiology programs toward standardization of terminology referring to the services they provide: the mounting emphasis on accountability and our increasing reliance on fees for services. Both factors require clear and consistent designation of whatever services have been provided. Furthermore, particularly in larger institutional contexts, the nomenclature used must be comprehensible to other professionals, to administrators, to clerical personnel, and to the clients served. Since this information is increasingly processed through automated systems, it must, in addition, be already coded or lend itself to coding.

Fewer standard systems have been devised for procedure coding than for diagnostic coding. Nevertheless, as with diagnostic codes, in some settings speech-language pathologists and audiologists may be required to report information according to an overall system adopted by the institution in which they are employed. In other instances, they may adopt a system exclusively designed to cover our professional services. Two standard systems for institutional applications will be considered here: *Standard Terminology for Curriculum and Instruction in Local and State School Systems*, a system developed for application in schools; and *Physicians' Current Procedural Terminology* (CPT), which is used in health services programs. Since neither of these systems permits sufficiently discrete coding of our services, more specifically applicable, although nonstandard, procedures will also be considered.

Standard Terminology for Curriculum and Instruction

This system was developed under the auspices of the National Center for Educational Statistics as one aspect of a larger series of manuals to assist education agencies in the development of improved records and reports. The project was described as "the result of five years of cooperative effort by some 70 national organizations and the Office of Education." (ASHA was one of the participating organizations.) The system seeks to codify information about the organization, administration, content, resources, and processes of instruction offered by education agencies or by specific units within those agencies. The scope of the system extends far beyond designations of procedures and services offered, but specifications of data about procedures and services are included.

This system is divided into five major groups of items: (1) *Items describing a school system* (10000 Series): These items characterize an entire school system, including the age span served, the evaluation services employed, and the instructional and supportive services provided. (2) *Items describing a school* (20000 Series): These items describe a specific school within a system in terms of such factors as schedules, pupils served, and instructional and supportive services provided. (3) *Items describing a program of studies* (30000 Series): A "program of studies" is defined as a "combination of related courses and/or self-contained classes organized for the attainment of specific educational objectives" (including programs of special education for handicapped children). These items include scheduling, pupils served, requirements for admission, and programs provided. As described, the two remaining series, *items describing a self-contained class, course or co-curricular activity* (40000 Series) and *items describing a section or instructional service activity* (50000 Series), include no listings directly applicable to coding speech, language, and hearing services or other special education and related services. (There is no explanation as to the basis of accounting for self-contained special education classes as programs in the 30000 Series, rather than in the 40000 Series that presumably applies to "self-contained" classes.)

Within this broad framework, specific programs can be accounted for in two different ways: in terms of the types of pupils served and in terms of the services offered. A standard taxonomy is provided and coded. In the taxonomy, the first place is coded with an X. For example, "mentally retarded" is coded X0960.30 and "school psychological services" is coded X3223. When entered into a records system, however, the X is replaced with the appropriate digit from the five major groups. For example, to indicate that a particular school district serves mentally retarded pupils the code would be 10960.30, and to indicate that a school district provides psychological services the code would be 13223. On the other hand, if the same information were recorded about a specific school within the district, the codes would be 20960.30 and 23223, respectively.

Within the section of the taxonomy entitled "pupils served," there is a subsection entitled "pupils outside the normal range of ability and performance." (All codes within this section begin X0960.) Within that subsection there is a further division entitled "physically handicapped" (coded X0960.40). Included within this division are the codes for deaf (X0960.43), hard of hearing (X0960.44), and speech impaired (X0960.45).

Our professional services are covered within the section of "services supporting instruction" (X3200 Series). Hearing screening (X3222.12) is included among health services. Speech pathology services are coded X3224.10, and audiology services are coded X3224.20. Other services that might be provided by speech-language pathologists and audiologists are placement services (X3221.70), communication to parents about health problems in children (X3222.50), working with other staff members (X3223.50), referral for further clinical diagnosis and treatment (X3223.60), and providing in-service education (X3236).

Standard Terminology for Curriculum and Instruction obviously affords little opportunity for discrete coding of speech-language pathology and audiology services. On the other hand, as was proposed for the broad diagnostic coding systems, one can refine the codes and still preserve the integrity of the system. For example, to detail specific services provided by a school district audiology program, one could elaborate the general code designation 13224.20 by adding one or two digits to the standard code to refer to diagnostic hearing testing, hearing aid evaluation, acoustic analysis of hearing aids, or whatever. For broader accounting purposes, then, the standard code notation would show that audiologic services were provided, but for supplementary or internal reporting, the exact services would also be recorded.

ICD-9-CM Procedure Codes

Although the third volume of ICD-9-CM is devoted to the classification of diagnostic and treatment procedures, that system has not been as widely accepted in health services programs in the United States as the ICD diagnostic codes. This may be partially attributable to the lack of refinement in many areas of the ICD procedure codes. For example, the following codes are offered for the description of "nonoperative procedures related to hearing":

95.41 Audiometry
    Bekesy 5-tone audiometry
    Impedance audiometry
    Stapedial reflex response
    Subjective audiometry
    Tympanogram
95.42 Clinical test of hearing
    Tuning fork test
    Whispered speech test
95.43 Audiological evaluation
    Audiological evaluation by:
        Barany noise machine
        Blindfold test
        Delayed feedback
        Masking
        Weber lateralization
95.44 Clinical vestibular function tests
    Thermal test of vestibular function
95.45 Rotation tests
    Barany chair
95.46 Other auditory and vestibular function tests
95.47 Hearing examination, not otherwise specified
95.48 Fitting of hearing aid
95.49 Other nonoperative procedures related to hearing

Under a category for "speech and reading rehabilitation and rehabilitation of the blind" are the following ICD listings:

93.71 Dyslexia training
93.72 Dysphasia training
93.73 Esophageal speech training
93.74 Speech defect training
93.75 Other speech training and therapy

Physicians' Current Procedural Terminology (CPT)

The most widely used standard coding system for health services procedures is the *Physicians' Current Procedural Terminology* (CPT) published by the American Medical Association. The nature and purpose of the CPT is stated in the introduction (p. iii):

> Physicians' *Current Procedural Terminology* (CPT) is a listing of descriptive terms and identifying codes for reporting medical services and procedures performed by physicians. The purpose of the terminology is to provide a uniform language that will accurately designate medical, surgical and diagnostic services, and will thereby provide an effective means for reliable, nationwide communication among physicians, patients, and third parties.

Even though the CPT is intended for physician use and is clearly structured to serve that purpose, many speech-language pathologists and audiologists must become familiar with this system. Not only is familiarity important to those employed in health care institutions, it may be important for anyone who seeks to recover third-party payment from health insurance carriers, which may require the use of CPT codes on claim forms. In instances where it is not required, the likelihood of coverage may increase when CPT codes are used.

Unequivocally, CPT is intended for use by physicians to describe procedures they personally administer or are administered under their immediate supervision. This intent is patently clear in listings applicable to speech-language pathology and audiology found in the section entitled "special otorhinolaryngologic services." The introduction defines them as "those diagnostic and treatment services not usually included in a comprehensive otorhinolaryngologic evaluation or office visit." It further specifies that all of the listed services include a "medical diagnostic evaluation," explaining that "technical procedures (which may or may not be performed by the physician personally) are often part of the service, but should not be mistaken to constitute the service itself." These assertions, however, cannot be reconciled with some of the actual listings found in the section, where any physician participation would be extremely unusual. The otolaryngologic services section contains three listings referable to speech-language pathology services:

92506 Medical evaluation speech, language and/or hearing problems
92507 Speech, language or hearing therapy with continuing medical supervision, individual
92508 Group session

Elsewhere in the CPT, in the neurology section, a listing occurs that is also referable to speech-language pathology services:

95880 Assessment of higher cerebral function with medical interpretation; aphasia testing

Among the otorhinolaryngologic procedures is also found a listing of audiologic procedures:

Basic Audiometry

92551 Screening test, pure tone, air only
92552 Pure-tone audiometry (threshold), air only
92553 Pure-tone audiometry (threshold), air and bone
92555 Speech audiometry, threshold only
92556 Speech audiometry, threshold and discrimination
92557 Basic comprehensive audiometry (92553 and 92556 combined) (pure tone, air and bone, and speech, threshold and discrimination)
92559 Audiometric testing of groups

Audiologic Tests

92560 Bekesy audiometry, screening
92561 Bekesy audiometry, diagnostic
92562 Loudness balance test, alternate binaural or monaural
92563 Tone decay test
92564 Short increment sensitivity index (SISI)
92565 Stenger test, pure tone
92566 Impedance testing
92567 Tympanometry
92568 Acoustic reflex testing
92569 Acoustic reflex decay test
92571 Filtered speech test
92572 Staggered spondaic word test
92573 Lombard test
92574 Swinging story test
92575 Sensorineural acuity level test
92576 Synthetic sentence identification test
92577 Stenger test, speech
92578 Delayed auditory feedback test

Special Audiometric Function Tests

92580 Electrodermal audiometry
92581 Evoked response (EEG) audiometry
92582 Conditioning play audiometry
92583 Select picture audiometry
92584 Electrocochleography
92585 Brainstem evoked response recording
92589 Central auditory function test(s) (specify)
92590 Hearing aid examination and selection; monaural
92591 Hearing aid examination and selection; binaural
92592 Hearing aid check; monaural
92593 Hearing aid check; binaural
92594 Electroacoustic evaluation for hearing aid; monaural
92595 Electroacoustic evaluation for hearing aid; binaural

Other Procedures

92599 Unlisted otorhinolaryngological service or procedure

In addition to the wide direct applications of the CPT, it has served as the basis for the development of other procedural coding systems, for example in the relative value scales developed by local and state medical associations and the services accounting and billing procedures used by individual health care institutions.

NONSTANDARD SYSTEMS FOR CODING SPEECH-LANGUAGE PATHOLOGY AND AUDIOLOGY PROCEDURES

Applying such medical systems as CPT to procedure coding for our professional services incurs at least two important risks. First and foremost, acceptance of such a system may well imply acceptance of its premise that the procedures are appropriately considered as services provided by a technician under the direct supervision of a physician. This premise is unacceptable to most members of our profession. Second, at least with respect to audiologic procedures, it focuses exclusively on tests, implying that the test used represents the hallmark of the procedure, and, by implication, that the tests listed are acceptable and others are not.

Approximately 10 years ago, an ASHA task force developed a detailed procedural coding system for speech-language pathology and audiology services. Regrettably, because of extraneous circumstances, that system failed to receive the recognition it deserved. The system was devised to support the development of relative value scales (an approach discussed in a later chapter). In view of some important questions about the legality of professional association relative value scales, the task force disbanded and the project was abandoned. Nevertheless, the task force made a notable contribution in preparing, for the first time, a comprehensive coding system for speech-language pathologists and audiologists entitled "Guidelines for Speech and Hearing Services" (1973):

Professional Services

Code No.	Service
10.00	Basic hearing evaluation
10.01	Bilateral speech reception threshold
10.02	Bilateral auditory discrimination
10.03	Bilateral pure-tone audiometry (air and bone)
10.04	Bilateral hearing screening (nonthreshold air)
20.00	Site of lesion hearing evaluation
20.01	Bekesy audiometry (sweep frequency)
20.02	Bekesy audiometry (fixed frequency)
20.03	Short Increment Sensitivity Index (SISI)
20.04	Loudness balance (alternate binaural)
20.05	Loudness balance (monaural bifrequency)
20.06	Tone decay test
20.07	Sensorineural acuity level (SAL)
20.08	Filtered speech tests
20.09	Competing message tests
20.10	Tympanometry
20.11	Evoked response audiometry (ERA)
20.12	Electronystagmography (ENG)
20.13	Modified Weber test for lateralization
20.99	Report of site of lesion hearing evaluation results
30.00	Validation of organicity hearing evaluation
30.01	Doerfler-Stewart test
30.02	Electrodermal audiometry (EDA)
30.03	Stenger test (pure tone or speech)
30.04	Shifting voice test
30.05	Delayed auditory feedback
30.99	Report of validation of organicity test results
40.00	Preschool hearing evaluation (birth to 6)
40.01	Observation of behavior to auditory stimuli
40.02	Conditioned orienting response (COR)
40.03	Tangible Reinforcement of Operant Conditioned audiometry (TROCA)
40.04	Play audiometry
40.99	Report of evaluation
50.00	Hearing aid selection evaluation
50.01	Prescriptive hearing aid recommendation resulting from user performance evaluation
50.01.1	Repetition of 50.01 within 3 months
50.02	Prescriptive hearing aid recommendations without user performance evaluation
50.02.1	Repetition of 50.02 within 3 months
50.03	Evaluation of user performance with hearing aid
50.99	Report of evaluation
60.00	Auditory rehabilitation (audiological habilitation)
60.01	Hearing aid orientation (individual, 1 hour)
60.02	Hearing aid orientation (group, 1 hour)
60.03	Auditory training (individual, 1 hour)
60.04	Auditory training (group, 1 hour)
60.05	Speechreading (individual, 1 hour)
60.06	Speechreading (group, 1 hour)
60.07	Speech conservation of hearing impaired (individual, 1 hour)
60.08	Speech conservation of hearing impaired (group, 1 hour)
60.09	Extended counseling
60.99	Report of rehabilitation
70.00	Speech, voice, and language evaluation
70.01	Speech evaluation

70.02	Voice evaluation
70.03	Language evaluation
70.99	Report of evaluation
80.00	Speech, voice, and language rehabilitation
80.01	Speech therapy (individual, 1 hour)
80.02	Speech therapy (group, 1 hour)
80.03	Voice therapy (individual, 1 hour)
80.04	Voice therapy (group, 1 hour)
80.05	Language therapy (individual, 1 hour)
80.06	Language therapy (group, 1 hour)
80.99	Final report of therapy
Technical Services	
500.00	Hearing aid-related duties
500.01	Assessment of electroacoustic hearing aid response
500.02	Trouble-shooting for hearing aid mechanical failure
500.03	Cleaning and adjusting hearing aid
500.04	Cleaning earmold
500.05	Provision of hearing aid accessories
500.06	Provision of loaner aid
500.07	Earmold impression (one ear)
500.08	Earmold impression (two ears)
500.09	Providing and fitting earmold
500.10	Providing and fitting hearing aid

These procedure codes have obviously not been updated since their publication a decade ago. Some procedures are omitted that are now in use; some that are included are no longer in common use. Nevertheless, it remains a useful model for one approach to procedure coding. This approach, however, should be used only for internal coding procedures, i.e., for analyzing those procedures conducted within a particular program or facility. It has many inherent hazards when applied to any external professional, administrative, or regulatory entity as the basis for developing fee schedules or for preparing data. This contention is based on four considerations:

1. Because of its technical terminology, the procedure listings can be understood only by people who are familiar with the field of speech-language pathology and audiology. Most members of other professions—let alone administrative and clerical personnel—do not understand these designations. Not only does this impede communication, it can also have serious economic consequences for speech-language pathologists and for their clients. Most decisions as to whether a particular service is to be covered by third-party payers—both public and private—are made by professionals and clerks who know little about our field. It is essential, therefore, that procedures be identified in terms that they can understand.
2. The system is overdetailed, making it unnecessarily complex. For example, is it really necessary to differentiate between hearing aid orientation (60.01) and counseling (60.09)? Or how would one code an aural rehabilitation session that included auditory training (60.03), speech reading (60.05), and speech conservation (60.07)? Or would a therapy session for a child with phonologic problems and other language problems be coded as speech therapy (80.01) or language therapy (80.05)? Whatever small advantages accrue from such detailed procedure designations do not justify the confusions that are inevitable, both in recording and interpreting data—particularly when the interpreter is not a member of our profession.
3. In its emphasis on specific techniques, rather than on the total professional service delivered, such a system of procedure designations can place speech-language pathologists and, in particular, audiologists in untenable positions. Many delivery systems, especially health care systems, assign the privilege of authorizing speech, language, and hearing services to members of other professions. These privileges are institutionalized in all manner of policies and regulations, most particularly in those policies and regulations determining payment for services. If we provide these other professionals with a standard vocabulary of procedures based on specific techniques, they have no choice but to specify the technique to be employed when they authorize a service.
4. Although the time spent in providing a particular service is one feature to be considered in defining procedures, designations should not specify exact times. Such specification is most likely to occur in designations of therapy sessions. If the exact times are mentioned in procedure codes, two problems may arise. First, when a member of another profession must authorize the service, he or she will be empowered to determine the length of the sessions that will be authorized. Furthermore, the speech-language pathologist or audiologist providing the service may be required to account, to the minute, for the time spent, instead of exercising professional judgment as to how long a particular client can cooperate and be productively engaged in therapeutic activities.

A preferable procedure coding system, then, is one that permits categorization of our primary professional services, is reasonably understandable to other professionals and clerical personnel, and permits referral for and authorization of services without dictating the way in which the service is to be carried out. The following system meets these criteria:

01 *Hearing Screening*

This category covers the audiologic procedures that are carried out to identify clients who should be seen for more complete hearing evaluations. These screening procedures may be administered to individual clients or to groups of clients. (When necessary it may be divided into two procedure designations: hearing screening, individual and hearing screening, group.)

02 *Basic Hearing Evaluation*

This category includes those procedures routinely carried out to describe a client's hearing function. In usual practice this includes pure-tone audiometry (air and bone), speech reception and speech discrimination testing, and impedance measurement. It may also involve one or more screening techniques to determine whether further special diagnostic procedures should be administered. This evaluation also involves taking a case history, interpreting test findings, and making recommendations.

03 *Children's Hearing Evaluation*

This category assumes that the client has not reached the level of development where he or she can participate in the standard procedures that comprise a basic hearing evaluation. The goal remains, nevertheless, to achieve as much of the information yielded by those standard procedures as possible. Usually more time is required, special testing procedures are employed, and a second audiologist or test assistant participates. This procedure also entails discussions with families to obtain case histories and to interpret findings and recommendations. It also frequently involves contacts with school agencies and other community services.

04 *Special Diagnostic Hearing Evaluation*

This category includes those more extensive and specialized procedures used in the identification of sites of lesions in the auditory system, to differentiate organic versus functional components in the results of basic hearing evaluations, or to further assess clients who are unable or unwilling to cooperate in the voluntary procedures incorporated in categories 02 and 03. In usual practice, these procedures supplement those included in the previous two categories and are pursued on the recommendation of the audiologist who provided those preliminary evaluations. The tests employed in special diagnostic hearing evaluations may range from Bekesy audiometry and tone decay testing to auditory evoked response measurement. Case history data have customarily been acquired as a part of the previous evaluations, but detailed interpretations of findings is usually required.

05 *Follow-up Hearing Evaluation*

This category is used to designate those procedures of greater magnitude than screening but less detailed than those described by 02, 03, and 04. It may be applied in instances where one or more additional visits are required to complete one of the previously designated procedures. Or it may be applied in instances where abbreviated testing sessions are scheduled to assess the results of surgery or medical treatment, or to determine the pattern and extent of fluctuating hearing impairments.

06 *Hearing Aid Selection Evaluation*

This category encompasses all procedures employed to make recommendations about the use of amplification, including whether it should be used at all, and the specification of characteristics of the amplification that may be beneficial (sometimes identifying the specific instrument by make and model). It also includes considerable counseling of clients and families.

07 *Hearing Aid Selection Follow-up*

This category covers all follow-up services provided in visits following those described by 06. It includes assessment of the electroacoustic characteristics of the hearing aid and the client's performance with and adjustment to amplification. Orientation to hearing aid use, as well as other counseling, is provided in this category. These procedures are distinguished from the follow-up procedures described by 05 and the counseling procedures defined in 08 for practical reasons. Many third-party payers specifically exclude hearing aid-related services from coverage; hence, it is wise to identify clearly those services conducted in connection with hearing aid selection, fitting, and orientation.

08 *Audiologic Counseling and Therapy, Individual*

This category covers counseling services that extend beyond those usually included with evaluation procedures. It also covers all therapy sessions that focus on helping hearing-impaired children and adults to improve their communication.

09 *Audiologic Counseling and Therapy, Group*

This category resembles 08, except that the services are provided to groups of clients rather than to individuals.

10 *Speech-Language Screening*

This category includes procedures administered for the purpose of identifying people who should be seen for further speech-language evaluations.

11 *Speech-Language Evaluation*
This category covers all formal and informal assessment procedures employed for the description of speech and language disorders to arrive at recommendations for management. It also involves the interviews required to complete a case history and the interpretation of findings and recommendations. It often entails contacts with schools and other community agencies.

12 *Speech-Language Follow-up Evaluation*
This category covers any subsequent visits required to complete the evaluation described by 11, or it may be used for abbreviated re-evaluations (e.g., for re-evaluating clients previously discharged from therapy).

13 *Speech-Language Therapy, Individual*
This category embraces all procedures used to assist individual clients in the amelioration of communication problems associated with speech, language, and voice disorders.

14 *Speech-Language Therapy, Group*
This category includes all procedures in which two or more clients are simultaneously engaged in programs seeking the amelioration of communication problems associated with speech, language, and voice disorders.

When used as the basis for the development of fee schedules or for the analysis of services provided by a facility or by individual staff members within a facility, these categories may be too broad. For example, the Special Diagnostic Hearing Evaluation category may apply to comparatively brief testing sessions or to complete auditory brainstem response (ABR) testing. These procedures may differ substantially, both in terms of time requirements and in the amount of special equipment required. Or the Speech-Language Therapy category might cover brief sessions conducted at bedside for stroke victims during early recovery and also cover hour-long sessions for fully cooperative clients, provided on an outpatient basis. It is usually necessary, therefore, to further delimit these broad categories. As a rule, this is best effected by using, as needed, the subcategories, *brief, limited,* and *extended.* Thus, using the same examples, a facility might use the procedure designation 041 Special Diagnostic Hearing Evaluation, Limited to denote an evaluation that included a battery of three or four tests commonly used to identify sites of lesion, and use the designation 042 Special Diagnostic Hearing Evaluation, Extended to cover such instances of extensive testing as ABR. Or a facility might use the procedure designation 131 Speech-Language Therapy, Individual, Brief to cover the abbreviated bedside session; 132 Speech-Language Therapy, Individual, Limited to cover sessions of approximately 30 minutes' duration; and 133 Speech-Language Therapy, Extended to cover sessions of 50 minutes or longer.

Facilities that use procedure designations such as these usually define what the designations signify in the procedure manuals that are required by most accrediting agencies and by many third-party carriers. Furthermore, and particularly when third-party payers are involved, client records should clearly show that the established criteria have been met for whatever procedure designations are applied.

Even with these three modifiers, however, this procedure coding system may lack sufficient precision for internal analyses of speech-language pathology and audiology programs. In these instances, further refinements, such as use of decimal coding, can be introduced (for example, reflecting the specific testing procedures employed in the course of a child's hearing evaluation or a special diagnostic hearing evaluation, or in documenting whether a follow-up evaluation was a postoperative study or monitoring someone being treated with an ototoxic drug). In these instances only the major procedure designations would be used for general accounting or billing procedures or for other external reporting. When more detailed analyses are needed, the refined or elaborated procedures codes can be used.

SUMMARY

Human services systems, particularly health care systems, are increasingly using standardized coding systems to denote diagnoses and clinical procedures. Such systems serve two major purposes. They offer nomenclatures that facilitate inter- and intraprofessional communication and serve administrative functions. They also meet the vocabulary requirements of modern information-processing technologies.

Regrettably, the major standardized systems for coding diagnoses and clinical procedures have many shortcomings for application by speech-language pathologists and audiologists. Most can, however, be adapted or expanded for our use. There is, nonetheless, an urgent need for the development of codes for accurate recording of clinical data in speech-language pathology and audiology.

References

American Medical Association: *Physicians' Current Procedural Terminology*. Chicago, American Medical Association, 1981.

American Speech-Language-Hearing Association: *CASE Information System*. Rockville, MD, American Speech-Language-Hearing Association, 1976.

American Psychiatric Association: *Diagnostic and Statistical Manual of Mental Disorders*, ed 3. Washington DC, American Psychiatric Association, 1980.

Guidelines for speech and hearing services. *ASHA* 15:351–352, 1973.

Iowa Quality Assurance Program: *Manual*. Cedar Rapids, IA, Iowa Speech and Hearing Association, 1977.

National Conference of Nomenclature: *Standard Nomenclature of Diseases and Operations*. New York, McGraw Hill, 1961.

The Rehabilitation Codes. New York, The Rehabilitation Codes, Inc., 1967.

United States National Center for Health Statistics: *International Classification of Diseases, 9th Revision, Clinical Modification*. Ann Arbor, MI, Commission on Professional and Hospital Activities, 1978.

United States Office of Education: *Standard Terminology for Curriculum and Instruction in Local and State School Systems*. Washington DC, United States Government Printing Office, 1970.

PART 3

The Economics of Delivering Speech-Language Pathology and Audiology Services

CHAPTER NINE

Computing the Costs of Speech-Language Pathology and Audiology Services

I once participated in a conversation with a group of colleagues who worked in programs supported primarily by client fees. We were joined by an audiologist who was employed by a county health department. After listening for a while to our concerns about our financial problems, he commented, "I'm certainly glad I work in a program where services don't cost anything!"

The audiologist's economic naïveté is regrettably prevalent among members of our profession. Presumably, he received a salary check each month. The secretary who made his appointments and typed his letters and reports was also paid. Someone bought the equipment he used and the supplies he consumed in conducting his program. Someone also paid the rent, the mortgage, or had made capital construction outlays to provide the facilities in which he carried out his practice. Yet, since his clients paid nothing for the services he provided, he concluded that no costs were entailed.

A business person who confuses the price—what is paid for a product or a service by a consumer or by some agent in behalf of the consumer—with cost—what the provider pays to make possible delivery of the product or service—will soon file for bankruptcy. The ultimate future of any similarly confused professional is not likely to be much brighter.

An old saying deplores people who consider "the price of everything and the value of nothing." Equally deplorable are professionals who consider the value of everything and the cost of nothing. Too frequently, professionals who participate in the human services delivery system consider what they do to be so meritorious that it should be immune from examination for cost effectiveness. But even in this "era of limits" we are still seeing escalation in costs within some segments of that system that outstrip any other inflationary spiral. No longer can any human services profession, agency, or organization claim immunity from rigorous financial accountability. Furthermore, everyone who delivers human services, whatever the setting in which he or she works and whatever his or her responsibilities within that setting, must maintain personal accountability for the cost of those services.

SOME BASIC CONSIDERATIONS IN COST COMPUTATION

Regardless of the setting in which speech-language pathology and audiology services are delivered, the essential similarities in cost computation outweigh the differences. However, three different factors may obscure those similarities. First are semantic factors, that is, the vocabularies employed in cost computations (for example, the vocabulary employed by a school administrator may be quite different from the vocabulary of a hospital administrator). Second is the amount of insulation between a clinician and direct involvement in cost-related matters. Whereas a solo private practitioner may hourly confront decisions related to out-of-pocket expenditures, a speech-language pathologist in a mammoth general hospital or a large school district may hear discussions of cost factors only at occasional staff meetings or through sporadic administrative bulletins. Third, the form of cost analysis may vary according to the purpose served. Cost analyses in private practice and in many private health services may primarily serve in the establishment of fee schedules. In school settings, analyses may serve as the basis for budget requests, applications for excess cost reimbursement, and in efforts toward new legislation. In community agencies, they serve as the basis for initiating budget requests to funding sources and for seeking new sources of support, particularly for new programs.

It is in this third respect that cost-price confusions are most likely to occur. Cost analyses must be conducted quite independently of considerations of how those costs are to be covered, i.e., of what prices are to be affixed to the services to be delivered (in this context "price" refers both to fees for individual services and to grants or allocations to cover entire programs of services). Nevertheless, a cost analysis must always provide the basis for affixing a fair price to each service.

To this end, cost analysis must clearly differentiate between *direct* costs and *indirect* costs. As applied to clinical services, direct costs represent those that can be allocated differentially among various services. Indirect costs are those that are shared equally by all services. For example, assume that a speech-language pathology and audiology program includes among its services speech-language therapy for adult clients, hearing aid evaluations, and special audiologic assessment procedures involving auditory brainstem response measurement. Each of these procedures differs significantly in terms of the professional time involved, the facilities used, the equipment employed, the supplies consumed, and the professional and clerical staff time involved for preparation of reports and other follow-up procedures. These factors figure in the computation of direct costs. On the other hand, the costs of overall administration of an agency, costs for basic records maintenance, and costs for billing, insurance claims processing, or otherwise seeking financial support are generally independent of the particular service being offered and must be shared equally, as indirect costs, among all services.

The emphasis on clear differentiation between direct and indirect costs may seem precious, but this differentiation can have crucial implications. As will be discussed later, many hospital-based speech-language pathology and audiology programs fail because they are held accountable for extortionate indirect costs. Without this clear distinction it may be impossible to derive fee schedules that can be defended against inquiries by third-party payers. Increasingly, financially beleaguered school districts are demanding precise delineations of costs to determine whether specific programs should be abandoned, provided jointly with other districts, or contracted out to independent providers. In each of these instances, the survival of a speech-language pathology and audiology program may depend upon scrupulous cost analysis procedures that accurately differentiate between direct and indirect costs.

Programs differ in the terminology applied to designate cost categories. Most, however, use some version of these five categories: *personnel*, *facilities*, *equipment*, *supplies*, and *other expenses*. Cost analysis usually involves two steps. First, costs are allotted among these categories. Second, costs are functionalized, i.e., costs are assigned according to the various functions of the agency or institution.

Personnel

In any clinical services program, the largest cost item should occur in connection with supplying the personnel required to deliver those services. Depending on the program, personnel costs may be allotted according to a one-stage or a two-stage procedure. The first stage involves allotting costs as direct or indirect expenses. The second stage involves functional allocation of direct costs. Programs in which all staff members carry essentially similar clinical responsibilities may employ only the first stage. When substantially different responsibilities are carried by various staff members, the two-stage procedure is necessary to achieve a fair allocation of personnel costs.

Five different personnel categories can be defined: *direct services professional personnel, direct services support personnel, professional supervisory personnel, administrative personnel*, and *clerical personnel.* The first category is self-explanatory, consisting of professionals who are directly engaged in the delivery of speech-language pathology and audiology services. Direct services support personnel consist of those employees who are paraprofessionals or aides, also directly engaged in the delivery of services (e.g., therapy assistants, audiometric assistants). Professional services supervisory personnel refer to the employees engaged in the supervision of professional staff and of whatever support personnel deliver clinical services (sometimes this includes students). Administrative personnel are involved in the planning and facilitation of services but are not directly involved in services delivery. Clerical personnel engage in activities directly related to clinical services (preparing reports, making appointments, etc.) and in activities that relate to overall administrative functions (billing, accounting procedures, records maintenance, etc.).

In all but the largest programs, a single employee's responsibilities may be allotted into two or more categories. For example, a single staff member may carry administrative responsibilities, supervise other staff, and provide direct clinical services.

To illustrate the first stage of personnel cost analysis, consider the example of a speech-language pathology department in a rehabilitation center. The department employs four speech-language pathologists, Brenda Callister, Sigrid Nordstrom, Wendell Slater, and Sheila Cohen. One secretary, Sylvia Stevens, is employed full time by the department; another, Jerry Barrett, spends half time in speech-language pathology and half time in another department. Analysis of previous years' schedules showed that vacation and professional leave, attendance at administrative staff meetings and in-service education programs, and other activities that were not directly assignable to clinical services delivery accounted for an average of 25% of all staff members' time. In addition to this time allotment, Ms. Callister functions as department head, accounting for another 35% of her time. Ms. Nordstrom occasionally assists Ms. Callister in administrative activities and supervises Ms. Cohen, who is completing her clinical fellowship this year; together these responsibilities account for 25% of her time (15% for administrative and 10% for supervision). Of the two secretaries, Ms. Stevens devotes 50% of her time to activities referable to direct clinical services, and Mr. Barrett spends about 45% of his total work week in direct clinical service-related activities in the department. Table 9.1 shows the completion of the first stage of personnel cost analysis for the department.

The second stage of analysis of personnel costs entails allocation of direct costs to each of the clinical services provided. Dif-

Table 9.1.
Direct/Indirect Personnel Cost Allocation

Category	Staff Member	Total Salary and Benefits	Direct Cost		Indirect Cost	
			% Time Allocated	Salary Allocated	% Time Allocated	Salary Allocated
Direct services professionals	Callister	$40,960	40	$16,384	25	$10,240
	Nordstrom	34,193	50	17,097	25	8,548
	Slater	31,304	75	23,478	25	7,826
	Cohen	22,618	75	16,964	25	5,655
Professional supervisory personnel	Nordstrom	34,193	10	3,419		
Administrative personnel	Callister	40,960			35	14,336
	Nordstrom	34,193			15	5,129
Clerical personnel	Stevens	18,462	50	9,231	50	9,231
	Barrett*	16,304	45	7,337	5	815
Total				$93,910		$61,780

* Half-time, also assigned to another department.

ferent services require different amounts of professional time and clerical support. In addition, more experienced, hence higher salaried, staff members may be assigned to different services than are less experienced staff members. The services assigned to less experienced professional staff or to support personnel will, on the other hand, require greater allocation of supervisor time. A functional personnel cost analysis requires consideration of each of these factors.

Table 9.2 illustrates this second stage of analysis on the same speech-language pathology department analyzed in Table 9.1. That department provides three different services: speech-language therapy for individual clients, group speech-language therapy, and speech-language evaluations. The functional analysis is based on the previous year's experience when 2,592 individual therapy visits, 956 group therapy visits, and 514 evaluations were provided. Each staff member's schedule for that year was then analyzed, and the approximate distribution of time among each of the three services was estimated. The secretarial time that was directly assignable to each procedure was also estimated. These time estimates were then converted into cost estimates so that direct personnel costs for these services could be computed.

Different approaches can be used to allocate indirect personnel costs. Although no system is entirely equitable, the fairest involves allocation of indirect costs in proportion to direct costs. Returning to the same example, in Step 1 (Table 9.1), direct personnel costs totaled $93,910. Step 2 showed that 49% of those direct costs were allotted to individual speech-language therapy; 12% to group speech-language therapy; and 39% to speech-language evaluations. Applying those same proportions to indirect costs, which totaled $61,780, would allot $30,272 in indirect personnel costs to individual speech-language therapy, $7,414 to group therapy, and $24,094 to speech-language evaluations. Finally, then, total personnel costs (both direct and indirect) can be allotted to these procedures at $76,220, $18,846, and $60,625, respectively.

As described here, personnel cost computations are based on the previous year's allocation of staff responsibilities. Obviously, this approach cannot be applied when significant changes in assignments occur or when new services are added. In these instances one simply makes educated guesses about the implications of these changes and computes costs accordingly. Many clinical services programs create serious financial problems by enthusiastically

Table 9.2.
Functional Allocation of Direct Personnel Costs

Category	Staff Member	Total Salary and Benefits	Individual Therapy (2,592 Visits)		Group Therapy (956 Visits)		Evaluations (514 Visits)	
			% Time Allocated	Salary Allocated	% Time Allocated	Salary Allocated	% Time Allocated	Salary Allocated
Direct services professionals	Callister	$40,960	18	$ 7,373			22	$ 9,011
	Nordstrom	34,193	22	7,522	6	$ 2,052	22	7,522
	Slater	31,304	38	11,896	15	4,696	22	6,887
	Cohen	22,618	50	11,309	10	2,262	25	3,393
Professional supervisory personnel	Nordstrom	34,193	5	1,710	2	684	3	$ 1,026
Clerical personnel	Stevens	18,462	20	3,692	5	923	25	$ 4,616
	Barrett	16,304	15	2,446	5	815	25	4,076
Total direct personnel costs				$45,948		$11,432		$36,531

instituting new services without sufficient consideration of economic implications. When instituting new services it is usually best at the outset to overestimate costs and to underestimate utilization of the services. This will facilitate conservative financial planning.

Facilities

This category includes all expenses related to acquiring, adapting, and maintaining the facilities used for the delivery of clinical services. These costs are usually accounted for by rent or by payments for amortization of construction or purchase costs over a period of several years. Amortization may be in the form of mortgage payments or payments to retire construction bonds (as in the case of most tax-supported facilities). When the costs of remodeling and adapting facilities have been substantial, these costs are also usually amortized over several years.

Particularly in larger programs, it is again important to distinguish between direct and indirect facilities costs. Direct costs relate to those facilities used for the conduct of clinical services. Indirect costs relate to facilities used for supportive functions: offices, records storage facilities, waiting rooms, corridors, etc.

In computing facilities costs, the first step once again involves allocation of total costs into direct and indirect expenses. Direct expenses are then allotted by function. From a practical standpoint, most speech, language, and hearing services facilities can be differentiated into two functional categories: facilities used for speech-language evaluations and therapy and for hearing therapy, and the facilities used for hearing evaluation procedures. Occasionally, when educational programs for children with hearing impairments or language disorders are also offered, a third facilities category may be distinguished. To functionalize direct facilities costs, an annual per-square-foot cost is established for each facility type. The use of those facilities is then determined by each service and the facilities costs assigned.

To illustrate, two speech-language pathologists and one audiologist have incorporated a group private practice and have leased a suite in a professional building. The suite includes an office (which serves as the reception area, business office, and records storage facility) with an adjoining waiting room that, together, occupy 600 square feet. There are two smaller therapy rooms and one larger room that occupy a total of 400 square feet. The audiologist's hearing-testing facility occupies 450 square feet. Since the audiologist dispenses hearing aids, she has set aside a small room of approximately 80 square feet for the hearing aid inventory and for the other equipment used in her dispensing program. Each clinician also has a small private office, together totaling 200 square feet. Internal corridors account for another 130 square feet.

The rent for the suite is $2,400 per month or $28,800 per year. The group pays $3,600 annually to a janitorial service for maintenance. The utility bills total $1,300 per year.

The building's owner repainted and carpeted the entire suite at the beginning of the lease so that no remodeling or refurbishing was required. However, the group secured a 10-year loan to cover the cost of a prefabricated sound-isolated hearing-testing facility. The payments on that loan total $3,600 annually.

For the facilities occupied by the group, then, two different base rates must be computed, one covering the hearing-testing facilities, the other covering all other facilities. The rent, maintenance, and utility charges assignable to the entire suite total $33,700 per year. Since the suite occupies 1,860 square feet, the basic annual facilities cost is approximately $18.00 per square foot. Adding the cost of the hearing testing facility brings the cost of that specific area to $26.00 per square foot.

In the first step—allocation of indirect versus direct costs—the cost of the reception-office-waiting room areas, staff offices, and corridors (totaling 930 square feet) accounts for an annual indirect facilities cost of $16,740. The second step involves allotting costs by function. The three clinicians provide seven different services: speech-language therapy, speech-language evaluations, basic diagnostic hearing evaluations, pediatric hearing evaluations, hearing aid evaluations, hearing aid dispensing, and hearing therapy. Through review of the previous year's schedule, the amount of time each room was used for each service was estimated. Then, as shown in Table 9.3, the direct facilities costs (based on the per-square-foot cost of the rooms used) were estimated for each procedure.

Once again, there is no completely equitable basis for allotting indirect facilities costs. Two approaches are possible. In one approach, these costs are divided equally among all client visits. Therefore, if the group in our example together accommodated an average of 3,200 client visits during a year, an indirect facilities cost of $5.00 would be assigned to each visit. This approach is somewhat inequitable because the client who is seen for a 1-hour visit is assigned the same share of the indirect facilities costs as the one seen for a 3-hour visit. Alternatively, indirect costs can be assigned on the basis of the average time spent to deliver a particular service. Here, a 2-hour evaluation session would carry twice the indirect cost allocation of a 1-hour therapy session. This approach is not entirely fair either because it is based on the dubious assumption of a direct relationship between utilization of facilities covered by indirect expense and the time spent for the delivery of a service. The only possible solution is effecting a compromise that seems sensible in the particular situation.

Many speech-language pathology and audiology programs are not required to pay directly for their facilities through rental or mortgage installments. Some have been given the buildings in which they conduct their programs. Others, such as most col-

Table 9.3.
Functional Allocation of Direct Facilities Costs

Service	Therapy/Eval Room 1 (100 sq. ft.) Total Cost = $1,800		Therapy/Eval Room 2 (100 sq. ft.) Total Cost = $1,800		Therapy/Eval Room 3 (200 sq. ft.) Total Cost = $3,600		Hearing Test Suite (450 sq. ft.) Total Cost = $11,700		Hearing Aid Room (80 sq. ft.) Total Cost = $1,440		Total Direct Cost
	% Use Allocated	Cost	% Use Allocated	Cost	% Use Allocated	Cost	% Use Allocated	Cost	% Use Allocated	Cost	
Individual speech/language therapy	70	$1,260	50	$900	60	$2,160					$4,320
Speech/language evaluation	30	540	30	540	30	1,080					2,160
Basic diagnostic hearing evaluation							40	$4,680			4,680
Pediatric hearing evaluation							20	2,340			2,340
Hearing aid evaluation							30	3,510			3,510
Hearing aid dispensing							10	1,170	100	$1,440	2,610
Hearing therapy			20	360	10	360					720

lege and university clinics, are permitted to use facilities at no cost to the clinical services program. Still others are charged for facilities use—often on a per-square-foot basis—but at rates that are substantially less than are charged in the private sector. In computing the costs of clinical services, however, it is usually advisable to compute facilities costs as though the program were paying for them at prevailing rates in the community. The difference between those costs and what is actually paid by the program is then shown as a contribution among the sources of income to the program. There are three reasons for this approach. First, every program should maintain a realistic accounting of its costs, regardless of the sources of support for those costs. Second, as funds become limited, more and more parent institutions are assigning increasing financial liabilities to the various activities within those institutions. Such situations are dealt with more easily when they can be reflected as changes in financial support (which they actually represent), rather than as changes in program costs. Third, many public and private sources of support for speech, language, and hearing services only underwrite portions of the costs of delivering those services. They expect the program to seek other sources of support also. When the true costs of contributed facilities are shown, the program may appear in a more favorable position in seeking grants and other contributions to maintain clinical services.

Equipment

Distinguishing between direct and indirect equipment costs is usually a fairly straightforward procedure. Direct costs relate to the equipment used to deliver clinical services. Indirect costs relate to the equipment—typewriters, files, office furniture, etc.—that is used to support the delivery of those services. Occasionally, as in the instance of computers and computer-related hardware, equipment may be used both in services delivery and for supportive functions and thus be divided between the direct and indirect costs.

Equipment costs usually represent a combination of the expense of acquiring the equipment initially and of maintaining it throughout its useful life. Equipment may be acquired in one of three ways: it may be purchased outright from available financial reserves, grants, or contributions; it may be purchased from funds obtained through loans; or it may be leased. The approach used to annualize equipment costs will differ, depending upon the way it is acquired originally.

Even though the initial purchase of equipment is subsidized, programs must often finance replacement when that equipment becomes obsolete and add new equipment to support new or expanded services. Even when all equipment purchases—new and replacement—are subsidized, it is usually advisable to include equipment expenses in the computation of total services costs. As noted with respect to donated facilities, expenses should be noted among program costs and the funds provided for equipment purchase among sources of financial support.

When equipment is initially purchased outright, two approaches may be used to annualize the costs. The first, and generally the best, involves amortization of the *replacement cost* of each piece of equipment over its estimated useful life. For example, a conservative estimate of the useful life of an audiometer is 8 years. Thus, each year one-eighth of the replacement cost would be included among equipment costs. Notice that the factor is replacement cost, not purchase cost, since replacement cost allows for inflation. Ideally, one should add 10% per year of the estimated life of the equipment to the purchase price to predict replacement costs. From a practical standpoint, however, 8% per year is about all most budgets can tolerate. At that rate, the replacement cost at the end of 8 years of an audiometer purchased for $8,000 would be $13,711. The cost of the audiometer, then, would be annualized as $1,714.

This approach seems to make no provision for the purchase of other than replacement equipment. In practice, however, it usually provides enough leeway so that funds may be "borrowed" for the purchase of new equipment. Fortunately, if equipment is well maintained, its useful life often substantially exceeds its estimated life. Furthermore, replacement may be obtained at less than the projected cost. These factors provide some cushion for prudent purchase of supplementary equipment.

The second approach involves making annual contributions to an equipment replacement fund which, although proportionate to the total complement of equipment owned, is not based on a strict replacement formula. Although commonly used by clinical services programs, this approach is risky. At best, it involves sheer guesswork. Moreover, since no logical premise is involved, an equipment replacement fund is always vulnerable to invasion in times of financial stress when such funds can be diverted to meet more immediate demands; thus, they will not be available when equipment must be replaced.

The other two options for acquiring equipment—purchase through loaned funds and leasing—are used most frequently by smaller clinical programs and by private practitioners and in other instances where capital for initial equipment purchases is not available. Since loan payments and lease payments are always computed on either a monthly or yearly basis, they are easily annualized for cost analyses. Some leases involve annual payments for a period of years, with an agreement to pay a fixed amount to purchase the equipment at the end of the lease. In these instances, the annual cost estimates must include both the lease payments and the accumulation of a reserve to pay for the equipment at the end of the lease period.

Lease options have been used frequently by audiologists to establish private practices. These options are generally managed by leasing companies which purchase equipment from manufacturers and subsequently realize a profit by leasing that equipment to individuals. Although once a readily available option, such lease plans have become relatively rare. As interest rates skyrocketed, leasing companies serving individual professionals have become less profitable, and those companies have turned to more lucrative investments.

Supplies

In most clinical programs, supplies include those consumable items that are used in the delivery of clinical services and in the various activities that support those services (reporting, record keeping, billing, etc.). Test kits and certain therapy program materials may fall somewhere between equipment and supplies in terms of definition. Even though they are not consumable in the same sense as test forms, tongue blades, and earmold impression compound, it is cumbersome to deal with them as equipment for the purpose of cost analysis. Most clinical programs, therefore, define these materials as supplies and allot a total sum for purchase among annual costs.

Supply costs can also be expressed as direct and indirect expenses, again differentiating on the basis of use for clinical versus supportive functions. Similarly, when a program offers a wide range of services with distinctly different supply requirements, it may be advisable to allot direct supply costs among those services.

Other Expenses

Although individual speech-language pathology and audiology programs may have unique categories of other expenses, most fall into one of the following:

1. *Travel.* Direct travel expenses include those that are incurred by getting staff to the various locations where services may be delivered: to the various schools with speech, language, and hearing services programs; to extended care facilities when contract services are provided; to clients' homes when services are provided in connection with home health services; to various facilities for participation in conferences regarding specific clients, etc. Indirect travel expenses primarily include those related to program administration.
2. *Telephone.* This expense is usually a very substantial item in the budgets of most clinical services programs, where commercial rather than residential rates apply.
3. *Insurance.* Most clinical services programs carry at least two types of insurance. They carry the

same kind of insurance coverage carried by any property owner or commercial enterprise for protection against theft and fire and to cover liability for any injuries sustained by the public on the program's premises. They also carry professional liability insurance to cover instances of alleged malpractice or other misadventures that occur in connection with professional services. This latter insurance must provide not only coverage of claims that may be awarded, but also coverage for legal defense against those claims.

4. *Taxes and license fees.* Although many speech-language pathology and audiology programs function as nonprofit hence tax-exempt agencies, some are conducted on a profit-making basis. These programs incur essentially the same tax liabilities as any commercial enterprise. Sometimes local and state business license fees also apply, particularly when services include dispensing hearing aids or other appliances. When states license speech-language pathologists and audiologists, their licensure fees may also be included among program expenses.
5. *Staff education expense.* Many programs consider the support of staff attendance at certain professional meetings, conferences, institutes, and short courses to be essential to the maintenance of high-quality clinical services. Therefore, these expenses are included among program costs.
6. *Public relations and information.* Speech, language, and hearing services seldom succeed without some continuing effort to alert the public about the importance of communicative disorders and about the services the particular program provides. Some expenses are usually associated with these efforts.
7. *Accounting costs and bad debts.* Sometimes billing and accounting services are purchased, rather than managed by employed clerical staff, and hence incur other expenses. Every program that involves fees for services must include bad debts as one of the costs of providing services.

With the exception of travel costs, it is usually difficult to allot these other expenses to specific clinical services. Therefore, most are simply considered as indirect expenses and assigned by some reasonably equitable approach among all services.

COST COMPUTATION IN DIFFERENT SERVICES SETTINGS

In a general sense, the various aspects of cost analysis covered in the previous section apply in all settings. However, the relative importance of each aspect may differ among settings.

Cost Computation in School Programs

For an era of 20 years or so, during the middle of the 20th century, our society seemed to have such a commitment to serving children with special needs that there appeared to be almost unlimited funds to support those services. This era culminated in the passage of PL 94-142. It was probably inevitable that some re-evaluation of that idealism would occur. A part of that re-evaluation has been a closer scrutiny of the exact costs of providing special educational services, with the resulting figures to serve as a basis for evaluating the demand for additional expenditures. Furthermore, states are requiring a more precise accounting of expenses when they share program costs with local education agencies.

The Comprehensive Assessment and Service Evaluation (CASE) system (American Speech and Hearing Association, 1976), described in Chapter 6, offers a specific and detailed approach to the computation of costs in school speech, language, and hearing services programs. This cost analysis procedure first involves completion of a Program Budget and Expenditure Report which reveals direct and indirect costs. "Staff costs" are defined as including salaries, equipment and materials/supplies, and travel. Student transportation costs are added to the total staff costs to complete the direct cost category. Indirect costs (consisting of costs assignable to facilities occupancy and maintenance, costs assignable to providing and receiving in-service education, etc.) are then added to achieve a grand total.

After total costs are determined, they are then functionalized. The first step in this process involves completion of a Monthly Staff Time Distribution Report. This report examines direct and indirect "service activities." Among the direct service activities are screening, assessment, staffing/

placement, intervention (further distributed by the types of problems served: articulation, language, voice, fluency, hearing, and communication differences), case management planning and record keeping, and consultation. The indirect services activities include in-service provided; in-service received; research; travel; program development, organization and evaluation; and other program activities.

The Monthly Staff Time Distribution Reports serve as the basis for preparation of a Staff Information Analysis and Time Distribution Report which, in turn, is compiled to complete a Cost Allocation of Aggregate Staff Hours. Finally, the accrued information is summarized in an Expenditure Allocation Summary Report. One section of this report allots direct and indirect costs by program, i.e., language and speech versus hearing. Another section allots direct and indirect costs by direct service activity, again using the breakdown of screening, assessment, staffing/placement, intervention, case management planning and record keeping, and consultation.

A more inclusive approach to analyzing the costs of all special education services was developed by the Rand Corporation in connection with a study conducted on contract from the United States Department of Education. Their report, entitled *The Cost of Special Education* (Kakalik et al., 1981), analyzed the added costs of special education services, that is, the costs of special educational and related services that are over and above the costs of educating all children. Although some of the conclusions of this study have been disputed, the cost categories established seem useful. Among the categories used were: instructional costs for employing special education teachers and aides; costs for related services personnel; screening costs; assessment costs; admission and Individualized Education Program (IEP) development costs; staff in-service education costs; technical assistance costs; transportation costs; and the added costs for special instructional supplies, texts, and equipment; additional administrative and secretarial support; special supervision; food service; facilities operation and maintenance; new facility construction; facility modification and improvement; and debt service.

The Rand Corporation report examined the costs of speech-language pathology services among the costs of related services. They used a twofold approach to that analysis. One approach distributed costs into such conventional categories as personnel costs, facilities, equipment, supplies, staff travel, and overhead (this category essentially resembles our earlier definition of indirect expenses). They also used a functional analysis approach employing six categories:

1. Instructional and therapeutic services to handicapped children.
2. Screening services to detect potential handicaps.
3. Admission of children to special education, placement, and individual education program development.
4. Staff in-service training.
5. Consulting with other professionals relative to special education.
6. Providing services for other target population programs such as those for disadvantaged and bilingual children.

Traditionally, school speech, language, and hearing specialists have been in an anomalous role with respect to the costs of the services they provide. On the one hand, they have few opportunities to participate in cost analyses and to make decisions about regulating expenditures within cost categories. On the other hand, they are held strictly accountable for expenditures and are frequently exhorted to limit costs. There are few more precarious positions than being held accountable without being held responsible. Let us hope that as school programs are increasingly required to effect economies in speech, language, and hearing services, the clinicians who provide those services will be increasingly involved in determining the allocations of whatever resources are available. Current trends, however, do not give rise to great optimism that this will, in fact, occur.

Cost Computation in Health Services Settings

Two particular aspects of cost computation deserve special attention from speech-language pathologists and audiologists in health service settings: indirect cost allocation, and cost computation as a basis for third-party reimbursement. Administrators commonly diffuse the impact of maintaining costly programs, facilities, and services by prorating what they define as indirect costs across all departments within the institution. In other words, instead of assigning only those indirect costs that can be fairly attributed to the department, all indirect costs for all departments are lumped together and distributed equally (on the basis of square feet assigned to the department, number of client visits provided, professional staff size, or some other factor). Furthermore, they are often imprecise in the determination of what constitutes indirect costs; costs that are actually assignable only to certain departments are assigned to all departments. These indirect cost allocation procedures may make financially feasible such costly programs as intensive care units, organ transplant centers, and facilities for exotic diagnostic procedures. But they may also make the costs of providing inherently less expensive procedures intolerable. Speech-language pathology services are usually among the least costly services provided in health care settings. Although somewhat more expensive, audiology services are modest compared to many health-related services. When speech-language pathology and audiology programs are allotted extortionate overhead expenses, they often fail because they can never become economically feasible. Consequently, when working in health care settings, one must maintain close surveillance over indirect cost allocations and over the procedures employed to arrive at those allocations.

Speech-language pathologists and audiologists in health care settings, particularly in inpatient facilities, must also be careful about the establishment of clear and complete cost analysis procedures because many third-party carriers base their reimbursement rates directly on those cost analyses. Outpatient services are usually covered through payment of fees for services. Inpatient care, on the other hand, is often covered on cost-based reimbursement formulas. (For example, Part A Medicare coverage, i.e., the coverage for inpatient services, is usually defined through cost-based formulas.) Therefore, when speech, language, or hearing services are provided in the context of inpatient care in an acute hospital or an extended care facility or, in some instances, through a home health agency, it is essential that the professionals providing those services be able to furnish exact cost analyses.

Cost Computation in Private Practice

In no other setting is the precise and continual monitoring of costs as essential as in private practice. In other settings when costs are underestimated some kind of bailout is usually available, if only temporarily. In private practice, however, when costs exceed the available resources to cover those costs, the practice is usually headed toward dissolution.

Private practitioners face some unique quandaries with respect to cost considerations. Success in private practice usually entails the availability of attractive and accessible facilities, preferably in a neighborhood where other human services professionals practice. Most audiologists, and those speech-language pathologists who depend substantially on medical referrals and who serve many clients with organically based disorders, find it particularly advantageous to establish offices in buildings that house several physicians or in professional office buildings adjacent to medical centers. But in most communities, rental rates in those facilities are among the highest.

Furthermore, private practitioners must primarily serve clients who are accustomed to assuming financial responsibility for their own care. These clients usually expect to receive that care in well furnished and appropriately commodious surroundings. They also expect the practitioners to have available whatever equipment is necessary to provide high-quality services. Unfortunately, then, although private practitioners may, at least initially, be in the poorest financial position to cover these costs, they may also be under the greatest pressure to make such expenditures. Beginning private practitioners must usually walk an extremely fine line between maintaining an appropriately professional environment and overextending financial resources so excessively that success is impossible.

Another unique aspect of cost computation in private practice relates to calculating personnel costs, i.e., the private practitioner's expected net earnings from the practice. Two approaches are possible. The first is preferable for new practitioners but is also used by many established practitioners. It involves computing personnel costs on the basis of what comparable human services professionals earn in that community. Notice that these costs should be "based on" rather than "equivalent to." Because of the additional risks they assume, private practitioners have the right to expect substantially higher earnings than the notoriously underpaid speech-language pathologists and audiologists in many clinical services programs. This salary-based approach is most practical when—as usually happens—a new practitioner must rely on other earnings to augment income during the period the practice is being established. It permits allocation of personnel expense in proportion to the time spent, essentially as one would for a part-time employee.

The other approach, used in many established practices, is that of replacing the estimated personnel costs for the services provided by the private practitioner (but not for any employees of the practitioner) with an estimated margin of profit. This procedure is comparable to that used in any small business. All costs, with the exception of the practitioner's earnings, are computed. A margin of profit is then added before the expenses of the practice are projected.

Because of restrictions, imposed by some third-party payers, forbidding direct payment for speech-language pathology services provided by private practitioners (to be discussed in detail in the next chapter), those professionals have been increasingly compelled to enter into contractual arrangements with various health care facilities. These contracts, too, must be based on scrupulous cost-accounting procedures or they can easily lead to disastrous financial consequences for the private practitioner.

Cost Computation in Community Agencies

The most frequently used guide to cost analysis for community agencies is a manual entitled *Accounting and Financial Reporting: A Guide for United Ways and Not-for-Profit Human Services Organizations* (United Way of America, 1974). Although published by the United Way of America primarily for use—often mandatory use—by member agencies, it has also been adopted by community agencies that are not funded by United Way campaigns. This cost analysis approach involves a two-dimensional allocation of expenses. The first involves establishment of "object expense classifications." These classifications resemble the categories employed in any cost analysis: salaries, supplies, occupancy, equipment, etc. The second dimension involves "functional classification" of expenses, i.e., assigning the object expenses into functional categories. Two broad functions are specified: program function and support function, essentially synonymous with what I have differentiated into direct and indirect expenses.

Program function costs (i.e., direct expenses) are allotted according to the *United Way of America Services Identification System* (UWASIS). UWASIS aspires to offer "a chart of human efforts to deal with ourselves and our circumstances" (p. 18), classifying services within a "comprehensive conceptual framework" of: (1) *broad human goals* for overall human betterment; (2) *services systems* designed to achieve those goals; (3) *services*, identified as major logical components of each services system; and (4) *programs*, identified as major logical clusters of activities—each cluster of activities having a common purpose for providing a given service.

UWASIS defines six broad human goals into which services can be classified:

I. Adequate income and economic opportunity (including employment and other income maintenance services, consumer protection, etc.)
II. Optimal environmental conditions and provisions of basic material needs (including food, nutrition and housing services, transportation, environmental and public protection, etc.)
III. Optimal health (including health and mental health maintenance and care, mental retardation and rehabilitation services, etc.)
IV. Adequate knowledge and skills (including formal and informal educational services)
V. Optimal personal and social adjustment and development (including family services, social adjustment and development, cultural services, etc.)
VI. Adequately organized social instrumentalities (including community organization, resource development, equal opportunity services, etc.)

Most speech-language pathology and audiology services would be categorized under goal III, primarily under rehabilitation services systems, specifically under the services category of "therapeutic services for the handicapped." Or specialized speech-language pathology services might be categorized within the mental retardation services system that also falls under goal III. Some services might be categorized under goal IV, within the "informal and supplementary services system," specifically under services to the disadvantaged.

Like all omnibus systems, UWASIS contains problems for categorizing specific services such as we provide. Nevertheless, its objectives are commendable, i.e., to relate the cost analysis of human services to broad goals for improving the lives of the members of the community an agency serves.

In addition to the usual elements of indirect expense, the support function analysis includes fund-raising expenses, an area of cost analysis that distinguishes community agencies from most other services settings. Most community agencies must engage in some form of fund raising—direct solicitation of funds from the public, or sponsoring benefits or other special events—in order to support their programs. All such efforts entail expenses through investment of staff time or retention of outside fund-raising specialists and in underwriting the costs of whatever activities are pursued.

There are, unfortunately, prominent examples of supposed human services agencies that engage in expensive fund-raising efforts which do little more than pay for the fund-raising efforts. Telethons, certain mail campaigns, and so-called "boiler-room" benefits are notorious for profiteering fund raisers, but they yield little return for the causes they espouse. Increasingly, however, state attorneys general offices are scrutinizing the fund-raising costs of nonprofit agencies. Fund-raising costs are also scrutinized when agencies turn to united givers' funds, to private foundations, and to other philanthropies for additional support. Fund-raising costs, like all costs, continue to escalate. Nevertheless, when they exceed about 25% of the gross receipts from the fund-raising effort, an agency courts serious criticisms.

COST CONTAINMENT

One admonition has been reiterated throughout this text: the steadily rising cost of the delivery of human services is a matter of personal concern to every provider of those services. Some people derive satisfaction from proposing that the money spent by our nation on particular human services is trivial compared to our nation's expenditures for battleships, cigarettes, or cosmetics. But these pious comparisons are specious and merely obfuscate the reality that there will always be limits to the resources our society will allocate to human services. Cost containment, therefore, remains an important concern in every segment of the human services delivery system and to every professional working in that system.

As the segment with the greatest acceleration of costs, health care has been the target of the most vigorous official efforts toward cost containment. At first, these efforts were proposed as preliminary to instituting a national health insurance program, in the belief that such a program must be preceded by a federally regulated system to control health care costs. This was a major impetus behind the passage of the National Health Planning and Resources Act of 1974 (PL 93-641). Although this legislation was also intended to facilitate improved health care to underserved Americans, a major thrust sought cost containment through reduction of duplication of services and better utilization of already available community resources.

During the period between the end of World War II and the passage of PL 93-641, there was a proliferation of new and expanded health care facilities, particularly hospitals, primarily financed by federal funds. This proliferation, together with improved approaches to the prevention and treatment of disease, led to serious underutilization. (Many communities now support hospitals with occupancy rates of less than 50%.) This underutilization became a substantial factor in the rapid growth of health care costs.

The same era saw the development of many new approaches to medical diagnosis and treatment. Notable among these were computed tomography (CT), sophisticated radiation therapy techniques, kidney dialysis, and organ transplant programs. These approaches revolutionized many aspects of health care, but they were also fantastically expensive. Underutilized hospitals that were already competing for patients launched drives to acquire the equipment and facilities necessary to offer these new services. Eventually, particularly in urban areas, there was such a proliferation of highly specialized medical services that these services, too, became seriously underutilized.

Under PL 93-641, the nation was divided into something over 200 regions for health planning, each to be served by a Health Services Agency (HSA). These HSA's were charged with the responsibility to review existing services and institutions in the light of the area's needs. The Act also charged governors to identify an agency in their state to coordinate HSA efforts. In addition to their advisory roles, HSA's were given the authority for determining the expenditure of federal health care funds within their regions.

Ostensibly, HSA's were intended to effect cost containment by increasing the efficiency of health care services through fuller utilization of existing facilities, through improved cooperation among those facilities, and through the channeling of federal dollars to areas of greatest need. Their effectiveness has varied considerably throughout the nation, but, in general, the salutary effects of PL 93-641 have probably fallen far short of its proponents' aspirations. However meritorious, many provisions are impractical. Furthermore, most of its fundamental tenets are anathema to organized medicine, which unwaiveringly promotes the sanctity of free enterprise, and organized medicine remains a formidable political force. The moves away from governmental regulation that have characterized the early 1980's have further weakened the influence of HSA's. For the present, at least, HSA's cannot be regarded as a major force in cost containment.

Although lacking the force of law of HSA's, utilization review has become a more important force in health care cost containment efforts. Utilization review programs may have the surface appearance of voluntary efforts by health care institutions, but in actuality they are mandated by accreditation and licensure requirements and by many third-party payers. Thus far, utilization review has focused primarily on inpatient acute care, although long-term care and outpatient services are increasingly being included within its purview. Two major areas have been scrutinized: admissions for and durations of hospitalizations, and the diagnostic and treatment procedures ordered while patients are hospitalized. The ultimate objective is to reduce costs by limiting hospital stays to what is absolutely necessary and by encouraging physicians to order only essential diagnostic and treatment procedures.

Whatever success has been achieved by utilization review is probably attributable to its emphasis on assigning to physicians the final authority for regulating medical practices. Although other health care professionals, primarily nurses, participate on utilization review committees, all ultimate decisions are inevitably made by physicians. This same characteristic may also reduce the effectiveness of this approach to cost containment. Its critics often cite the analogy of assigning to the fox the responsibility of guarding the chicken coop.

Thus far, neither comprehensive health planning nor utilization review programs have exerted nationwide impact on the delivery of speech-language pathology and audiology services. Nevertheless, some local impact has been apparent. In specific communities, HSA's have reviewed the establishment of new speech, language, and hearing services programs within health care agencies. Occasionally, utilization review committees scrutinize physician requests for diagnostic services provided by speech-language pathologists and audiologists. To date, however, these represent isolated examples.

Official efforts toward cost containment in human services areas other than health care have wielded much greater influence in our field. These efforts, in such areas as special education and rehabilitation, have been far less complex but much more vigorous. They include drastic reductions in total allocations for services, redefining eligibility so that fewer clients can be served, and imposing "caps" or limits on the total number of clients that may be served by a program.

Whether we work in settings subjected to official cost containment efforts or not, we must always effect economies wherever possible. Ingenuity in developing our own strategies for cost containment may well be the best protection from unacceptable regulations or indiscriminate reduction in allocations by governmental agencies, by administrators, and by groups representing other professions. Every factor that accounts for the costs of our services must continually be subjected to dispassionate self-scrutiny by every practitioner of our profession.

Containing Personnel Costs

As the source of the largest expenditures in any speech-language pathology and audiology program, cost containment efforts must first consider expenditures for personnel. A simplistic approach to cost containment might view salary limitation as the route to reduced personnel expenses. This notion is deceiving and shortsighted. In general, salaries of speech-language pathologists and audiologists already compare unfavorably with salaries of other human services professionals with comparable, or even less stringent, educational requirements. This factor influences the caliber of individuals entering our profession, their longevity within the profession, and the level of committment and aspiration of many of its practitioners. Therefore, the economies that appear to be effected by low salaries may be more than offset by the amount of supervision required, by the expense of orienting new personnel when there are frequent staff turnovers, by high absenteeism, by loss of clients who are ineptly managed, and by discouraging referral sources when they do not obtain the help they are seeking for their clients. In the final analysis, it may be more economical to expect high levels of productivity from capable, mature, and experienced professionals who are appropriately remunerated for the services they provide. There are, nevertheless, several approaches to personnel cost containment that deserve careful attention.

EXPANDING PROFESSIONAL PRODUCTIVITY

"Productivity" is a euphemism commonly applied to describe a professional's primary responsibilities, i.e., activities that yield income to the professional or to the employer of the professional. In most human services professions, productivity implies either direct client contacts or the pursuit of other activities in behalf of individual clients, since these contacts and activities determine income. (That income may be in the form of fees for services or of overall program subsidy.)

In general, there is a direct relationship between productivity and cost containment. When personnel expenditures are held constant, the higher the professional productivity, the lower the cost of each service provided by those professionals. Several approaches can be proposed: *increasing client contacts*, *reducing secondary responsibilities*, *reducing cancellations and failed appointments*, *using support personnel*, and *reducing professional staff absenteeism.*

Increasing client contacts. It may be true that in some settings, especially in the public schools, members of our profession have been expected to manage such large caseloads that high-quality services become impossible. However, the situation may be quite different in other settings. Aleo and Pece's (1977) survey of hospital and community speech and hearing centers showed that scheduled client contact hours averaged 23.8 and 22.5 hours per week, respectively, out of total weekly schedules approximating 37 hours per week. The survey may have used too narrow a view of productivity, since such activities directly related to client services as preparation time and participation in conferences regarding clients were excluded. Nevertheless, these data probably compare unfavorably to the characteristic productivity of other human services professionals.

Another approach to expanding staff productivity involves increasing the number of clients served by a single clinician within a given time interval, primarily through working with clients in groups. This approach has been exploited more fully by mental health professionals and by such rehabilitation professionals as physical and occupational therapists than by speech-language pathologists and audiologists, excepting the members of our profession who work in school settings. Perhaps because of the common practice in school programs of accommodating excessive caseloads through group therapy, our profession has too readily concluded that group services are inferior to individual services. Consequently, we have not been particularly adventurous in exploring new approaches to working with several clients at the same time and fully exploiting the therapeutic benefits of group interaction. Conceivably, such programs can both improve the quality of services to certain clients and at the same time increase professional productivity.

Reducing secondary responsibilities. Aleo and Pece's (1977) survey showed that in the programs they studied speech-language pathologists and audiologists spent almost 40% of their time in meetings, staffings, preparation, record keeping, and other activities that did not involve direct client contact. In some centers, these activities occupied over 50% of staff time. Although it is impossible to cite an optimal time allocation applicable in all settings, cost containment can be effected through reducing the time spent on these activities.

However meritorious, the concept of "teamwork" that has been so enthusiastically embraced in most human services delivery systems entails an almost endless variety of conferences, staffings, and other efforts at face-to-face inter- and intraprofessional communication. The form of these meetings is essentially ritualized: each member of the team reports his or her findings, conclusions, and recommendations, followed by a general discussion leading to formulation of plans. This process may be valid and the outcomes useful, but a dispassionate evaluation of most sessions leads to the conclusion that they are repetitive, unfocused, and otherwise uneconomical, and that much of the reported information will have little bearing on the client's care. Yet these meetings add substantially to the costs of human services programs. Any program that devotes significant portions of staff time to these sessions should scrutinize them carefully to determine whether the same objective cannot be achieved through briefer, carefully structured and skillfully chaired meetings, and with less frequent reviews of the same client.

Many school clinicians have wryly observed that one consequence of PL 94-142 is that they now spend their days attending meetings rather than working with children. In some instances a meeting is held to compile information about a child and to plan an initial evaluation. Then a second meeting is scheduled to review the initial evaluation and to determine whether further evaluations are necessary. Finally, a meeting is scheduled to prepare and approve the Individualized Education Program (IEP). Thereafter, annual meetings occur to review the previous IEP and to prepare a new IEP for the next year. It is not surprising that the earlier-mentioned Rand Corporation study attributed an average cost of $103 per child per year to the cost of admission, placement, and IEP development, an amount approximately equal to that spent on all assessment services. This item accounted for approximately 3% of the total cost of special education per handicapped child in the 1977–1978 school year. The overall quality of educational programs may have improved through this added emphasis on intraprofessional communication; nevertheless, one must again question cost effectiveness.

When meetings involve professionals in different locations, the cost of travel time must also be considered. The teleconference technique described by Vaughan (1976) (see Chapter 3) may be quite economical. This approach is often used by home health agencies when the various professionals concerned with a single client are scattered throughout an extensive area.

Many speech, language, and hearing services programs participate in providing training experiences for future professionals. These efforts may consist of observational experiences for beginning students, clinical practicum for more advanced students, or clinical fellowship year opportunities for recent graduates. Although obviously essential to the future of our profession and to the continued availability of the services we provide, all of these activities make extensive demands on staff time. University training programs are seldom able to reimburse agencies for expenditures in providing observational and clinical practicum experiences; host agencies may, therefore, need to impose rigid limits on these contributions.

Clinical fellows can, however, often participate in revenue-producing services. Furthermore, the stipends offered to clinical fellows may be significantly reduced to offset the costs of supervision.

The economics of report writing and record keeping have been discussed in earlier chapters. It will suffice to reiterate here that these are expensive procedures and must be constantly reviewed from the standpoints of cost effectiveness and personnel cost containment.

Reducing cancellations and failed appointments. One of the most pernicious sources of waste in clinical services programs occurs when clients do not appear for scheduled appointments. The potential cost of this problem can be derived from one case mentioned in the Aleo and Pece (1977) report. One community center revealed that when the rate of client absenteeism was added to the other factors that reduce clinician-client contacts, their speech-language pathologists averaged only 2.8 hours per day and their audiologists only 1.7 hours per day in client contacts. It seems highly unlikely that any program could continue with this rate of professional productivity.

Some programs attempt to hold clients financially liable for last minute cancellations and failed appointments, but these attempts are seldom successful. Among other reasons, third-party payers will cover only services that are actually delivered. Nevertheless, most programs do impose strict limitations on the number of unexcused absences that will be allowed, but even this practice involves substantial waste before any remedial action is taken.

The first approach to reducing failed appointments is to examine the conditions under which the appointments are made. Frequently, clients and potential clients accept appointments they do not intend to keep because it is easier than overtly refusing to accept what has been recommended. Referral sources may be so eager to facilitate their recommendations that they make appointments for clients who have not really accepted those recommendations. Moreover, appointments are often made for clients with no real consideration of the clients' ability to accommodate the appointments in their schedules, to travel to the facility, or to pay for the service. Any of these factors may lead to no-shows.

Even when clients appear for evaluations, they may not follow through on appointments for whatever additional services are recommended. Clients seeking quick cures for speech problems often fail to appear for recommended therapy sessions. Clients who expect audiologists to conclude that their hearing problems are too mild to require amplification often fail to appear for hearing aid evaluations. Parents who are coerced into accepting evaluations for children they consider to be normal often do not keep further appointments. Regardless of how urgent or essential a professional considers services to be, in the final analysis each client determines whether he or she wishes to accept those services and whether he or she will keep whatever appointments have been made.

Failed appointments may be more prevalent in programs that serve low-income clients than in programs serving clients with higher incomes. Bar (1975) published an account of efforts to reduce the no-show rate in an urban speech and hearing clinic that predominantly served clients from low-income Puerto Rican and black families from Harlem. Over a 4-year period, the clinic reduced its no-show rate from 70% to 16%. Among the problems attacked were misdiagnoses of ethnic speech and language characteristics as pathologic problems, poor appointment systems that offered clients little opportunity to arrange appointments to their convenience, poor follow-up on no-show clients, long waiting lists, and cumbersome and unnecessary medical referral requirements. The amelioration of each of these problems simultaneously improved the quality of client care and the productivity of the professionals staffing the clinic. Such experiences lead to the inevitable conclusion that programs with excessive no-show rates should first examine the quality of their professional practices.

In their discussion of ways for improving productivity, Schultz and Burkhart (1978) offered another approach to limiting failed appointments. They executed a professional productivity agreement with each staff member, specifying 27.5 hours of weekly client contact with no allowance for failed appointments. In other words, when clients failed appointments, clinicians had to schedule additional appointments to compensate for the time lost. This led the staff to be more vigorous in their efforts to reduce the prevalence of no-shows.

In other programs, where staff members share directly or indirectly in clinic revenue through incentive programs, they also share the income loss from failed appointments. Although this approach may encourage agressiveness in reducing the frequency of no-shows, and although such agressiveness may offend the professional sensibilities of some members of our profession, it is distinctly preferable to the possible alternative of bankruptcy.

Using support personnel. One notable recent development throughout the human services system is the increased involvement of paraprofessionals. The presumed economic impact relates to utilizing lower salaried support personnel to absorb the more menial and routine responsibilities of higher income professionals. Such efforts are typified by physicians' assistants, physical and occupational therapy assistants, and teacher aides.

With the exception of utilization of paraprofessionals in hearing conservation programs, some use of test assistants in audiology programs, and the occasional use of therapy aides in public school speech, language, and hearing services programs, paraprofessionals have been utilized less in the delivery of speech-language pathology and audiology services than in other areas of human services. There are many explanations. In the first place, the generally low salaries of the members of our profession leave little leeway for cost savings by the employment of aides at salaries that are only slightly lower. The inevitable supervision requirements may reduce the productivity of professional staff to an extent that few savings are realized. Furthermore, in many settings it is difficult to manage schedules so that professionals and paraprofessionals can be productively occupied at all times.

It is likely, nevertheless, that the use of paraprofessionals has not been fully exploited in many speech, language, and hearing services programs. Such personnel may be used most effectively in programs where clients are potentially available at many times during the day, as in residential facilities, in inpatient rehabilitation centers, and in extended care and day care facilities. Less frequent client contacts with professionals may be augmented by paraprofessionals carrying out programs defined by the professionals. Sometimes professionals and paraprofessionals may work in teams with groups of clients, one carrying out activities with the group while the other pursues an individualized activity with a single client.

The American Speech-Language-Hearing Association (1981) published guidelines for the preparation and supervision of paraprofessionals. Several states that license speech-language pathologists and audiologists also require registration of speech-language pathology and audiology aides. Despite these efforts, the utilization of paraprofessionals as an approach to cost containment within our fields of service remains virtually unexplored.

Reducing professional staff absenteeism. I know of no data that quantify rates of absenteeism among speech-language pathologists and audiologists. Although the overall rate is probably considerably lower than is characteristic in business and industry, absenteeism remains a potentially expensive problem in many speech, language, and hearing services programs. Typically, rates of absenteeism are substantially higher among certain staff members. Several potential solutions are possible.

The concept of "flex time" has not as yet been widely applied to clinical services programs. This concept permits an employee to distribute his or her work in some other pattern than five 8-hour, 9:00 a.m. to 5:00 p.m. work days. An employee may, for example, elect to spend four 10-hour days on the job. Obviously, flex time cannot be accommodated in settings where speech, language, and hearing services schedules must adhere to the schedule of a total agency, as for example in schools or in many outpatient medical centers. On the other hand, the services of many programs might be enhanced by the ability to offer early morning, late afternoon, or evening appointments. Conceivably, then, offering greater worktime flexibility to staff may, in some circumstances, both reduce absenteeism and extend clinical services to previously difficult-to-serve clients.

Job sharing is another scheduling concept that is increasingly prevalent in business and industry. Here, two employees share what was formerly a position held by one full-time employee. Job-sharing involves some special problems for employers, but it may, in some instances, be an antidote to absenteeism and may enable mature and experienced staff members to continue work despite time-consuming family responsibilities.

Overuse of sick leave benefits, typically on the basis of one day at a time, can also constitute absenteeism. To combat this problem, some agencies do not differentiate between vacation and sick leave, offering instead a fixed amount of leave that may be applied as the staff member chooses. Incentive pay plans, in which a staff member's income is partially or entirely determined on the basis of the revenue he or she generates, may also be a deterrent to absenteeism.

Recently, there have been frequent discussions about the problem of "burnout" in the human services professions, referring to the effects of the demanding yet often routine responsibilities that characterize many of these professions. Absenteeism may be one symptom of burnout. Among the possible approaches to prevention and treatment may be extended leave provisions, ongoing continuing education opportunities, changes in assignments, and greater participation in agency decision-making processes. Peculiarly, as a profession that is presumably geared to dealing sensitively with our clients and to helping them feel successful as they struggle to achieve, we too seldom extend the same consideration to our professional colleagues and to the professionals we supervise.

OTHER APPROACHES TO CONTAINING PROFESSIONAL PERSONNEL COSTS

Most efforts toward containing costs of professional personnel relate to productivity, but two other areas deserve attention: *limiting overspecialization* and *containing employee benefit costs.*

Limiting overspecialization. Overspecialization can seriously curtail the efficient and economical utilization of professional staff. The question of how much specialization constitutes overspecialization can only be answered in terms of the magnitude of a program and the kinds of clients it serves. A staff member whose primary expertise and exclusive interests concern adults with acquired language disorders may be invaluable in a Veterans Administration speech and hearing clinic but difficult to accommodate in a two-person department in a general hospital outpatient clinic. Because of the breadth of our professional practices, many universities encourage specialization among students, even at the beginning of graduate programs. Although there are many quite rational arguments to support this approach, it does not always coincide with the demands of our services delivery system.

In all but the largest, most specialized settings, a staff of reasonably versatile professionals can contribute significantly to the economical operation of a clinical program. The wider the range of competencies of each staff member, the more efficient the use of the entire staff is likely to be.

Containing employee benefit costs. In many clinical services programs, the magnitude of employee benefit packages has grown much more rapidly than employee salaries. The cost of these packages may range between 20% and 30% of total salary allocations. Typically, benefits are given to all employees whether they want them or not. Obviously, benefit packages contribute substantially to the costs of services.

When speech-language pathology and audiology programs are conducted within large agencies or institutions, they may have no control over benefit packages. The same may obtain when staffs belong to unions or other collective bargaining units. In the instance of public institutions, retirement contributions may constitute a particularly pernicious problem. Typically, speech, language, and hearing services programs employ many junior-level professionals who remain only long enough to acquire sufficient experience to move on to more lucrative positions. In most public retirement programs, on leaving the system, an employee is reimbursed for all of his or her contributions, but the employer's contributions remain in the system. Often, then, the substantial annual contributions made by the employer to these programs—contributions that substantially increase the costs of services—actually provide few employees with benefits from those retirement programs.

In many settings, the answer to the question "What can be done to contain employee benefit costs?" is "Nothing". In other settings, some options are available. At one extreme, smaller agencies and private practitioners may contract for staff as independent agents rather than as employees. Usually, this entails offering the staff member a share of the income he or she generates. Although that share may seem to be substantial, it may amount to less than an appropriate salary plus benefits. The staff members then make their own Social Security contributions in the form of a self-employment tax, and contribute to whatever other retirement and insurance programs they choose. Actually, in the current economy, employees can keep greater benefits through independent investing than through contributions to institutionalized retirement and insurance programs.

In some agencies where employees are salaried, although Social Security contributions are mandatory, the employees may be offered the choice of salary differentials in lieu of benefits. Since this approach is antithetical to most group retirement and insurance programs, however, the option is available in fewer and fewer instances.

CONTAINING CLERICAL STAFF COSTS

In many speech-language pathology and audiology programs, the important cost-related issue is not the containment of expenditures for clerical staff, but, instead, profligacy in squandering valuable professional staff time on tasks that should be carried out by clerical staff. Nevertheless, most programs can effect economies in their utilization of clerical staff time. Once again, the earlier discussions of economical approaches to reporting and record keeping apply. Wordy reports are wasteful both to the writer and to the clerk who must type them. Poorly organized records result in squandering clerical staff time in entering and retrieving information. Searching for mislaid or misfiled records is also expensive. Efficiency in these functions, therefore, serves not only good client care, but economy of operation.

It is frequently shortsighted to communicate by written reports or letters when communication by telephone—even long distance—may be at least as effective and is usually far less expensive than the per-hour cost of report typing.

Because of their apparent up-front costs, human services agencies often shy away from the current computer and word-processing technologies that have effected substantial savings in clerical services for business and industry. It is discouraging to recognize that, despite the tremendous changes that have occurred in information recording and transmittal, most clinical services programs use essentially the same methods they used 50 years ago, even though those methods are inherently wasteful.

Containing Facilities Costs

Allusions have been made here regarding the quandaries faced by private practitioners in seeking facilities that project the prosperous image that may be essential to success and, at the same time, keeping the costs of those facilities within manageable limits. To some extent, this is also true of other speech-language pathology and audiology programs.

Two major factors should influence the selection and planning of facilities: the demographic characteristics of the population from which clients are drawn, and the kind and scope of services that are to be offered. All too frequently, facilities providing short-range advantages lead to long-range economic disasters. As an example, human services agencies may acquire property in urban redevelopment areas at bargain rates, but soon discover that clients who can pay for their own care will not come to those neighborhoods to obtain services. In other instances, individual practitioners or groups of practitioners may be offered facilities within physician group practice complexes or in private medical clinics at favorable rates. They are all too often disappointed to learn that the association with a specific group of physicians precludes referrals from all other physicians. Or, location within or immediately adjoining acute medical facilities may appear advantageous to speech, language, and hearing services programs, but it may soon be evident that this represents the most expensive of all types of accommodation. Furthermore, this kind of space is often pre-empted by physicians—who are always higher in the pecking order—necessitating expensive moves. All of these examples underline the need to select facilities carefully, on the basis of detailed considerations of all possible evaluations. They emphasize that what initially may seem the least costly facilities may not, in fact, be the most economical.

Other aspects of facilities cost containment relate to the utility and versatility of the quarters that are selected. Speech, language, and hearing programs are often housed in mansions donated by benefactors or purchased in distress sales. However grand and commodious, most mansions are ill adapted to clinical services programs. Because of the inevitable waste of unusable or poorly adaptable space, the per-square-foot costs of facilities acquisition and maintenance may be exorbitant when functionalized over the activities that can actually be carried out.

Waste may even be apparent in buildings that are presumably designed for the programs they house. The most common problem is analogous to the earlier-mentioned inefficiencies of staff overspecialization, i.e., facilities overspecialization. Architects usually make detailed analyses of the specific activities carried out by programs before designing facilities to house those programs—often with the enthusiastic encouragement of the program staff. They then design facilities uniquely adapted to each activity, failing to recognize that those adaptations may seriously restrict the use of the particular space. Even when these facilities begin operations, many areas may be underutilized because of the unique design. As programs grow and change, moreover, the space will become even less usable because of its inflexibility. Except for the obvious unique requirements for the units in which hearing tests are administered or in which special educational programs—particularly for preschoolers—are conducted, the best facilities are those that can be used for the delivery of virtually any of our professional services.

Any discussion of facilities cost containment must also recognize the escalation of building costs that have occurred in recent years, a trend that is not likely to be reversed in the forseeable future. Although regrettable, it seems almost certain that spacious therapy rooms, private staff offices, and extensive storage facilities will be luxuries no longer available to most speech, language, and hearing services programs. Ideal facilities, created especially for the programs they house, may become mere dim recollections of earlier days. Future programs will probably need increasingly to adapt themselves to whatever facilities they can afford.

Containing Equipment and Supplies Costs

A walk through the exhibit area of the annual convention of the American Speech-Language-Hearing Association would convince any skeptic that manufacturing the equipment used in the delivery of our professional services has become very big business indeed. The degree to which much of that equipment is effectively used by most clinical programs is another matter. Just as Americans are devoted to equipping their automobiles with supplemental gadgetry and their kitchens with all manner of exotic appliances, American clinicians are often inordinately attracted to hardware. There is a special mystique about imposing instrumentation between the clinician and the client, as though the instrumentation lends credibility to all proceedings.

Without question, many procedures can be accomplished only with well designed and well maintained equipment. It is equally true, however, that much of that equipment offers capabilities that are seldom if ever used. Many programs are equipped with several full-capacity $8,000 clinical audiometers, when one or two such instruments would suffice, complemented by audiometers with more limited capabilities. Speech-language pathologists often use recording equipment that would serve commercial studios, when their purposes would be as well served by modest portable recorders. Videotape recorders are now often considered an essential clinic tool, but in many programs they gather dust in store-rooms. Each year brings a new kind of clinical gadgetry: to monitor loudness in clients with voice problems, to display acoustic information visually to speakers with profound hearing impairments, or to assist in pediatric hearing evaluations. But after initial enthusiasms subside, much of this equipment is used only to entertain visitors.

The first step in containing equipment costs, then, is to purchase only that equipment which is clearly destined for regular use and which has only the capacities necessary to meet normal demands. Most programs should equip themselves to provide whatever services are required by 80% to 90% of their clients, openly admitting that clients requiring services which entail more specialized equipment will be referred elsewhere. Currently, auditory brainstem response (ABR) testing has become the audiologic sine qua non. (Although less costly, ABR is to speech, language, and hearing services as CT scanners are to hospitals—something that no one should be without, whether effectively used or not.) Despite the unquestionable value of the procedure, every audiologist in private practice and every audiology program cannot sensibly aspire to offer this service.

First and foremost, then, containing equipment costs involves careful planning. Purchases should be planned on sounder premises than the fact that someone on the staff wants it, a neighboring clinic has it, or its glories are extolled in the latest edition of some professional journal.

Also important to this aspect of cost containment is extension of the life of already purchased equipment. The respect accorded to any instrument during its daily use is a major determinant of its longevity. In training students and professionals to use equipment, we seldom train them to use it carefully. Yet, respectful use can substantially reduce maintenance and replacement costs. False economies may also be attempted by scrimping on equipment maintenance contracts, when, once again, skillful maintenance can at least double the life of most instruments.

The proliferation of published tests and therapy materials in our field far outstrips even the proliferation of new equipment. But, more often than not, the tests that sound promising when announced by their publishers add little to the batteries that clinicians trust. After occasional use, many new therapy materials are stored away and forgotten. Two remedies seem sensible. First, there should be a well defined budget for purchasing materials and supplies, with the entire staff participating in decisions as to how those funds are spent. Second, preferably as part of the quality assurance program, the needs for tests and materials should be defined in terms of deficient services. For example, when reviews of evaluation procedures reveal inadequate consideration of particular areas of behavior or function, the staff should consider whether any published tests are available to assist in overcoming those deficiencies. Therapy materials should also be selected to fill demonstrated needs. Decisions to purchase tests and materials should be based, therefore, on some reasonable assurance that they will satisfy a demonstrated need, rather than on the basis of their attractiveness in catalogs or convention commercial exhibits or of glowing reviews in professional journals.

COST-BENEFIT RATIOS

In most areas of commerce and government, estimations of cost-benefit ratios have long been used as bases for decision making. Expressed simply, the estimation of a cost-benefit ratio involves comparison of the cost of a product or service with the benefit accrued. The benefit can be assessed from the perspective of the provider or from the perspective of the consumer. In the first instance, a provider considers whether the cost involved in delivering a product or service is justified by the return, usually expressed as financial return. In the second instance, a consumer considers, or someone considers in the consumer's behalf, whether the cost of securing a product or service is justified by whatever advantages are afforded.

Cost-benefit ratios of speech-language pathology and audiology services can also be viewed from the perspectives of provider benefits and consumer benefits. The first, i.e., appraisal of benefits accruing to programs and agencies, is more easily assessed. One can, for example, conduct a straightforward assessment of whether the costs of the delivery of a particular service are offset by the income (in the form of fees for services, grants, or other financial support) yielded by that service. Often, however, such assessments are complicated by the need to consider benefits that are less easily quantified than financial return. These benefits may include increased visibility within the community or within the larger institution served by a speech, language, and hearing services program; access to new referral sources; and access to previously underserved populations. Therefore, even though the immediate financial return from a particular service may not seem to justify its cost, the overall advantages may warrant initiation and continuation of the service.

The second perspective for estimating cost-benefit ratios, that is, from the standpoint of benefits accrued to clients, may involve two different considerations. One inquires whether the overall benefits that accrue for the client are justified by the cost of providing the services. The other inquires whether the same benefits might accrue from less costly approaches to delivering whatever services are required. Both of these issues have been widely discussed under the rubric of "accountability."

Few speech-language pathologists and audiologists would be so naïve as to assume that they should be exempt from all forms of accountability. On the other hand, assuming that it is easy to establish the criteria on which to base accountability may be even more naïve.

In many instances, formats for accountability are established by people with little understanding of our professional services or, for that matter, of the complexity of most human services. Virtually always, some form of quantification is involved. At one extreme, communication behaviors are parceled out and counted (various authorities have referred to this as the "beads-on-a-string" or "building-block" approach, in which complex communication behaviors are fractioned into discrete quantifiable units). Changes are then computed on the basis of increases or decreases in whatever numbers are derived. At the other extreme, all communicative behaviors may be massed together, or roughly classified into broad categories such as "articulation," "language," "voice," and "fluency." An overall rating, usually on a 0 to 5 scale, is then assigned.

The first approach may seem to have some theoretic merit because of its apparent reliance on scientifically respectable methodology, but it has two major shortcomings: It can only deal with things that can be counted and measured; and, at least for the present, many important aspects of communication can be neither counted nor measured. Furthermore, it assumes that the quantitative expressions derived from observing individual behaviors can be summarized to accurately reflect total communicative proficiency. Siegel (1975, p. 797) commented about this approach:

> There is an implication in the demand for accountability that what counts in clinical service is what is countable. It is obviously worthwhile to have objective, quantitative ways of dealing with communication disorders. What must be avoided, however, is the corollary implication that it is only those events that are countable that are important. The emphasis on tallying and charting responses is consistent with the cost-accounting approach to speech and language correction, but it is not the only way of describing behavior. Numbers are useful devices. When we use them, however, we do so at the cost of some loss of detail.
>
> Numbers must be used with great care when they form the base for judgments of clinical accountability. The child who makes 10 misarticulations is not necessarily twice as handicapped as another who makes only five errors. Some forms of stuttering are far more disabling and distracting than are others, so that stuttering severity must involve more than a count of stuttering moments. It is not always the case that the more response the child has made the more productive the therapy session. Nor are the steps in an intervention program likely to be separated by equal difficulty throughout the program of a given child or when comparing different children. There are qualitative factors involved in the determination of severity of a disorder and difficulty of remediation that are not readily accounted for by simple enumeration. Charting and accounting are useful ways of representing some of the data of therapy, but by no means can all of the essential information concerning a client's performance be captured by these devices.

A pernicious influence of overemphasis on counting and measuring approaches to accountability is manifested in therapy planning. Understandably, clinicians who are to be held accountable for quantitative changes in measures of particular behaviors will concentrate on those behaviors, whether they have any ultimate benefits or not. For example, we can design auditory training programs that increase a client's ability to distinguish a target word from three foils that differ by only one phoneme. Yet there is no evidence to support the relevance of this achievement to speech comprehension in real-life situations. Or those children with language disorders who score poorly on tests purporting to assess auditory memory may be drilled in short-term memory for sentences with successively increasing numbers of words, morphemes, or whatever. But again, there is no established relationship between these tasks and linguistic competence.

The second approach to quantification, i.e., through summary ratings of broad aspects of communication, may be even more vicious. After months of diligent efforts, clients may achieve notable progress in communication without warranting the revision of a rating of "moderate" to a rating of "mild." Yet, when this approach to accountability is employed, successful clients can be excluded from services merely because the system is so insensitive in reflecting whatever achievements occur. These systems particularly militate against clients with more serious disorders.

There can be little doubt that we sorely need improved approaches to describing and quantifying what we do, better vocabularies for describing relevant baseline communicative behaviors, and better ways for documenting changes in those behaviors. But for the present, if we surrender to pressures to trivialize, fractionate, or distort communicative behaviors merely to satisfy demands for accountability, we are clearly guilty of unprofessional conduct. Complex behaviors cannot be summarized simply. It helps no one to pretend that they can. Recognizing that simplistic criteria for accountability do not work in our areas of service does not mean that we consider ourselves above accountability. To account for what we do, we must often resort to qualitative assessments of what our clients have achieved. If we admit this to the people to whom we are accountable, we are not uncooperative or unscientific. There is nothing more scientific than telling the truth. Siegel (1975, p. 797) summarized his concepts of accountability in these words:

The speech clinician has important tasks to accomplish. Of course we must be accountable, not in the sense that the word has become a slogan, but in our continuing efforts to recruit bright and talented people in this field; in the insistence on high standards in graduate education; by continued support for applied and basic research; by our insistence that the clinician is more than a technician and must have time and encouragement to think and study and grow. Accountability can serve as a call to critical and reasoned self-evaluation. These are the attributes of mature professional practice and dedicated service. They arise from our collective desire to understand and perform more effectively as speech, language, and hearing clinicians, and not in response to the implication that we have already been judged and found wanting.

SUMMARY

Every speech-language pathologist and audiologist must assume some direct responsibility for the costs of the services he or she delivers. Furthermore, the development and maintenance of all speech, language, and hearing services depends, in part, upon precise cost computations. Depending upon the setting in which those services are delivered, there may be some differences in the methods applied to analyzing costs and the vocabulary employed in allotting those costs. Nevertheless, the essential similarities far outweigh the differences.

Not only are all professionals in some measure responsible for the costs of the services they provide, they are also responsible for containing those costs. For the forseeable future at least, cost containment may be the single most important factor in determining whether our services will continue to be available to the children and adults who require those services.

References

Aleo EL, Pece CO: Review of time allocation and professional fees of speech-language pathologists and audiologists. *ASHA* 19:755–758, 1977.

American Speech and Hearing Association: *Comprehensive Assessment and Service Evaluation Information System.* Rockville, MD, American Speech-Language-Hearing Association, 1976.

American Speech-Language-Hearing Association: Guidelines for the employment and utilization of supportive personnel. *ASHA* 23:165–169, 1981.

Bar A: Decreasing the no-show rate in an urban speech and hearing clinic. *ASHA* 17:455–456, 1975.

Kakalik JS, Furry WS, Thomas MA, et al: *The Cost of Special Education.* Report N-1792-ED, Santa Monica, CA, The Rand Corporation, 1981.

Schultz MC, Burkhart MC: Professional productivity: a case study. *ASHA* 20:963–964, 1978.

Siegel G: The high cost of accountability. *ASHA* 17:796–797, 1975.

United Way of America: *Accounting and Financial Reporting. A Guide for United Ways and Not-For-Profit Human Services Organizations.* Alexandria, VA, United Way of America, 1974.

Vaughan GR: Tel-communicology health-care delivery system for persons with communicative disorders. *ASHA* 18:13–17, 1976.

Supplemental Readings

Alpiner JG, Ogden JA, Wiggins JE: The utilization of supportive personnel in speech correction in the public schools: a pilot project. *ASHA* 12:415–417, 1970.

American Speech and Hearing Association: *Determining the Cost of Speech and Hearing Services.* Rockville, MD, American Speech-Language-Hearing Association, 1971.

Dempsey V: Planning for health planning. *ASHA* 18:348–352, 1976.

Hester EJ: Health planning agencies and speech-language pathology. *ASHA* 23:85–92, 1981.

Irwin JV: Supportive personnel in speech pathology and audiology. *ASHA* 9:348–354, 1967.

Kamara C, Kamara AS: Computer billing, service analysis, and financial reporting in a hearing and speech agency. *ASHA* 18:229–231, 1976.

Lawrence CF: Public Law 89-749. Comprehensive health planning. *ASHA* 9:261–266, 1967.

Northern JL, Suter AH: Supportive personnel in audiology. *ASHA* 14:354–357, 1972.

CHAPTER TEN

Paying for Speech-Language Pathology and Audiology Services

There can surely be no question at this point of my conviction that speech-language pathology and audiology is an independent profession in the human services delivery system. Yet there is an inherent incongruity between our declarations of professional independence and our overwhelming dependence upon public institutions. This concern was explored by Feldman in his 1981 presidential address to the American Speech-Language-Hearing Association (p. 942):

> Our professional service delivery system has evolved, as do all others, from one history. Contrary to the independent heritage in many phases of health care, our roots are more deeply entrenched in education. Our professional services have been, and continue to be, provided in sheltered governmental or other institutionally supported agencies such as public schools, universities, community nonprofit facilities, and hospitals. Though constituting the largest entity within the profession, the clinical practitioner in our field is seldom an independent entrepreneur.
>
> This lack of fiscal autonomy cannot help but diminish the view of the profession as autonomous. Despite our cries to the contrary, our actions often depict us as a dependent rather than an independent profession. Why must services be subsidized? Aren't they important enough to be paid for directly?

In an earlier chapter I proposed that the key to the flourishing of our profession during the past three decades lay in our ability to prosper in such a diversity of human services settings. To some extent, that diversity has also entailed the development of new sources and patterns of payment for speech, language, and hearing services. As Feldman observed, however, the vast majority of those services depend upon governmental or other institutional support. Nevertheless, despite that history, it seems likely that the key to our continued professional prosperity during the next decade will lie in our capacity for developing new, more diversified, and less institutional sources of financial support for the delivery of our clinical services.

Throughout this text I have reiterated my concerns that because of accelerating changes in public policies some sections may be outdated by the time it is published. At this writing, the precise form of imminent policy changes is unpredictable. But one thing is certain: governmental agencies—federal, state, and local—will proportionately reduce their financial support of speech-language pathology and audiology services. These changes have at least two implications. First, those concerned should ascertain what subsequent changes may have occurred in statutory programs. Second, nonpublic sources of support are becoming increasingly important. Therefore, particular attention should be paid to discussions of these sources even by those who practice or plan to practice in settings traditionally supported by public funds.

Support for speech-language pathology and audiology services may be in two different forms. In one form, it is based on the provision of services to individual clients; generally, fees are paid by the client or by some other individual or agency in the client's behalf. In the other form, support is provided to an overall program. Thus, support may be provided to an entire program for speech, language, and hearing services, as in public school programs, or it may be provided for a specific set of services within a larger program (e.g., a preschool program for hearing-impaired children may be underwritten within an agency that provides all other services on a fee basis). Sometimes, both types of support are combined to serve the same clients. For example, many university speech and hearing clinics receive a combination of token fees paid by clients combined with overall program funding from the university. Traditionally, the second form, i.e., overall program support, has been the dominant pattern of support for our professional services. Reliance on fees for services is a growing trend; that growth will almost certainly accelerate.

SUPPORT BASED ON INDIVIDUAL CLIENT SERVICES

In the final analysis, any pattern of payment that is strictly related to the exact type and number of services provided to clients is based on fees for services. Broader program support formulas may sometimes be based on the number of clients served and the type and extent of services provided, but a one-to-one relationship between services delivered and payment accorded seldom applies.

In planning services that are to be individually supported, the first step is establishment of a schedule of fees for services. This schedule will apply whether a client is responsible for paying those fees, whether a third party covers them, or whether payment is shared between clients and third-party payers.

Developing Fee Schedules

One fundamental principle must underlie the development of a fee schedule for speech-language pathology and audiology services: the schedule must be developed primarily on the basis of the cost of providing those services. As will be noted later, certain practical considerations may lead to compromising that principle, but it should always remain primary. Agencies or professionals who apply what they assume their clients can afford as a major determiner in establishing their fee schedules take the first step toward financial disaster. What services cost and what clients can or are willing to pay for the service, or what a third party allows in payment, must always be treated as separate issues. When client or third-party payments fall below cost-based fees, services must obviously be subsidized. In these instances, the fee schedule should remain as a realistic expression of costs, but the subsidies should be displayed as sources of income support to the program. This practice should obtain even when virtually all services are subsidized.

Four different approaches to establishing fee schedules will be described: *the unit of service approach*, *the functional approach*, *the relative values approach*, and *the pragmatic approach*. The merits of each approach depend upon the requirements of the program that is developing the schedule. All depend, to some extent, upon the cost analysis procedures described in the previous chapter.

THE UNIT OF SERVICE APPROACH

This approach is straightforward and generally the simplest of the available options. It assumes that the time expended in providing a service is the primary determiner of the fee. Preparation of such a fee schedule involves the following steps:

Step 1. The agency analyzes its schedule of clinical services to discover the smallest block of time that is normally scheduled for the delivery of any service, and that block is designated as one unit of service. For example, in many speech, language, and hearing services programs, a 30-minute therapy session represents the smallest block of time that is usually scheduled.

Step 2. Each service that is to be included in the fee schedule is expressed in terms of units of service on the basis of time typically allotted to provide the service. For example, if a 30-minute therapy session represents one unit of service, an evaluation session for which 2½ hours are allotted would represent five units of service. When more than one professional staff member is involved in providing the service, units are adjusted accordingly. For example, if two staff members are scheduled to participate in each 2-hour pediatric hearing evaluation, the procedure would be assigned eight units of service. When a group of clients are served simultaneously, this is also reflected in the units assigned. For example, in our illustrative agency, when two or more clients participate in a 1-hour group therapy session, only one unit might be assigned.

Step 3. Previous years' schedules are analyzed to estimate the total units of service provided annually by the agency.
Step 4. The agency then totals all expenses in its current budget that are attributable either directly or indirectly to maintaining its clinical services program. (In an agency that is primarily devoted to the delivery of clinical services, this will probably represent the total budget. If other educational or consultative services are provided, those costs will be deducted from the total budget.)
Step 5. Total expenses are divided by the estimated total of units of services provided to derive the cost per unit of service.
Step 6. The units of service assigned to each procedure on the fee schedule are multiplied by the cost per unit of service to determine the fee for each procedure.

The unit of service approach may be satisfactory when an agency offers a relatively limited range of services in which the only variable considered is time. The approach is inequitable, however, when a wide range of services must be covered. As was discussed earlier, these services may differ substantially in terms of the expertise of the staff participating, the equipment and facilities required, the supplies consumed, and the reporting entailed. When the unit of service method is used, all costs beyond professional time are distributed equally. Therefore, the client who receives a 1-hour service with modest overhead costs pays the same as one who receives a service of the same duration with high overhead costs. Despite its essential simplicity, then, the unit of service approach to establishing fee schedules is unsatisfactory for most comprehensive speech-language pathology and audiology programs.

THE FUNCTIONAL APPROACH

Although more complex than the unit of service approach, the functional approach attempts a fairer allocation of costs, basing fees on estimates of the actual costs of providing particular services. This evolves logically from the basic approach to functional cost analysis described in Chapter 9.

Step 1. The agency develops a functional cost analysis following the procedures described in the previous chapter.
Step 2. Previous years' schedules are analyzed as a basis for estimating the number of times a particular procedure is scheduled during a year. (When a new procedure is to be added, its probable frequency and total costs are estimated.)
Step 3. The fee for each service is determined by dividing the estimated functionalized cost for the procedure by the estimated frequency of scheduling.

The functional approach obviously requires more elaborate cost-accounting procedures than the unit of service approach, but it is probably the most equitable of all approaches and the most easily supported when questions from clients or third-party payers arise.

THE RELATIVE VALUES APPROACH

This approach also seeks to establish fees that fairly reflect the cost of delivering a particular service. Although in many respects it is similar to the functional approach, it also resembles the unit of service approach in its establishment of units which are converted into fees. The fundamental concept underlying the relative values approach is that, regardless of the many factors that may affect the actual dollar value of a service, the relative costs of delivering various services remain essentially constant. For example, if the cost of conducting a hearing aid evaluation, because of the time spent and equipment required, is twice the cost of conducting a basic hearing evaluation, that relationship will remain the same. Thus, even though the costs of providing those services may be significantly less in a small Midwestern community than in a large Northeastern city, it will probably still cost approximately twice as much to provide a hearing aid evaluation as to provide a basic hearing evaluation in both communities. Furthermore, within a single agency, we can predict that, because of inflation, the costs of providing each of these services will probably increase significantly over the next 5 years. Nevertheless, the relationship between the costs of the two procedures will probably remain essentially constant. In each of these instances, then, when a relative values approach is employed, the fee charged for the hearing aid evaluation will always be twice the fee for the basic hearing evaluation, regardless of actual dollar amounts.

The following procedure is used to establish a fee scale based on relative values:

Step 1. One service is selected as the basis for computations. That service should be the one among the most frequently offered services that involves the least demand for special equipment and facilities, expensive materials, and supportive staff. The cost, then, should be primarily attributable to professional staff time, to the minimum of other direct costs that must be borne by any service, and to a reasonable apportionment of indirect costs. (In comprehensive speech-language pathology and audiology programs, individual speech-language therapy sessions most often qualify as the most suitable service to use as a basis for relative values computation.) The service selected is then assigned a value of 1.0.

Step 2. The estimated costs for providing other services are then analyzed much as in the functional approach. This analysis leads to comparisons of the relative costs of each service with the costs of the base procedure that has been assigned the value of 1.0. If the cost of providing a particular service were estimated to be half the cost of the base service, it would be assigned a value of .5; if the cost were twice that of the base service, it would be assigned a value of 2.0, etc. On this basis, then, a relative values scale is developed that covers each item to be included on the fee schedule.

Step 3. To assign actual fees, a conversion factor must be computed. Once again, annual schedules are analyzed for each procedure's frequency, these frequencies are converted according to the assigned values, and a total is computed. Thus, if 3,000 speech therapy sessions were provided and each session had a relative value of 1.0, and 600 speech-language evaluations were provided, each with a relative value of 3.5, the total would be 5,100 units (3,000 for the therapy sessions and 2,100 for the evaluations). The entire budget covering all costs assignable to clinical services is then divided by that total to determine the conversion factor. (In our illustration, if the aggregate costs assignable to the delivery of those services were $265,000, then by dividing that amount by 5,100, we would arrive at a conversion factor of approximately $52.00.)

Step 4. The fee schedule is devised by multiplying the assigned relative value for each procedure by the conversion factor. (In our illustration, the fee for a therapy session would be $52.00 and the fee for a speech-language evaluation would be $182.00.)

As described, the relative values approach may seem an unnecessarily cumbersome way to establish a fee schedule. Actually, it is probably seldom if ever used independently by a single program in establishing its fee schedule. On the other hand, the relative values approach is frequently used to establish comparable fee schedules among several different providers. Specifically, it is often used by physicians to establish their fees and, in turn, by third-party payers to establish their rates of reimbursement. The most frequently identified model is the relative values scale developed and published by the California Medical Association.

The more widespread application of relative values scales has been halted by a declaration by the Federal Trade Commission (FTC) that such scales are illegal because they represent price fixing. There are, however, growing pressures to exclude professional practices from the purview of FTC regulations; therefore, the use of these scales may become more prevalent. It may even be advantageous for speech-language pathology and audiology programs in different regions to join in the development of relative values scales for their services, primarily to be used as guides to third-party payers. Although each program should maintain the right to establish its own fee schedule, third-party reimbursement might well be facilitated if those schedules were established on the basis of the same relative values scale.

THE PRAGMATIC APPROACH

The fourth category of approaches to establishing fee schedules is not parallel to the three just described. There are, however, factors that must often be considered which are neglected in those approaches. Despite the earlier dictum that fee schedules should be based strictly on the costs of services rather than on what clients are willing and able to pay for those services, programs can seldom adhere absolutely to that dictum. This final approach, therefore, is not strictly a system for establishing fee schedules but, rather, a concession to some pragmatic factors that are likely to be considered regardless of the systematic approach applied.

Three factors are most often considered:

1. *Prevailing community fees.* No private practitioner or program is likely to succeed when their fee schedules substantially exceed charges for comparable services in comparable facilities elsewhere in the community. Physicians, psychologists, and other human services professionals who are establishing new private practice offices are usually advised to set their fees at the 90th percentile of prevailing fees in their communities.
2. *Duration of services.* Many clients and families can cover fees for short-term services but are unable to pay for prolonged services. Similarly, many third-party payers limit coverage to short-term services. Consequently, some programs establish proportionately higher fees for services that are likely to be of short duration. For example, proportionately higher fees may be set for evaluation services than for therapy, since therapy programs can be of long duration.
3. *Third-party coverage.* Most third-party carriers would be aghast at the suggestion that covered services commonly bear proportionately higher fees than noncovered services; yet this is true in virtually all health care programs. It would be unfortunate to imply that this factor is a major determiner in setting fees for our professional services; nevertheless, it cannot be ignored. The most obvious example is found in setting fees for audiology services. Although most public and private health insurance plans cover hearing evaluations to establish medical diagnoses, most specifically exclude all audiologic services connected with hearing aid selection and fitting. This is particularly unfortunate since most hearing aid services are provided to oldsters on limited incomes. Commonly, then, audiology programs set proportionately higher fees for diagnostic hearing evaluations than for hearing aid-related procedures.

None of these pragmatic considerations should be sole determiners of fee schedules. On the other hand, no matter which procedure is applied to develop a fee schedule, that schedule should be reviewed with these factors in mind. Adjustments to accommodate these factors are completely legitimate when judiciously applied.

Third-party Payment

During the second half of the 20th century, the costs of human services have increased so rapidly that fewer and fewer Americans are able to pay for them directly. This is especially true of health care services. Two solutions have emerged. The first solution has developed through people joining together to share the risks of expensive services. By accumulating premiums in insurance funds, the costs of caring for people who require many expensive services are pooled with the costs of providing care to people who require few services. Through this pooling of costs, then, care presumably becomes affordable to all subscribers to the insurance plan. In many instances, the premiums are paid, either partially or entirely, by employers as a part of "fringe benefit" packages.

The second solution has developed to assure services to people whose incomes are so limited that they are unable to pay for services even on a shared-risk basis and to people representing other special populations. This solution involved the development of various governmental third-party payment programs that either cover all services costs or share those costs with the consumers.

The term "third-party payment" has been used so frequently throughout this text that a definition may now be unnecessary. Nevertheless, to preclude any possible confusion, as I have used it, third-party payment refers to any plan or program in which payment of fees for services comes from someone other than the client, the client's family, or some other private individual. In most instances, third-party payment is synonymous with payment by a public or private insurance program. Furthermore, with occasional exceptions, third-party payment is based on coverage of fees for services.

There are essential similarities between private insurance and governmental third-party payment programs. Ostensibly, these similarities grow out of efforts to provide "mainstream" care to beneficiaries of governmental programs, i.e., care that is no different from what is available to people who can afford to pay for it. In reality, however, the similarities also result from the persistent political efforts of several powerful organizations of health care providers to preserve free enterprise in our nation's health care system. Despite these efforts, legislators are repeatedly questioning whether government can any longer afford the costs of mainstream health care.

Even though there are many similarities between private and governmental third-party payment programs, there are also important differences to providers in general and to speech-language pathologists and audiologists in particular. These differences are discussed separately in succeeding sections of this chapter.

PRIVATE INSURANCE

With rare exceptions, the only private insurance plans to provide for payment of speech-language pathology and audiology services are covered by the rubric of health insurance. History's first health insurance policy is said to have originated around 2000 B.C., when members of the Chinese aristocracy paid physicians retainers so long as they, the aristocrats, stayed healthy, but executed them when illnesses proved fatal. Modern health insurance programs began in the 1920's when a few pioneer prepaid hospital and group practice plans were introduced locally in the United States. Group health insurance plans proliferated during World War II. At that time, wages were often frozen to prevent "runaway inflation." Consequently, benefits packages became an increasingly important factor in the negotiation of labor union contracts.

The two giants of private health insurance, Blue Cross and Blue Shield, began in the years immediately following World War II. Blue Cross plans are usually organized as nonprofit corporations. They are restricted to the coverage of the costs of hospitalization and of some limited out-of-hospital services immediately following hospitalization. Blue Shield plans are also commonly incorporated on a nonprofit basis and cover costs of physician services and certain related services. Relationships between Blue Cross and Blue Shield plans may range from complete separation to total unification.

Even though Blue Cross and Blue Shield plans enroll far more subscribers than any other private insurer, many other plans are currently available. Some are provided by companies that offer several different types of insurance, others by companies specializing in health insurance.

While private health insurance plans are almost infinitely variable, some constant factors can be defined. All professionals who provide health-related services should be cognizant of these factors whether they are directly paid by insurance plans or not.

Types of health insurance. Health insurance can be characterized from two different standpoints: functional and organizational. Six different types of health insurance can be defined from a functional standpoint:

1. *Hospital expense insurance.* This type of insurance is essentially intended to cover expenses sustained while a client is in a hospital. Coverage may include admissions to both acute care facilities and extended care facilities. Increasingly, because it is a less expensive alternative to hospitalization, home health services are covered by hospital expense insurance when those services are provided immediately following discharge from a hospital.
2. *Surgical expense insurance.* In recent years surgical expense coverage has been incorporated with other health insurance policies. Nevertheless, separate surgical insurance policies remain available. As the name implies, this type of insurance covers expenses directly related to surgical treatment.
3. *Physician expense insurance.* This type of insurance is designed to cover fees for services provided by physicians or carried out by direction of and under the supervision of a physician. With the growing involvement of so-called "allied professionals" in the health care system, definitions of professional services covered by this type

of insurance have often broadened to cover the services of certain nonphysician providers. Many plans require physicians to bill for services delivered by other professionals working under their supervision. Other plans permit direct payment to these nonphysician professionals but still require that their services be ordered by a physician, with review and recertification by that physician at regular intervals.

4. *Major medical expense insurance.* Major medical coverage is designed to provide broad substantial coverage against large and unpredictable medical expenses. Originally, such coverage was intended for people who wished to protect themselves only against catastrophic situations or to supplement plans with more limited coverage. Currently, however, virtually any situation requiring hospitalization has become so expensive that major medical coverage has become less distinguishable from other types of coverage. Although separate major medical plans are still available, basic hospital and physician expense plans now often include what amounts to major medical coverage.
5. *Disability income protection.* This type of insurance does not, in the strictest sense, pay for professional services (although some disability insurance plans are coordinated with other health insurance plans that pay for certain rehabilitative services). It is intended to protect a subscriber against income loss during periods of extended, but still temporary, illness or disability. Usually, such plans are written to cover the period between exhaustion of whatever sick leave is offered by an employer and the point at which the client can return to work or is declared permanently disabled (thus becoming eligible for Social Security or other benefits.)
6. *Dental expense insurance.* Dental care is specifically excluded from virtually all insurance plans covering fees for health care services. As the cost of dentistry has increased, dental plans, based on the same share-the-risk principles as other health insurance plans, have become increasingly popular. Employee groups have increasingly included dental plans in their benefit package negotiations. Dental plans essentially resemble physician expense plans in their organization and operation.

Private health insurance can also be categorized according to three different organizational patterns:

1. *Individual plans.* In individual plans, clients deal directly with an insurance carrier to purchase coverage for themselves and their families. Rates will depend upon such factors as the scope and extent of the covered services and the ages and health histories of the subscribers.
2. *Group plans.* These plans are characterized by several clients banding together to negotiate—or to have negotiated in their behalf—health insurance coverage. Groups typically consist of the employees of a particular company or other institution or the members of a trade union. Frequently, the distribution of costs between employees and employers and the extent of coverage provided by the insurance are negotiated as a part of employee contracts.

   As with individual plans, the extent of coverage will depend upon the amount the premium payer is willing to pay. Furthermore, that coverage may depend to some extent on the relative actuarial risks of the group being covered. When employees are responsible for payment of all or a portion of the premiums, they may have options as to the extent of coverage they wish to pay for. Sometimes employers pay for basic coverage, but employees may extend coverage at their own expense.
3. *Health maintenance organizations* (HMO's). Health maintenance organizations were described among the models for delivering health care services in an earlier chapter. As noted, HMO's are characterized by prepayment for health care services from specified providers rather than by reimbursement for fees from virtually all qualified providers. Strictly speaking, of the two types of HMO's—prepaid group practices and foundations for medical care—only the second should be included in this discussion of third-party payment of fees for services. Remember that foundations for medical care are usually comprised of groups of individual practitioners who agree to provide specified services to HMO subscribers at agreed-upon rates, thus qualifying within the definition of private third-party payment.

   HMO foundations for medical care resemble other private insurance plans in that subscribers may exercise some options as to the extent of services to be covered. Subscribers will then assume personal liability for uncovered services. HMO plans are usually available to both individual subscribers and to groups. In the latter instance, the group negotiates the amount and extent of coverage and the amount of membership fees.

Coverage. Theoretically, health insurers should be willing to offer any benefits for which the insured is willing to pay, with risks defined in terms of the likelihood that payment will occur and the amount of financial liability that may be assumed. For example, coverage against tuberculosis for a group of middle-class Americans entails a very small risk for a health insurer, even though extended treatment for that disease might be very expensive. On the other hand, the coverage of maternity, newborn, and well-child care for a group of subscribers that include many people in their twenties and thirties is quite a different matter.

In reality, however, no private insurance plan covers all health care costs. Actual coverage can usually be defined within five different areas:

1. *Where the service is provided.* This limitation was immediately apparent in the earlier-defined classification in which hospital expense insurance was distinguished from physician expense insurance. The first category specified that services be provided in an acute hospital, an extended care facility, or through a home health agency. Formerly, many insurance plans covered only expenses incurred during hospitalization. This led to overutilization of hospitals, i.e., physicians would hospitalize people for diagnostic and treatment procedures that could as well be provided on an outpatient basis. More and more health insurance plans now cover outpatient services; however, many specify that those services must be provided in a physician's office or in a laboratory or other facility that is directly supervised by a physician.
2. *The type of service rendered.* Virtually all health insurance plans distinguish between covered and noncovered services. Among the commonly excluded services are dentistry, routine eye care and eye glasses, hearing aids and services related to their selection and fitting, and cosmetic surgery. Formerly, most plans excluded psychiatry and all other mental health services; however, recent years have seen the inclusion of more of these services, but usually with strict limitations imposed.
3. *The condition for which the service is required.* Health insurance plans commonly exclude specific conditions from coverage. Most often specified are conditions which pre-exist the effective date of the insurance and conditions stemming from alcohol or drug abuse and self-inflicted injuries. Many policies also exclude congenital disorders and conditions acquired during early neonatal life, even though the family was insured on the date of the child's birth.
4. *The provider of the service.* Health insurance policies often restrict payment for services provided by another professional, technician, or paraprofessional working directly under the physician's supervision. When direct payment for services provided by members of other professions is allowed, those professionals are usually specified and their qualifications defined—primarily on the basis of licensure and certification.
5. *Maximum liability.* Nearly all health insurance plans establish a financial cap on their coverage and pay for no services after that limit has been reached. Such caps may specify that no more than a given amount of money will be expended during a particular time interval (per period of hospitalization, per year, etc.) and also establish a limit for expenditures during the client's lifetime. In addition to time-defined limitations, there may be maximums specified for specific types of coverage, such as inpatient hospital care, home health services, and psychotherapy.

Other important factors. Some other factors are significant in understanding health insurance coverage. Among the more important are: *deductibles, methods of payment, assignment of payment, co-insurance,* and *co-payment.*

1. *Deductibles.* The concept of deductibles is probably most familiar with reference to automobile insurance. Here, the insured agrees to pay the first $100, $150, $250, or whatever, of all bills for accidental damages to his or her automobile (thus the policies are described as $100 deductible, $150 deductible, $250 deductible, etc.). Understandably, since the liability of the insurance company for paying claims increases with lower deductible amounts, the insurance premium is higher. Most health insurance plans also have deductibles. The subscriber agrees to pay the first $100, $250, $500, or whatever, of his or her health care costs each year, making the insurance carrier liable for costs exceeding the agreed-upon deductible. As with automobile insurance, the higher the deductible, the lower the premium.
2. *Method of payment.* Health insurance carriers adhere to one (or occasionally to a combination) of three methods for determining the amount to be paid for a particular service: on the basis of usual, customary, and reasonable charges (UCR); according to fee schedules; or by relative values scales.

   In the UCR method, insurance carriers establish profiles of prevailing fees for particular services among providers in a community. Ostensibly, these profiles are fixed at the 90th percentile of prevailing fees. As costs have escalated, however, UCR profiles are often well below the fees charged by many, if not most, professionals in a community. Once kept strictly secret by insurance carriers, UCR profiles are now often available under the Freedom of Information Act when they are applied for reimbursement under such public programs as Medicare.

Some insurance carriers establish their own fee schedules, simply allowing whatever they choose to pay for particular services. Although, presumably, these fees should to some degree reflect prevailing charges, they may be established quite arbitrarily.

The relative values approach was described earlier in this chapter. When applied by insurance carriers, a conversion factor is established for determining the dollar value of covered procedures that presumably reflects the cost of service delivery in the community where the provider practices.

3. *Assignment of payment.* Health insurance plans generally pay claims in one of two ways; often the subscriber and the provider may choose between the two. In one instance, payment (in the amount determined by one of the above methods and adjusted for deductibles, co-payment, or co-insurance) is paid directly to the client, who is then billed for the service by the provider, using the provider's own fee schedule. Thus, the client is responsible for payment of the fee but is reimbursed by the insurance carrier for at least a portion of that payment (assuming it exceeds the deductible). In the second instance, the carrier pays the professional directly for the service (again adjusted according to the previously specified factors). Many professionals accept whatever the carrier allows as full payment (some carriers require this), except, of course, that the client is always responsible for deductibles, co-payment, and co-insurance.

   Many confusions about health insurance coverage derive from assigning payment. Clients may be surprised to receive bills from providers when they assume that they are fully covered by health insurance. When insurance covers only a portion of the fee—as for instance, when the plan calls for paying 80% of charges, or when the carrier pays claims according to fee schedules or UCR profiles that are well below usual charges—clients may accuse professionals of charging exorbitant fees. When professionals accept assignment of payments, they often encounter major problems in collecting uncovered fees from clients. Any professional who serves clients covered by health insurance is well advised not only to determine the extent of coverage but also to be certain that the client understands the exact terms of coverage and what his or her personal liability may be.

4. *Co-insurance.* Many health insurance plans specify that the insured maintains responsibility for a percentage of all charges. (Once again, these are charges beyond the deductible and those based on the fee levels permitted by the carrier.) Commonly, plans covering outpatient care specify that the client is responsible for payment of 20% of these charges.

5. *Co-payment.* Occasionally, plans specify a flat amount to be paid by the client for each unit of service. Currently, co-payments are most often found in HMO plans in which clients frequently pay a set fee (usually modest) for each visit or service, with the remainder of the cost for services covered by HMO. Co-payment is often established as a deterrent to overutilization.

Coverage of speech-language pathology and audiology services. The coverage of our professional services by private health insurers is problematic from several standpoints. First and foremost are persistent questions as to whether speech, language, and hearing disorders constitute health problems and as to whether speech-language pathologists and audiologists are health professionals. In his 1973 analysis of the coverage of our services by commercial health insurance, Marvin Brantman, then chairman of the Health Insurance Council's Rehabilitation Services Committee, wrote (p. 183):

> There are some things about the professions of speech pathology and audiology which set them apart from just about all other professions covered by health insurance policies. Speech pathologists straddle a fuzzy borderline between health care and education with some of the services provided falling on either side of this indistinct line. This is evident in the occupational patterns in the profession with some employed by educational systems, some working in hospitals or clinical programs and some in private practice.

Not only are there confusions in our status as providers of health versus educational services, there is even confusion as to the nature of the health care services we do provide, i.e., are we engaged in the treatment of the consequences of organic impairment, or are we providers of mental health services? These confusions exist not only in the minds of other professionals, of insurance companies, and even of the public at large, they are even expressed by the members of our profession.

Brantman (1973, p. 184) wrote further:

> Traditionally health insurance covers primarily medically oriented treatment for loss due to accident or sickness. We have not covered general or special education. Where do we draw the line

> in considering speech therapy with reference to what is loss due to sickness and what is education?
>
> It is obvious that aphasia due to stroke is clearly a sickness. It is also quite obvious that elimination of a foreign dialect should not be considered loss due to accident or sickness. But what about disorders with no demonstrable organic cause such as stuttering or certain kinds of voice or language problems? When are these services medically oriented and when are they the responsibility of our public school system?
>
> There does not seem to be any easy answer to these questions. We will ultimately include in our policies the services which the public wants and for which they will pay. We will leave out payment for services which do not require any individual protection because society has decided to assume the cost through our school system collectively.

A second problem relates to the lack of uniform definition as to who are qualified providers of speech-language pathology and audiology services, i.e., exactly who should be reimbursed for providing those services. Specifically, this problem derives from the absence of nationwide licensure laws. Brantman stresses that "Speech pathologists and audiologists are perhaps the only professionals providing therapeutic health care services, often in medical settings, who are not generally regulated by licensing laws." He explored the problem of identifying qualified speech-language pathologists and audiologists further (p. 185):

> As long as there are so few licensing laws, we can use any educational requirements we want in our definition, but we cannot mandate a voluntary certification program. We can require that the eligible practitioner meet the requirements for the Certificate of Clinical Competence, but while such certification remains voluntary, we cannot require that he actually take the examination and become certified, nor can we eliminate those practitioners who do meet certification requirements but for one reason or another have not chosen to apply for certification. To do so would be considered either unconstitutional or unfair restraint of trade.

Had Brantman's statement been written today, he probably would not have used the words "so few licensing laws," but since we are far short of the goal of licensure in all 50 states, his conclusions remain valid. Furthermore, until the goal of nationwide licensure is achieved, there will continue to be serious deterrents to the improvement of coverage of speech-language pathology and audiology services through health insurance plans.

The third problem area derives from restrictions imposed by most health insurers as to which professional services are reimbursable. Ostensibly, to assure that services are health related and are essential within a total treatment plan, insurers usually require that services be prescribed or ordered by a physician and that they then be carried out under the physician's supervision. Although most speech-language pathologists and audiologists are pleased to receive physician referrals, they do not provide services by prescription. Moreover, in many settings there is not even tenuous physician supervision of our services. As more insurance carriers have covered speech-language pathology and audiology services, greater flexibility has emerged with respect to these restrictions. Most insurers accept a valid physician's referral in lieu of prescription and accept physician certification and recertification of treatment plans and progress reports as discharging supervision requirements. Nevertheless, there remain wide variances among insurers, and even among different offices of the same carrier, with respect to these requirements. There may even be inconsistencies in processing claims within a single office.

Brantman summarizes four generalizations with respect to coverage of speech-language pathology and audiology services by virtually all health insurance carriers (p. 186):

> 1. All covered services must be prescribed or recommended by a physician.
> 2. Most policies cover the expense of speech pathology for rehabilitation purposes where the disorder occurs from an organic disease such as brain damage due to a stroke, after normal speech has already developed.
> 3. Most policies do not cover speech pathology services directed against developmental speech defects which have no demonstrable organic cause. This category would indicate stuttering

and articulation defects unless due to a readily apparent organic cause such as cleft palate.

4. Most major medical policies exclude expenses for hearing aids and examinations for the purpose of prescribing hearing aids, but do cover audiometric examinations for other diagnostic purposes. Despite the commonly existing exclusions for hearing aids, some companies would pay for them administratively if the hearing loss was due to an accident rather than sickness.

Anyone who delivers speech, language, and hearing services to health insurance beneficiaries must live with uncertainties and inconsistencies. These uncertainties and inconsistencies relate in a large measure to the already noted disparities between requirements for covering the services we provide and the way we usually provide our services. Of at least equal importance, however, is the fact that, with rare and notable exceptions, our claims are processed by people with little or no information about communicative disorders or about the practice of speech-language pathology and audiology. These people may be clerical personnel or physicians or other health professionals of disparate backgrounds. To achieve coverage, then, we must acquire considerable skill in claims preparation, presenting those claims in such a way that uninformed evaluators can understand the rationale for including the services within the scope of covered benefits.

The following eminently practical tips for claims submission were formulated by ASHA's Task Force on Private Health Insurance (1980, pp. 48–49). (These were published with the disclaimer "In no way do they reflect ASHA policy concerning appropriate restrictions and conditions for reimbursement of speech-language pathology or audiology services in public or private insurance programs.")

Where the claim form asks for the client's diagnosis, indicate the *medical* diagnosis supplied by the physician as the primary diagnosis to which the speech-language pathology or audiology services are applicable, then list associated speech or hearing diagnoses.

Use diagnostic codes from the International Classification of Disease Adapted (ICDA) whenever possible.

When the medical diagnosis is a degenerative disease, specify that the client has stabilized or is in remission, when such is the case.

Make sure that a current treatment plan signed by the physician (if required) is submitted.

Use the term "treatment" in describing your activities; avoid the term "therapy."

Use the term "rehabilitation" where appropriate, not "habilitation."

In notes on treatment, restrict description to "treatment according to treatment plan" if this accurately describes your activities.

When treatment *is* described, indicate what *you* did, not what the patient did.

Use codes from the American Medical Association's "Current Procedural Terminology" instead of narrative description of treatment procedures whenever possible.

In describing the client's progress, show significant, practical improvement in objective, measurable terms (where such improvement has occurred).

In documenting improvement, indicate wherever possible how the client has applied the progress made in treatment sessions to situations outside of treatment.

If a client is ill or otherwise unable to engage in treatment, note that no treatment took place on that date.

Elsewhere in their report, the ASHA task force offered this summary to their discussion of coverage of speech-language pathology and audiology services by private health insurers (p. 48):

Insurance coverage of a service ultimately is a matter solely between the client and his or her insurer. However, speech-language pathologists and audiologists have a responsibility to their clients to fulfill their role in the insurance claims process in such a way that the clients are able to obtain the maximum coverage to which they are entitled.

GOVERNMENTAL THIRD-PARTY PAYMENT PROGRAMS

Many countries throughout the world provide health care to all citizens as tax-supported benefits. Such programs are typified by the national health programs of Great Britain and most Scandinavian countries. Although there are many advocates of national health plans in the United States, all such proposals are far from realization. In lieu of programs including all citizens, our nation has developed third-party payment programs to assist particularly needy and especially deserving people to secure the care they require. Many of these programs allow reimbursement for certain speech-language pathology and audiology services.

Medicare. On July 1, 1966, through the provisions of Title XIII of the Social Security Act, the United States instituted Medicare, its first massive effort to underwrite health care for a substantial segment of the population. The program offers hospital and medical insurance protection for people age 65 and older, and for certain disabled people under age 65, who receive cash benefits under the Social Security or Railroad Retirement programs. Medicare was fundamentally patterned after private health insurance plans, hence there is an essential similarity to the provisions of private third-party programs just described.

Medicare consists of two parts: *Part A* is hospital insurance and covers three types of care; (1) inpatient hospital care, (2) inpatient care in a skilled nursing facility, and (3) home health care. *Part B* is medical insurance and covers physicians' services, certain specified outpatient services (including rehabilitative services), laboratory tests, certain prosthetic appliances, and some medical supplies. Participation in Part B is voluntary, and subscribers must pay monthly premiums. To be eligible for reimbursement under either Part A or B, services must be delivered by a qualified provider and, except for the services of a physician and a few other health care providers, must be provided in a facility that is certified to provide Medicare services.

Medicare also resembles private health insurance plans in that deductibles are imposed; co-insurance and co-payment may apply; reimbursement (under Part B) is based on what is considered usual, customary, and reasonable; and maximum limits of coverage are defined. (Since all of these factors are determined by changing regulations, current Medicare bulletins should be consulted for specific details.) Furthermore, anyone working with Medicare beneficiaries must realize that all health-related services are not covered, that only a percentage of charges for covered services are reimbursed after the deductible is met, and that the fee profiles applied may not be comparable to current fees. Realizing that Medicare provides only partial protection against rising health care costs, many beneficiaries purchase supplementary health insurance to cover gaps in Medicare coverage.

Although a federal program, Medicare does not involve direct reimbursement to providers from a federal agency. Instead, the government has contracted with a group of *fiscal intermediaries*, who process claims and disperse payments to beneficiaries or directly to providers. Blue Cross remains the major intermediary for Part A, although some commercial insurers have assumed that responsibility in some states. Although Blue Shield often serves as the Part B intermediary (more correctly referred to as a "carrier" with respect to Part B), in many localities commercial insurers carry this responsibility.

Fiscal intermediaries must adhere to federal regulations in approving and reimbursing claims. There is, nevertheless, some leeway in interpreting these regulations. Moreover, there may be major procedural differences in processing claims. Consequently, specific details with respect to coverage and processing procedures may vary from one geographic region to another.

Medicare provisions for speech-language pathology services differ significantly from provisions for audiology services. Under Part A, speech-language pathology services may be provided in three different ways (in each instance, services must be provided by a qualified speech-language pathologist, with "qualified," as noted earlier, defined as holding ASHA certification, being engaged in the clinical fellowship year, or holding an appropriate state license): (1) services may be provided to hospitalized Medicare beneficiaries when those services are directly related to the treatment program being carried out; (2) services may be covered when a Medicare beneficiary is discharged from an acute hospital to a skilled nursing facility; (3) services may be provided as a home health benefit immediately following discharge from an acute hospital or a skilled nursing facility when those services constitute further treatment of the condition for which the client was hospitalized. All services under Part A must be provided in or through Medicare-certified facilities. Services provided by independent speech-language pathologists or by agencies with no contractual relationship to the certified facility may not be covered under Part A. Furthermore, all claims must be submitted by and will be paid to the certified facility. They may not be submitted directly by a speech-language pathologist. In Medicare parlance, the facility, not the speech-language pathologist, is the *provider* of services. The speech-language pathologist is defined as the *supplier* of the services.

Under Part B, outpatient speech-language pathology services may be provided in a hospital outpatient clinic, in a medical clinic, in a rehabilitation agency, or in a physician's office. Medicare regulations permit some speech and hearing centers to qualify for certification as rehabilitation agencies. Part B also covers speech-language pathology services to homebound clients as a home health service. Once again, independent speech-language pathologists may not be reimbursed directly. To qualify under Part B, these services must also be provided through and claims submitted by one of the specified types of health or rehabilitation agencies or through a physician's office.

Since Medicare is, after all, a health insurance program, the same regulations as to covered conditions exist as for private insurance. Speech-language pathology services are generally restricted to the treatment of conditions resulting from illness or injury. As with all health insurance plans, the need for services must be certified initially by a physician, and the need for continuing services must be recertified by a physician at regular intervals (in usual practice, every 30 days). Formerly, the law specified that the treatment plan must also be written by a physician. However, in 1980, the law was revised to specify that a treatment plan may be established by a physician or "by the speech pathologist providing such services." The requirements for initial physician referral and recertification remained unchanged.

Although the terms "audiology" or "audiologist" appear nowhere in the Medicare law, audiology services are covered in many instances. Under both Part A and Part B, audiologic evaluations may be covered when conducted at a physician's request to assist in formulating the medical diagnosis. Rehabilitative audiologic services can be covered when requested by a physician and when part of a treatment program for a condition requiring hospitalization or outpatient services in a physician-directed clinic. To qualify to provide services under Part A, an audiologist must be employed by or under contract to the hospital or skilled nursing facility where the beneficiary is being treated. However, independent audiologists may secure Medicare provider numbers to deliver diagnostic services under Part B and be reimbursed directly for those services. Again, however, all services must be requested by a physician.

All services connected with hearing aid selection and fitting are specifically excluded in the Medicare law. When billing for diagnostic services, then, audiologists are well advised to make it clear that the services were not related to hearing aid selection. Efforts to extend Medicare benefits to cover hearing aids and related services continue to be sponsored by various professional, trade, and consumer groups. For the present, at least, it seems unlikely that these efforts will succeed.

Medicaid. Title XIX of the Social Security Act, enacted in 1965, established a medical assistance program for low-income and otherwise needy individuals, subsequently known as Medicaid. The program is administered by each state according to fairly broad federal requirements and guidelines. It is financed jointly by federal and state funds.

Medicaid provides medical assistance to individuals and to families who are eligible to receive monthly cash payments under such welfare programs as Aid to Families of Dependent Children (AFDC) and Supplemental Security Income (SSI). Medicaid benefits may also be extended to people who have sufficient income to cover basic living expenses but insufficient funds to cover medical care. This latter provision is often invoked when people with moderate incomes encounter catastrophic health problems that are not covered or are insufficiently covered by health insurance. Some Medicare beneficiaries who live on meager incomes are also covered by Medicaid, receiving Medicaid funds to pay Part B premiums, to pay deductibles and co-payments, and to pay for certain services not covered by Medicare (in some states this includes hearing aids).

Although states may, through their Medicaid programs, cover other categories of services, five are mandatory: (1) inpatient hospital services; (2) outpatient hospital services; (3) physicians' services; (4) skilled nursing facilities and certain home health services for adults; early and periodic screening, diagnosis, and treatment of physical and mental defects in children; and family planning services; (5) laboratory and x-ray services.

Speech-language pathology and audiology services may be included within several of these mandatory categories. If such services are normally provided to a hospital's inpatients and outpatients or to the patients of a skilled nursing facility, they must also be available to Medicaid beneficiaries. In most instances, nonphysicians working under the "personal supervision" of a physician are included within the mandated coverage of physician services; this may include speech-language pathologists and audiologists.

In an effort to stress preventive services, particularly among children, Medicaid includes, as a mandated service, "early and periodic screening, diagnosis, and treatment" (EPSDT). While speech, language, and hearing screening may be included, speech-language pathologists and audiologists may not be reimbursed separately for these services. Such special screening services must be provided within a complete package and payment rendered for the package. Some state Medicaid programs offer no reimbursement for EPSDT services, but instead rely on other resources, such as public health programs, to carry out the mandate.

Medicaid also specifies certain optional services that may be provided by states. Those that may involve speech-language pathology and audiology are: (1) medical care, or any other type of remedial care recognized under state law, furnished by licensed practitioners within the scope of their practice as defined by state law; (2) home health care services (other than home health nursing) and home health aid services; (3) clinic services; (4) prescribed prosthetic devices (which may include hearing aids and nonoral communication devices); (5) other diagnostic, screening, preventive, and rehabilitative services; (6) intermediate care facility services; (7) physical therapy, occupational therapy, and services for individuals with speech, hearing, and language disorders. At first glance, this list might seem to cover virtually any service provided by a speech-language pathologist or audiologist. However, all states impose stringent regulations in the provision of whatever optional services their Medicaid programs offer. As with Medicare, Medicaid regulations virtually always require initial physician referral and physician recertification of continuing services. All states impose further limitations on covered services—limitations with respect to the amount, duration, and scope of both mandatory and optional services. Amount and duration of services may be limited on the basis of covered days of inpatient care or number of allowable outpatient visits. Scope of services may be restricted so that they are only provided in connection with episodes of acute illness.

Medicaid programs frequently require prior authorization for certain services. Often, diagnostic services provided by speech-language pathologists and audiologists may be covered without prior authorization (usually with the stipulation that these services must be connected with the establishment of medical diagnoses), but ongoing rehabilitation services may only be provided after prior authorization. Such authorizations usually cover a specified time interval or a specified number of visits, with reauthorization required for continued services.

States vary in approaches to payment of Medicaid claims for speech-language pathology and audiology services. Some adhere to Medicare restrictions with respect to direct payment to independent speech-language pathologists and audiologists and to freestanding speech and hearing agencies; others will pay claims directly to the individuals and agencies meeting specified qualifications. Some states also resemble Medicare in their use of fiscal intermediaries, whereas others administer their programs via state agencies. Some states cover usual, reasonable, and customary fees (so long as those fees do not exceed the amount paid for Medicare claims); others pay according to schedules of maximum allowances. State Medicaid programs are showing growing interest in participation in HMO's and other prepaid plans.

As in other third-party payment programs, there are frequent confusions with respect to which services should be covered by Medicaid programs and which should be covered by public education agencies. Some states preclude from Medicaid coverage virtually all speech-language pathology services to school-age children, presuming that these represent educational rather than health services. Although other states may cover some services for children, they may impose stringent restrictions as to the problems covered, the extent of that coverage, and the circumstances under which services may be provided.

Workers' compensation. By law, all states require that workers be insured by their employers for occupationally induced disabilities. Such insurance may be purchased by the employer from a private carrier, may be provided by the employer directly, or, in some states, a state agency functions as the insurer, collecting premiums from employers and paying claims to eligible employees.

Workers' compensation insurance provides benefits in three categories: cash benefits, either in the form of covering income loss during recovery from job-related physical impairments or in the form of lump-sum payment for irreversible impairments; medical benefits to cover diagnosis and treatment of those impairments; and rehabilitation to ameliorate the effects of irreversible impairments. Rehabilitation services may be delegated to other state agencies or to state-operated rehabilitation centers.

Our profession is most likely to be concerned with workers' compensation programs in connection with occupationally induced hearing impairment. Audiologists may participate in the initial diagnostic process, in the determination of the degree of disability, and in whatever rehabilitation measures are instituted. Workers' compensation policies frequently cover purchase of hearing aids for eligible beneficiaries.

Many criticisms have been leveled at workers' compensation programs with respect to coverage of job-related hearing impairment. Their policies may not only disparage the significance of handicaps imposed by hearing impairment, but may actually discourage workers from seeking needed services. These problems are particularized in Ginnold's (1979) detailed and critical analysis of state and federal provisions for occupational hearing loss.

In occasional instances of speech and language disorders consequent to job-related misadventures, speech-language pathologists may also provide diagnostic and rehabilitative services to workers' compensation beneficiaries. Such services are most likely to be provided in connection with clients who have suffered head injuries, trauma to the peripheral speech mechanism, or, rarely, laryngeal problems caused by the inhalation of caustic agents.

Rehabilitation services. All states provide rehabilitation services (sometimes called vocational rehabilitation services) according to federal regulations. These services are supported jointly by state and federal funds. Originally, rehabilitation services were focused exclusively on the objective of preparing the disabled to assume or, in the instance of acquired disabilities, to return to gainful employment. During the 1960's and 1970's, many states, encouraged by increased federal subsidies, expanded definitions of rehabilitation to include clients who could achieve higher levels of independence but who were not likely to secure gainful employment. Although aspects of this expanded mission remain in some states, recent years have seen increasing restrictions on eligibility for rehabilitation services. Not only is there again greater emphasis on rehabilitation for employment, there are also increasing mandates to emphasize services to severely disabled clients.

It is not entirely accurate to include rehabilitation services among governmental third-party payers. Although some state rehabilitation agencies do function as third-party payers, others provide overall program support to selected agencies and facilities, either in addition to or instead of providing third-party payment for individual client services.

When state rehabilitation services do function as third-party payers, they usually invoke some procedure to compensate providers of reimbursable services. Prior authorization is usually required if any kind of continuing therapeutic program is contemplated or hearing aids or other prosthetic appliances are to be purchased. Payment for all services is usually specified either by contractual agreement or by a published schedule of maximum allowances.

Profound hearing impairment represents the communicative disorder most frequently found among clients of most state rehabilitation services. Clients with less severe hearing impairments may also be included, with audiologists providing diagnostic and rehabilitative services. Hearing aids may be purchased, particularly when they are important to the achievement of a vocational goal.

In many states, it has become difficult to secure authorization for long-term speech-language pathology services for rehabilitation clients. Often, however, short-term services are authorized, again particularly when they serve a specific vocational goal. Speech and language services are usually readily authorized for the rehabilitation of working-age laryngectomees, but time-limited therapy programs for clients with other communicative disorders, such as language impairments, dysarthria, and stuttering, are also sometimes authorized.

State rehabilitation agencies assign to their rehabilitation counselors the primary responsibility for determining what is to be offered to a client and how his or her program is to be implemented. Although counselors' activities are restricted by specified policies and procedures, they remain pivotal in the determination of the nature and scope of programs available to individual clients. This kind of case management is found in no other governmental third-party payment program.

Crippled Children Services. When originally passed in 1935, the Social Security Act included, in Title V, authorization for financial aid to the states to assist them in the development of services to crippled children. These programs, usually referred to as Crippled Children Services (CCS) have been substantially modified and expanded during the ensuing years. As with rehabilitation services, it is not entirely accurate to include CCS among governmental third-party payers, since some state CCS programs provide programmatic support through grants to agencies and, in a few instances, have established networks for direct services. Currently, however, most state CCS programs function essentially as third-party payers.

Although broad guidelines for CCS programs are defined in federal laws and regulations, states are given substantial leeway in designing their own programs. In most instances, states supplement federal funds in underwriting CCS budgets. The majority of states administer their programs through health departments, but others designate welfare or education departments or, occasionally, independent commissions as the responsible agencies. Oregon and Iowa offer unique programs administered through their state universities.

CCS funds are intended to assist states in improving and extending services for locating children with handicaps or with conditions that may lead to handicaps, for establishing accurate diagnoses, and for providing needed care. Considerable discretion is granted in defining the precise conditions that are considered to be handicapping.

Most states include some audiologic services to hearing-impaired children within their CCS programs, often restricting those services to more severely impaired children. These services may include provision of hearing aids. Usually, speech-language pathology services are offered for children with cleft palate and children with cerebral palsy and other neurologic handicaps. There are, however, wide differences among the states in their policies regarding coverage of other speech and language disorders.

Financial eligibility requirements also vary considerably among the states. Some impose stringent limitations on family incomes for eligibility; others are more generous in their coverage. Some states require full or partial repayment for treatment and for prosthetic appliances when families have sufficient means but are unable to cover those costs immediately. Some states have effected cooperative agreements between their CCS and Medicaid programs, dividing financial responsibilities for children who are eligible for both programs.

When CCS programs function as third-party payers, their provisions resemble other third-party payment programs. Physicians must establish the diagnosis of a covered handicapping condition but may effect whatever referrals are required to establish that diagnosis. Treatment plans involving nonphysician providers must usually be initially approved and recertified by a physician. CCS programs often require prior authorization from state or regional offices before any service may be provided. They may also require more detailed direct reporting on all covered services than is typical for other third-party payers.

Recent legislative changes have altered the amount and pattern of federal involvement in CCS programs. Nevertheless, in most states the program remains a major source of assistance for the delivery of services to some children with communicative disorders. Every speech-language pathologist and audiologist who serves children, regardless of the work setting, should maintain current information about CCS policies and procedures in his or her state and community.

Civilian Health and Medical Program of the Uniformed Services (CHAMPUS). In general, active and retired military personnel and their dependents are eligible for care at medical facilities operated by the Department of Defense (DOD). In addition, however, the DOD offers the CHAMPUS program to provide for reimbursement (usually after a deductible) for covered medical services rendered in civilian facilities to wives and children of active military personnel, to retired military personnel, and to dependents of deceased military personnel (excluding, in each instance, individuals covered by Part A of Medicare). The program is intended to assist these beneficiaries to secure services to which they are entitled but who are unable to use DOD medical facilities because of distance, overcrowding, or unavailability of appropriate care.

The policies and procedures governing the operation of CHAMPUS tend to be complex, and their administration and interpretation are variable. Specific kinds of speech-language pathology and audiology services may be covered, but their coverage is problematic. Sometimes such coverage is initiated through referral from a DOD medical facility, although other procedures may also be invoked. Speech-language pathologists and audiologists should be aware of CHAMPUS as a potential source of third-party payment for eligible clients, but it is by no means a consistent source. Potentially eligible clients and families must usually institute requests for coverage themselves and investigate the likelihood of coverage under existing circumstances.

Contract Services

Supplying speech-language pathology and audiology services on contract has become an increasingly important source of revenue for both private practitioners and agencies. Such contract services may be provided to virtually any type of human services facility.

Several factors account for the increasing utilization of contract services. Many health care and rehabilitation facilities must qualify for accreditation and licensure under regulations that require the availability of speech-language pathology services. These facilities often consider it infeasible to employ members of our profession and, instead, arrange for those services on contract. At the same time, as noted earlier, many governmental and private third-party payers specifically prohibit payment of fees for services directly to individual speech-language pathologists. This requires these professionals to negotiate contracts with agencies that are authorized to function as providers of speech-language pathology services, so that the speech-language pathologists may, in turn, be paid as suppliers of these services.

Audiologists are in a somewhat different position with respect to contract services. Even though they are not under similar proscriptions against direct payment, their services may also be sought on a contract basis. The large initial financial outlay required for instituting audiology facilities often encourages health care or rehabilitation facilities to contract for those services, at least until they determine the likely demand for such services.

Recent trends have also encouraged public school districts to write contracts for speech-language pathology and audiology services. In many instances, PL 94-142 has been interpreted to mandate, or at least to allow for, contracting for these services to complete assessments and to provide special services specified in Individualized Education Programs when those services cannot be provided by school district personnel.

Another factor has led school districts—and some other types of public institutions as well—to seek contract services. As collective bargaining has been increasingly applied in negotiations, the costs of benefit packages have escalated. Administrators can, therefore, effect economies by arranging for services through contracts with private providers instead of engaging specialists as regular employees.

Although categorized here as one source of support to individual clients, contracts may occasionally call for programmatic services with payment unrelated to the precise number of clients served or to the number of services provided. For example, a Head Start program may contract for speech, language, and hearing screening of all children registered in the program. A contract is written and payment made on an aggregate basis, without regard to the exact number of children served.

Whether a contract calls for delivery of services to individual clients or for a whole program of services, certain factors should always be considered. The following seven factors should be covered in most contracts: *term of contract and conditions of termination; services to be provided; qualifications of personnel; facilities, materials, and equipment; reports, authorizations, and records; insurance and other liability; method of compensation.*

1. *Term of contract and conditions of termination.* The contract should always be written for a specified period of time, usually 1 year. When contractual arrangements are open-ended, all manner of problems can develop for both parties. Health care facilities have been known to write open-ended contracts in order to assure licensure or accreditation and to continue to use the name of the speech-language pathologist or audiologist even though no clients are ever referred. Annual expiration of a contract requires both parties to review their relationship at regular intervals. Most importantly, it is easiest to update financial arrangements at the time the contract is renewed. The contracts should also specify the procedures to be followed for termination before expiration. Usually these provide for cancellation by either party with appropriate notice.
2. *Services to be provided.* The contract should specify the exact services to be provided. These services should be specified in sufficiently precise terms to forestall misunderstandings. For example, if hearing screening services are offered, the nature and limitations of these procedures should be specified so that the contracting facility will not expect more extensive diagnostic services.

   It is usually advisable to specify at least limited services as offered continuously throughout the term of the contract rather than offering services exclusively on an as-needed basis. Skilled nursing facilities and home health agencies frequently write contracts with speech-language pathologists (again to discharge licensure requirements) and then make few if any referrals. This kind of exploitation is less likely when a contract specifies that regular services (screening, staff orientation, consultation, or whatever) will occur—if only on a brief once-monthly basis—and calls for payment for those services.
3. *Qualifications of personnel.* Contracting facilities have the right to expect that all professional staff meet all qualifications for legal practice and for third-party payment. Commonly, these requirements are stated in terms of ASHA certification, state licensure, and, sometimes, when the contractor is a school district, credentials issued by the state education department.

   When personnel provided under the contract include individuals completing clinical fellowship year requirements, that fact should be specified and provisions for supervision described. When supportive personnel are involved (as in contracts for hearing conservation programs), their training should be described and the responsibility for supervision specified.
4. *Facilities, materials, and equipment.* The contract should specify the space allocation that the supplier expects from the contracting facility. The allocation should consider the size of the room or rooms to be provided, accessibility, acoustic characteristics, and any other essential features. Any restrictions on availability of shared space should be noted.

   The contract should also assign responsibility for supplying materials and equipment. If that responsibility is shared, details should be specified. The responsibility for equipment maintenance should be assigned, covering financial responsibility and such matters as provision of replacement equipment when permanent equipment is under repair.
5. *Reports, authorizations, and records.* The contract should detail the reports that are to be rendered and assign the responsibility for preparing and duplicating these reports. It should cover the procedures to be followed in securing any required authorizations for service (for example, in instances where third-party payers demand prior authorization for services). It should also delineate procedures for securing physician referrals and recertification of treatment plans when required for third-party payment.

   The responsibility for records maintenance should also be specified. If maintained by the contracting facility, the general procedure for entering information and obtaining access to the records should be noted. If maintained by the supplier, the contract should define the facility's access to those records both during the term of the contract and after the contract terminates.
6. *Insurance and other liability.* The contract should clearly define responsibility for coverage for malpractice and other liability. The exact limits of that liability, both in terms of circumstances and dollar amounts, must be spelled out. The responsibility for legal defense in the event of litigation must also be defined. (Regardless of the coverage specified by the contracting facility, suppliers are well advised to maintain substantial personal insurance coverage as well.)

   When the supplier involves employees in providing contractual services, it is essential to define liability for those employees. That liability should consider all circumstances related to contacts with clients as well as claims by the employee in connection with work-related injuries or other problems.
7. *Method of compensation.* The contract should clearly specify the fees to be levied by the supplier, the terms of payment, and the circumstances under which the fees will be waived or refunded. Suppliers should avoid contracts that call for a payment of a percentage of fees col-

lected by a provider. (The prohibition of direct third-party payment to speech-language pathologists has led to profiteering by certified providers, who exact cuts of 50% or more merely for providing billing services.) Instead, contracts should state the fee to be charged for each service. Since the contracting agency is providing billing services and assuming other overhead expenses, those fees are usually less than are charged directly to clients served in the supplier's agency or private office.

The contract should define billing periods and specify the time limit for payment by the contracting agency. Here is another pitfall for suppliers. When no time limits are specified, contractors may impose lengthy delays on payment. Frequently, they defer payment until claims for the speech-language pathology or audiology services are paid by the third-party carrier, often after delays of several months. Since many contracting agencies depend on third-party carriers for major portions of their incomes, delays in payment of claims must be assumed within their total financial planning. However, speech-language pathologists and audiologists in private practice and many speech and hearing clinics cannot accommodate such delays within their financial operations, especially when a substantial segment of their services is provided through contracts.

Another practical matter concerning payment must also be covered in a contract: financial responsibility for retroactively disallowed claims. Because of lengthy procedural delays, speech-language pathologists often institute therapy programs before they are assured that a third-party payer will authorize payment. This occurs most frequently when the speech-language pathologist concludes that a client's condition requires immediate institution of therapy. In these instances, many sessions may have already been provided before claims are denied. If we insist that we should make all decisions as to whether particular services should be instituted, then we must accept all responsibilities—including financial—for those decisions. Therefore, in most instances, the contract must specify that fees paid to the supplier by the contracting agency will be refunded to the agency when claims are retroactively denied, unless some other source of payment is available.

These seven factors do not cover all eventualities. Specific provisions may differ depending upon the parties involved, the laws of the particular state, and the regulations of the fiscal agents involved. Unless a speech-language pathologist or audiologist is thoroughly experienced in these matters, legal counsel should be sought to forestall potentially serious financial, procedural, and professional problems.

Dispensing Products

Recent changes in attitudes about the appropriateness of professionals engaging in what was once considered commercial enterprise have led more and more members of our profession to consider dispensing products as an additional source of revenue. The involvement of audiologists in hearing aid dispensing has been discussed most extensively. However, conceivably, as more prosthetic appliances become available for speech-handicapped clients, speech-language pathologists will increasingly consider dispensing these products. Whatever the merits and demerits of speech-language pathologists and audiologists becoming involved in product dispensing, this area requires a rather different approach to professional economics and introduces some problems that differ markedly from those encountered in more traditional professional practices. Because hearing aid dispensing is most frequently at issue, this discussion will focus on that particular product. It seems likely, however, that the same principles will apply to dispensing other prostheses when they become more prevalent.

Hearing aid dispensing programs may be designed in several different ways. In some instances, dispensaries are established within or adjacent to audiology facilities but maintain financial independence from those facilities. In other instances, a dispensary is established as one of the services provided by the audiology facility, with one or more staff members (who may or may not be audiologists) employed exclusively within the dispensary. In still other instances, audiologists provide dispensing services as a part of their overall clinical responsibilities, and all aspects of dispensing are included within the overall financial structure of the agency or private practice. Loavenbruck and Madell (1981) discussed the many ramifications of these three approaches.

Among the many unique financial problems that are initiated by the introduction of product dispensing into a speech, language, and hearing services program are those related to *inventory maintenance*, *income and cash flow*, and *provision of supplies and repair services.*

INVENTORY MAINTENANCE

If one is to dispense products, the first step is to procure the products to be dispensed. With respect to hearing aids, Loavenbruck and Madell outlined three different approaches to procurement. The first option involves no inventory. Based on the initial hearing evaluation, potentially suitable hearing aids are ordered from the manufacturer. After the aid to be purchased is selected, the other instruments are returned to the manufacturer. (This procedure seems precarious at best since it makes unreasonable demands on manufacturers' return policies.)

The second approach involves purchase of a representative stock of hearing aids. These aids are used only for evaluations; they are never dispensed to clients. When an apparently suitable instrument is selected on the basis of a client's performance with a hearing aid from the trial stock, an aid of the same make and model is ordered from the manufacturer and dispensed to the client. This option offers some limitations on initial financial outlay, since only one each of a representative range of instruments is required, but it also presents some practical problems. Clients may object to time delays between selection of the aid and its availability for dispensing. The plan also requires an additional visit for the client to receive the hearing aid since it is unavailable when the recommendation is made, requiring additional time commitments from both client and professional staff. Furthermore, there are frequent performance disparities between the hearing aid in the trial stock and the one ordered for the client, even though they are of identical make and model. Therefore, the ordered aid may not suit the client as well as the aid used during the evaluation.

The third option involves maintaining a complete inventory of hearing aids. Aids used during evaluations are taken from this stock. When an aid seems satisfactory on the basis of the evaluation, that specific instrument is dispensed to the client. This option is generally preferable from the standpoint of quality of services. Its disadvantages lie in the required initial financial outlay to acquire the inventory, in the financial resources tied up in the inventory, and in the financial loss incurred from depreciation of the instruments in the inventory that are not ultimately dispensed to clients. All of these factors can be calculated in the costs of operating a dispensing program and offset in the fees and other income. Nevertheless, considerations related to inventory maintenance demand different kinds of financial planning than are required for other speech-language pathology and audiology services.

INCOME AND CASH FLOW

It is widely proposed that when a professional dispenses products, there should be a clear differentiation between fees for attendant professional services and the price of the product itself (sometimes referred to as "unbundling"). Unfortunately, this differentiation is not as simple as it might seem. When hearing aids are purchased through the usual commercial dispensing system a client pays a fixed sum of money (albeit frequently after some bargaining) that presumably covers the instrument and whatever services are provided by the dispenser in connection with selecting and fitting the instrument. Clients often expect the same approach when an audiologist dispenses the instrument. Yet, when there is no differentiation between purchase price and professional fees, the experienced hearing aid user who requires minimal services will be charged the same amount as the new "problem" user who requires extensive professional services. In usual practice, compromises are effected, with some differentiation of fees depending upon the extent of services required, but often the maximum fees do not actually cover the time expended.

Even though the professional time and overhead costs involved in selection and fitting procedures are covered through professional fees, several factors must be considered in establishing the actual price of the hearing aid. Among these factors are the cost of purchasing the instrument from the manufacturer, the cost of ordering the instrument, a share of the cost of maintaining the inventory and of purchasing and maintaining equipment for the dispensary, space occupancy, and other indirect costs. Naïve audiologists often propose that the cost of hearing aids to consumers would be substantially reduced if our profession were to assume total responsibility for dispensing. It has been amply demonstrated, however, that when audiologists must fully recoup all costs for time expended in attendant professional services and for maintaining an adequate inventory of instruments in a fully equipped dispensary, the actual consumer costs differ little from their costs in securing aids from many commercial dispensers. Any advantages we offer clients relate to quality and consistency of services, not to cost.

Ultimately, any audiologist or agency engaged in hearing aid dispensing may also face problems in cash flow that differ from the problems faced in connection with other services. When manufacturers sell instruments to dispensers, they must be paid promptly. If the instrument stays in the inventory, or if it is dispensed to a client who has not yet paid for it, the manufacturer must, nonetheless, be paid. Programs that stock large inventories or permit substantial accounts receivable for dispensed instruments can soon encounter major financial problems. Client convenience must often be sacrificed to economic practicalities. Agencies must usually restrict their inventories, including in them only the most frequently recommended instruments, even though clients may have to wait for a special order when another instrument is recommended. Furthermore, agencies often require payment on delivery to the client, with an agreement for full refund if the instrument proves unsatisfactory.

SUPPLIES AND REPAIR SERVICES

A dispenser's responsibility for a hearing aid does not cease when the client purchases it, because the instrument must be maintained throughout its useful life. This factor also introduces problems that are not encountered in other areas of professional practice. In dispensing hearing aids, some audiologists assume that maintenance is not included among their responsibilities. This attitude is unfair both to the client and to whomever the client may turn (usually a commercial dispenser) for maintenance services.

Hearing aid maintenance entails supplying replacement earmolds and batteries and repair services. New earmolds are usually dispensed at the time the hearing aid is sold. A separate fee is usually levied by the dispenser, covering the cost of taking the impression and the cost of fabrication, plus appropriate overhead. Replacement earmolds are usually dispensed on the same basis.

Most dispensers also maintain a stock of batteries for sale, either directly or by mail. Clients should be advised when more convenient sources for batteries are available, but it is important that they also recognize that the dispenser remains a source of ongoing assistance, even for such small services as providing batteries. Maintaining an inventory of batteries and dealing with the practical aspects of battery sales may be annoying and inconvenient, but in most situations this is a necessary component of an adequate dispensing program.

Few dispensers, whether commercial or professional, provide more than cursory hearing aid repair services. Instruments are usually returned to manufacturers for repairs, although other repair services are available in some communities. Usually, the fee for repair of the instrument is billed to the dispenser, who, in turn, charges the client an amount based upon the repair costs together with the costs of handling the instrument and arranging for its repair. Most dispensers maintain a stock of used instruments to be loaned to clients while their hearing aids are being repaired.

Professionals may make some of their most important contributions to dispensing practices through their role in maintaining their clients' hearing aids. Commercial dispensers often use the sale of supplies and arrangements for repairs as opportunities for selling new instruments. They may imply that a client's aid is superannuated or beyond repair when it is still satisfactory. Professionals who believe that hearing aid dispensing is best managed by professionals must manifest continuing concern for clients. That concern is best demonstrated through a willingness to assist clients in the day-to-day maintenance of the hearing aids they have dispensed.

PROGRAM-BASED SUPPORT

From their inception in the United States, speech-language pathology and audiology services have most frequently developed through program-based support. In this arrangement, services are funded on an overall programmatic basis rather than on the basis of covering costs of serving individual clients. Such support frequently entails specifications as to the scope of services to be provided, the number and type of clients to be served, the qualifications of providers, and other criteria that must be met to receive initial and continuing support.

The precise level of support may be constant, it may be renegotiated at intervals—usually annually—or it may fluctuate according to the volume of services provided during a particular time interval (in the latter instance, program-based support may be essentially indistinguishable from third-party payment). Program-based support may cover all costs, a portion of the costs, or, occasionally, may be provided in the form of subsidies to cover financial deficits.

One of the oldest examples of program-based support for services to clients with communicative disorders is the college or university speech and hearing clinic. Here, a college or university, whether public or private, provides funds to support clinical services, ostensibly because they are an essential component of a training program for speech-language pathologists and audiologists. Universities may also subsidize speech-language pathology and audiology programs in their medical centers, which serve to train physicians and other health professionals. Sometimes, college and university clinics are completely underwritten by their parent institutions. In other instances, these institutions make up the deficits between the costs of operating the clinics and the income from patients, third-party payers, or other sources.

Program-based support may be of two general types. It may be continuing support that will presumably be available so long as the services are needed and the program continues to meet whatever criteria have been established, and so long as funds are available. Or support may be time-limited, with funding offered to support services during a specified time interval. Usually, time-limited support is offered to assist in the establishment of new programs. Often these are considered to be innovative or demonstration programs, i.e., demonstrating the needs for particular services or innovative approaches to delivering services to previously underserved populations. Both continuing and time-limited program support may be provided by governmental and private agencies.

Governmental Agency Support

The same principle underlies governmental support for human services programs as underlies governmental support for human services to individuals. A free, humane society is responsible for meeting certain special needs of its citizens. Attitudes change from one political era to another as to the nature and scope of those responsibilities and as to how they should be carried out. Nevertheless, it is highly unlikely that our nation will ever completely abandon this basic principle.

Governmental support for programs is provided in at least as many forms as governmental support for individual services. The dominant example of support for speech, language, and hearing services programs is obviously found in the public schools, but other examples can also be cited.

SUPPORT FOR SCHOOL SERVICES

One fundamental premise has guided the development of financial support for special educational services in our public schools. It presupposes that local education agencies will be encouraged to offer these services if state education departments share the expense. Therefore, reimbursement plans are designed to pay all or part of the costs that exceed what the local education agency spends in educating any child. In other words, although the financial responsibility for providing regular education programs is assumed to rest with local education agencies, the cost for modifying or supplementing education programs to accommodate handicapped children is borne, at least partially, by the state education agency. In recent years this same principle has been extended so that states have been reimbursed by the federal government for a portion of their expenditures for special education.

Once again, it is difficult to be specific in discussing this aspect of service delivery in the schools because each state presents some unique features in its approaches to support of school services. Some states may even apply different approaches depending on the size of the school district, its organizational structure (e.g., county versus city, unified versus independent), and the type of services offered. In general, however, three different patterns of support can be defined: *unit reimbursement*, *per-pupil reimbursement*, and *special reimbursement* (Jones and Healey, 1975).

Unit reimbursement. In this pattern of reimbursement, a state pays a fixed sum or a percentage of the total cost for each special class or special program that meets specified standards. For example, a state may pay a local school district a given amount for each special class for hearing-impaired children that qualifies within standards of minimum and maximum enrollment and is assigned to a properly credentialed teacher. Or, a state may pay a local school district X dollars per annum for each speech, language, and hearing services program when that program carries a caseload within a specified range and is conducted by a credentialed specialist. (In one variation of unit support for speech-language pathology services, a "unit" is defined as a given number of pupils, e.g., one state specifies a unit as 24 pupils. Under this system a single clinician may be responsible for two or even three "units" and generate reimbursement accordingly.)

So long as equitable formulas are applied, unit reimbursement is probably superior to other plans in programmatic terms. The local education agency is encouraged to develop programs that meet specified standards and is reimbursed accordingly, regardless of the number of children enrolled within each program (assuming, of course, that the number exceeds specified minimum enrollments). The approach can be disadvantageous to speech-language pathologists who function within a system that permits them to carry several units, resulting in pressure to enroll an excessive caseload. Occasionally, this system may also encourage school districts to meet minimum enrollment criteria by registering children inappropriately in special classes. This can occur in programs for hearing-impaired children, in which children with moderate impairments are grouped with children who have profound impairments in order to meet minimum class size requirements.

Per-pupil reimbursement. Here, a local education agency is compensated for each pupil receiving special services. The precise amount may be established on the basis of the nature of the disability and the type of services delivered. One widely applied version of per-pupil reimbursement is compensation on the basis of average daily attendance (ADA). In this system a school is paid a specified amount for each "unit of ADA" reported. When applied to full-time special placements, the formula reimburses on the basis of the average daily attendance in that class. (Thus, if a class for severely hearing-impaired children has an average daily attendance of 5.4, compensation would be based on 5.4 times the amount of money the state allows per unit of ADA.)

When applied to speech-language pathology services, ADA formulas are adapted to recognize that each child is served during only a portion of the school day. Therefore, each child enrolled in a speech-language pathology program generates a fraction of ADA support. As a rule, formulas are applied that differentiate between individual and group therapy sessions.

Once again, standards as to class size and teacher/specialist qualifications are usually specified as criteria for reimbursement. Nevertheless, per-pupil compensation does tend to emphasize quantity rather than quality. Particularly during the present era of declining support to education, administrators often pressure specialists to work with larger and larger numbers of children in order to generate more and more money.

A further disadvantage of per-pupil reimbursement is found in states that insist that all pupil counts be unduplicated. In other words, if a child is generating ADA support because of placement in a class for severely handicapped children, he or she may not also generate ADA support when served by a speech, language, and hearing specialist. This situation can deter the availability of supplementary special services to children who are enrolled in special education programs.

Special reimbursement. From time to time, state education departments offer special reimbursement plans. Usually, these plans serve to complement unit or per-pupil reimbursement. They may also be used to encourage the development of new programs, often as "demonstrations." Or special reimbursement may be offered to solve problems encountered by certain school districts in providing special services (e.g., rural districts, districts serving children from central cities or non-English-speaking children). Special reimbursement may also be provided on a regular basis to facilitate activities and services that are not covered within the provisions of other reimbursement systems (e.g., medical, psychological, and social work services, summer sessions, residential schools). Special reimbursement is usually offered either on the basis of a fixed sum grant or on the basis of compensation to a local school district for all or a portion of their expenditures in connection with a particular service or activity.

Jones and Healey (1975) identified nine categories in which special reimbursement may be provided: (1) instructional materials and equipment; (2) transportation; (3) facilities; (4) research and experimentation; (5) personnel training; (6) pupil assessment; (7) residential care; (8) extended school year; and (9) specific personnel such as administrators and supervisors, teachers and specialists, paraprofessionals, and such ancillary services personnel as physicians, audiologists, psychologists, social workers, etc.

OTHER GOVERNMENTAL SUPPORT

The outstanding example of federal program-based support for speech-language pathology and audiology services can be found in the network of programs sponsored by the Veterans Administration. These services were established immediately following World War II. Although most VA programs provide hospital-based in- and outpatient services, some exclusively outpatient clinics remain. The treatment of conditions related to military service-connected disabilities is the major emphasis of VA programs, but in some instances other clients are also served. Both speech-language pathology and audiology services are usually provided within the same program, but occasionally only one or the other is offered. The VA delivery system for hearing aids is particularly innovative and has been widely studied by many public and private groups (most notably by the Federal Trade Commission) that are seeking alternatives to the delivery system available to the public at large.

Another network of federally supported programs is found in DOD military facilities. Some, but by no means all, military hospitals offer speech-language pathology and audiology services. These programs may be staffed by military personnel or by civilians. Services are available to military personnel on active duty and to their dependents and to retired personnel and their dependents. As mentioned in the earlier discussion of CHAMPUS, DOD facilities establish priorities, so that dependents and retired personnel may not always be served immediately.

The federal government has also supported occasional speech-language pathology and audiology services through the Bureau of Indian Affairs. This agency has provided funds for construction of health care facilities, for continuing program support, and for the training of health care specialists to serve Native Americans of the continental United States and Alaska.

Speech-language pathology and audiology services have also been supported by various federal maternal and child health funds. Typical are maternal and infant care projects (primarily those aimed at "high-risk" mothers and infants) and children and youth projects aimed at the delivery of services to low-income families. The era of the "war on poverty" saw the rapid expansion of these programs and of other health and human services targeting low-income groups. The earlier-discussed Project Head Start was one such program. The increased commitment to services for the developmentally disabled that also characterized this era made substantial federal funds available for special program support. Succeeding years have seen the phasing out of many of these programs and the transfer of others to local jurisdictions, often with some level of federal support continuing. Other out-of-school services, supported by such state and local governmental agencies as health and mental hygiene departments, were reviewed in Chapter 3 because they represent models for service delivery as well as models for financial support.

In addition to providing ongoing support, governmental funds have also been available for the initiation of innovative programs, particularly for demonstrating new approaches to providing care for previously ill-served populations. Among the agencies that currently award such funds are the Bureau of Community Health Services, the National Center for Health Services Research, and the Administration on Aging (all component agencies of the Department of Health and Human Services); and the Division of Innovation and Development and the National Institute of Handicapped Research, which function under the Office of Special Education and Rehabilitative Services of the Department of Education. Generally, these funds are awarded to agencies that can offer some assurance of continuing local support after the demonstration period has passed.

Private Support

Support for speech-language pathology and audiology services—both continuing and time-limited support—may be provided by private benefactors. Although private support may come from an almost infinite variety of sources, most fall within one of four categories.

UNITED GIVERS FUNDS AND VOLUNTARY HEALTH AGENCIES

The first half of this century saw the emergence of many charitable organizations, each turning to the public for support through individual contributions. Many had drives for direct cash contributions through such avenues as the March of Dimes; some sponsored telethons; others engaged in the sale of Christmas seals or Easter seals. All of these organizations sought large donations from business and industry and from private philanthropies, but they also stressed the importance of more modest contributions from the public at large. Most were completely reputable, exercising stringent stewardship over their funds. A few, however, were less scrupulous, using the major portion of their incomes to cover fund-raising costs and other overhead expenses and allotting little to the services they purportedly offered.

Gradually, leaders in many communities became concerned about the proliferation of charity appeals and about the limited monitoring of the funds that accrued to these charities. In particular, executives in business and industry and labor union officials were distressed by the increasing solicitations of employee groups. They reacted by lending their support to the development of united givers funds. These funds have developed in different ways in our communities, but there are many essential similarities. Most are now affiliated with the United Way of America. United funds ostensibly offer communities, and businesses and industries within those communities, the promise that one gift will cover all affiliated community agencies. On the strength of this promise, most have achieved such important kinds of cooperation as payroll withholding of pledged contributions. In actual fact, however, few united fund-affiliated agencies receive sufficient support to forego other fund-raising activities, often including direct solicitation of contributions.

Typically, united givers funds establish detailed admissions procedures and standards for agencies seeking affiliation. Applications are reviewed by committees comprised of volunteer community representatives in consultation with professional staff. Because of financial limitations, relatively few new agencies have become affiliates of united givers funds in recent years.

Affiliated agencies present funding requests annually. These requests are reviewed by budget panels, which are also composed of volunteers representing the community. This review usually entails both appraisal of the services offered by the agency and scrutiny of financial operations. Ultimately, allocations to all member agencies are determined by a single budget committee. These allocations are intended, as a rule, to cover deficits that remain after all other public and private funding resources have been exhausted. Seldom, then, do united giver fund allocations provide the major support for member agencies' programs.

Organized united givers funds in some communities are affiliated with religious groups. These funds, typified by united Jewish appeals and Catholic charity drives, often exist concurrently with the secular united givers funds in a community.

United givers funds have provided direct support for many community speech and hearing centers. Frequently, other human services agencies that are beneficiaries of these funds either employ members of our profession or purchase speech, language, and hearing services from private practitioners or other agencies.

The voluntary health association is another charity phenomenon of the 20th century in America. Some—such as United Cerebral Palsy, the American Heart Association, the American Cancer Society, and Aid for Retarded Citizens—focus their efforts on serving clients with specific conditions and fund research in areas directly related to those conditions. Others, like the Easter Seals Societies for Crippled Children and Adults, serve broader client groups. Although some of these associations are affiliated with united givers funds in their communities, others maintain completely independent fund-raising efforts (some associations forbid affiliation with united funds).

Typically, contributions to voluntary

health associations are divided according to established formulas, with a portion being forwarded to national and state associations and the remainder assigned to the local affiliate. Associations that place major emphasis on research and public education require that a major share be forwarded to the national organization; those emphasizing delivery of direct services permit most of the money to remain in the local community.

Voluntary health associations have played a significant role in financing speech, language, and hearing services. Many support rehabilitation centers and other human services agencies that include our professional services among their offerings. Most notable among these are the Easter Seals Societies and local affiliates of United Cerebral Palsy. Local affiliates of the American Cancer Society have supported speech services for laryngectomees, and affiliates of the American Heart Association provide speech services to stroke victims who are aphasic. Although presented here as resources for programmatic support, voluntary health associations in some communities occasionally function as third-party payers, covering fees for services to clients who fall within their purview.

SERVICE CLUBS AND FRATERNAL ORGANIZATIONS

Another important source of programmatic funding in many communities is found among service clubs and fraternal organizations. Although these groups are formed to provide social opportunities for their members, most also are dedicated to carrying out human services projects in their communities. These projects may be modest in extent—conducted primarily by club members on a voluntary basis—but others may be of substantial magnitude, involving significant support for professional services. Usually, when extensive services are supported, individual clubs join together on a regional or statewide basis.

These organizations often designate nationally a particular area of service, and urge local and state groups to develop projects in that area. After many years of support to projects for the visually impaired, Lions International recently added a commitment to services for the hearing impaired and encouraged local Lions Clubs to support programs in that area. For several years Sertoma has encouraged support of programs serving children and adults with communicative disorders. Through its Major Projects, the Elks have developed programs for children with cerebral palsy and other severely handicapping conditions, which often include speech-language pathology services.

Many service clubs and fraternal organizations grant complete discretion to local groups in choosing areas of service. Most groups, therefore, can be considered as potential benefactors of speech, language, and hearing services. Again, although discussed here as providers of program support, these organizations can pay for services to individual clients. Furthermore, they may be available to assist in the purchase of particular pieces of equipment for individual clients or for services agencies.

Although organizationally quite different from other service clubs and fraternal organizations, the Junior League has assisted human services programs in many communities. They may occasionally provide long-range support, but most local Junior League groups emphasize time-limited funding of innovative projects. Their grants, which usually diminish over 3- to 5-year intervals, are awarded only with clear assurance of other support for continuing the program after the demonstration period is over.

Sorority alumnae groups have also provided services to children and adults with communicative disorders; some have even designated this area for emphasis at a national level. These groups are usually more available for limited support for individual clients and for assistance in the purchase of specific equipment and materials than for substantial program funding.

FOUNDATIONS AND OTHER PHILANTHROPIES

Encouraged by our nation's tax laws, there are literally thousands of private foundations in the United States. Some are multimillion dollar organizations offering sizable grants in many areas of human service. Others, based on small endowments, award limited amounts of money within narrowly defined areas. Private foundations remain a major source of programmatic support for human services programs.

Occasionally, private foundations provide continuing program support, but most make time-limited grants offering diminishing financial aid to cover a demonstration period (once again, assurance for continued funding from other sources can be a crucial requirement). With some notable exceptions, grants for community programs are most likely to be supported by local foundations in the same community.

Many large communities publish guides to local and regional foundations. These guides not only assist in identifying appropriate foundations, they also specify application procedures.

When a foundation employs a professional staff, the initial approach is often via personal interviews with staff members. Frequently, foundations request brief written summaries of proposals as a screening device. If that summary interests them, a full application is invited. Foundations differ widely in the kind of applications they prefer. Some request brief, concise proposals; others require long, detailed applications.

Most local foundations assign the responsibility for awarding grants to their boards of directors. Often, personal contacts with one or more members of those boards, preferably from a personal acquaintance, can be very influential.

A few local foundations set aside funds for direct payment for services to individual clients. Payment for speech-language pathology and audiology services is occasionally available.

Although tax laws have encouraged philanthropists to work through foundations, private philanthropy still exists. Community speech and hearing centers have particularly benefited from the generosity of affluent individuals. Many speech, language, and hearing services agencies have also benefited from bequests. These seldom arrive out of the blue; they are usually cultivated over long periods of time.

BUSINESS AND INDUSTRY

Support for speech, language, and hearing services can come from business and industry in two different ways. Such services may be provided for their employees, most frequently in the form of hearing conservation programs. Many—particularly larger—businesses and industries have established foundations that support a variety of activities in their communities. These corporate foundations constitute a further financial source for human services programs. Often, when a particular corporation actively supports the local united givers fund, it excludes member agencies from consideration for grants from their corporate foundation. In most respects, corporate foundations operate similarly to other private foundations and offer comparable resources for support for speech, language, and hearing services.

SUMMARY

During the past two decades many new sources have emerged for supporting speech-language pathology and audiology services. Some cover the costs of delivering services to individual clients. Typically, these sources are public and private third-party payment programs, essentially intended to cover the costs of health care services. Other sources of support cover all or portions of total program costs rather than covering fees for individual client services. These sources of program-based support may also be public agencies—departments of education, health departments, such federal agencies as the Veterans Administration, etc.—or they may be private agencies or individual philanthropists.

Despite the many new sources that have developed, as the costs of human services have escalated, there is increasing competition for securing payment for these services on either an individual or a programmatic basis. If speech-language pathology and audiology services are to be available to the people who need them, we must be increasingly enterprising in developing new sources of support. Furthermore, it is inevitable that, for the immediate future at least, consumers must assume increasing personal responsibility for paying for the services they receive.

References

American Speech-Language-Hearing Association Governmental Affairs Department: Medicare Supplement. *Governmental Affairs Review*, June 1981.

American Speech-Language-Hearing Association Task Force on Private Health Insurance: *A Report on Third Party Reimbursement of Speech-Language Pathology and Audiology Services*. Rockville, MD, American Speech-Language-Hearing Association, 1980.

Brantman M: The status and outlook for commercial health insurance: coverage of speech and hearing services. *ASHA* 15:183–187, 1973.

Feldman AS: The challenge of autonomy. *ASHA* 23:941–945, 1981.

Ginnold RE: *Occupational Hearing Loss: Workers' Compensation under State and Federal Programs*. Washington DC, United States Environmental Protection Agency, 1979.

Goates JS, Goates WA: Increasing third-party coverage of speech-language pathology and audiology services. *ASHA* 19:887–889, 1977.

Jones SA, Healey WC: *Project Upgrade: Guidelines for Evaluating State Education Laws and Regulations*. Rockville, MD, American Speech and Hearing Association, 1975.

Loavenbruck AM, Madell JR: *Hearing Aid Dispensing for Audiologists*. New York, Grune and Stratton, 1981.

Pines PL: Revised Medicare requirements. *ASHA* 23:357–358, 1981.

Prussin JA, Wood JC: Private third party reimbursement. *Topics in Health Care Financing* 2:1–89, 1975.

Stryker S: Procedures relating to Medicare and other third-party payments. *ASHA* 18:491–495, 1976.

PART 4

Protecting the Consumers of Speech-Language Pathology and Audiology Services

CHAPTER ELEVEN

Legal and Ethical Considerations in Delivering Speech-Language Pathology and Audiology Services

Substantial concern for client rights is a relatively new development in the field of human services. So long as their clients' lives, limbs, and psyches were not severely impaired, and so long as they generally filled the roles that society assigned to them, human services professionals were once granted essential immunity from close scrutiny. The protection of professional sovereignty was a major determiner of the laws that governed professional practices. It was an even more dominant element in the codes of ethics adopted by most professional associations.

During the mid-20th century, freethinkers asserted that consumers of human services, like all citizens of a free society, had inalienable rights. This mood infected students of our nation's educational system, patients in our health care system, and clients of our social agencies. The influence of this consumer rights movement was increasingly reflected in the laws and regulations adopted by federal and state governments. Gradually, professional associations re-evaluated the self-serving provisions of their codes of ethics, and—often to forestall legal action—shifted the focus toward preserving client rights.

From the outset, the profession of speech-language pathology and audiology has asserted greater concern for the protection of the consumers of our services than for professional self-protection. But this situation probably can be attributed to the patterns of our development rather than to our essential virtue. Since most of our early programs developed in the protected environs of educational agencies, there was little need to achieve precise legal definitions of our field. Furthermore, we seldom found ourselves in competition with other professions or, for that matter, with each other. Therefore, we had little need to legally define our professional territory or our interprofessional relationships or to dwell on intraprofessional relationships in our code of ethics.

In our public postures, we may have appeared more deeply concerned with consumer rights than were some other professions, but our private attitudes have not always been as scrupulous. Our use of individuals with communicative disorders in research and teaching, our abrupt termination of services to clients at the end of semesters and school years, our tolerance for inadequately trained personnel, our disregard for the costs of our services and of the recommendations we make are all prevalent practices that neglect our clients' best interests.

Clients of speech-language pathologists and audiologists have the same fundamental rights as the clients of all providers of human services. Many human services agencies have formulated and published formal statements of these rights. The following, adapted from several of these statements, is proposed as a Bill of Rights for consumers of speech-language pathology and audiology services:

A Client Bill of Rights

As you become a client of this program/department/agency, it is our duty to remind you that the services you receive are a cooperative effort between you as a client and the members of our professional staff. While you are receiving our services, someone will always be available to assist you in the decisions you must make and to help you understand your rights as a client. The following is a list of your rights. You should always advise us of any questions or concerns about any of these rights.

1. A potential client has the right to complete and accurate information regarding services available and procedures employed.
2. A client has the right to informed participation in all decisions regarding his or her care.
3. A client has the right to a clear, complete, and accurate evaulation of his or her condition and prognosis before being asked to consent to any procedure.
4. A client has the right to a clear, concise explanation, in layperson's terms, of all proposed procedures and their probability of success and will not be subjected to any procedure without his or her voluntary, competent, and understanding consent.
5. A client has the right to know the identity and professional status of all those providing services.
6. A client has the right to know when he or she is participating in teaching or research programs and to be informed of what alternatives are available in the community.
7. A client has the right not to be subjected to any test or procedure designed for educational purposes rather than for his or her direct personal benefit.
8. A client has the right to refuse any particular test or procedure.
9. A client has the right to privacy of both person and information with respect to the professional staff, other professionals, students, and other clients.
10. A client has the right to discuss his or her condition and care with a consultant specialist, at the client's request and expense.
11. A client has the right to all information contained in his or her record and to examine the record on request.
12. A client has the right not to be transferred or referred to another facility unless he or she has received a complete explanation of the desirability and need for the transfer or referral, the other facility has accepted the transfer or referral, and the client has agreed.
13. A client has the right, regardless of the source of payment, to examine and receive an itemized and detailed explanation of all bills for services rendered.
14. A client has the right to competent counseling to help in obtaining financial assistance from public or private sources to meet the expense of services.
15. A client has the right to timely prior notice of termination of eligibility for services or eligibility for third-party payment for those services or of any other circumstances that will influence the client's financial liability.

LEGAL VERSUS ETHICAL CONSTRAINTS

Our society has enacted laws, presumably to serve its best interests, that directly and indirectly regulate many facets of the delivery of human services. All organizations of human services professionals have also established codes of ethics that define acceptable standards of professional conduct. Although laws and codes of ethics may address similar issues, they apply quite different constraints. Laws and the regulations that elaborate those laws are enforced by exacting legal penalties for violations, penalties that can include the loss of the right to practice a profession, liability for fines, judgments requiring financial settlements, and the loss of public funds to support professional services. Violations of codes of ethics, however, involve less rigorous consequences. A code of ethics is adopted by an association and voluntarily subscribed to by its members. Therefore, it exerts influence only over those professionals who choose to belong to that association. Furthermore, the severest penalty that can be exacted for violations of a code of ethics involves revoking the culprit's membership in the association.

On the one hand, because of the graver penalties that may be exacted, laws are more effective regulators of professional practices. On the other hand, laws generally define the absolute limits of professional practices, beyond which they are clearly antithetical to the public interest. As voluntarily imposed standards of practice, codes of ethics are generally more stringent than laws and legal regulations.

The American Speech-Language-Hearing Association has adopted a Code of Ethics for the profession of speech-language pathology and audiology. That Code must be subscribed to by all members of ASHA and by all other holders of the ASHA Certificates of Clinical Competence. In its most recently revised edition, the Code describes the "fundamental rules of ethical conduct" in three categories: Principles of Ethics, Ethical Proscriptions, and Matters of Professional Propriety. There are six principles which serve as a "basis for the evaluation of professional conduct." The ethical proscriptions are "formal statements of prohibitions" that are derived from the principles. Matters of professional propriety present "guidelines of conduct designed to promote the public interest."

Ten broad aspects of the practice of our profession are addressed both in law and in ASHA's Code of Ethics. These are: professional qualifications; informed consent; confidentiality and the prudent management of clinical information; negligence and malpractice; use of clients in research and teaching; fees and other financial arrangements; advertising and public information; dispensing products; nondiscrimination and the right to services; and intra- and interprofessional relationships.

Professional Qualifications

An obvious first consideration in consumer protection is some assurance that professionals possess the basic qualifications to provide the services they offer. This consideration underlies both legal and ethical constraints.

LEGAL CONSTRAINTS

Approaches to defining legally who may provide speech-language pathology and audiology were discussed in some detail in Chapter 2. To recap, two general approaches are most frequently employed. The first involves state licensure. The second involves the definition in laws and regulations of qualifications to deliver services within public programs. The clearest example of this approach can be found in the laws and regulations of all 50 states, defining qualifications for providing speech, language, and hearing services in the public schools. It is also illustrated by provider regulations for such federal and state third-party payment programs as Medicare, Medicaid, Crippled Children Services, and departments of rehabilitation. (These regulations generally specify state licensure, or ASHA certification when no state licensure laws exist.)

When states license speech-language pathologists and audiologists, unlicensed practitioners are subject to prosecution. Unlicensed practice is considered a grave offense in some areas of human service—particularly in medicine—but thus far unlicensed speech-language pathologists and audiologists have not been dealt with severely. Although warnings may be issued, some kind of amicable agreement is usually reached.

Instances of forfeiture or suspension of licenses have been more common. As with all professions, however, such actions are usually precipitated by egregious offenses. Licensure statutes usually name, as bases for disciplinary action, malpractice and professional incompetence, mental and physical incapacity, and conviction for a state or federal drug offense or other crimes that impinge on professional practice. To result in legal disciplinary action, instances of malpractice and professional incompetence are usually so flagrant that the offenses are patently obvious. When less serious problems arise, license holders are usually warned by the agency that administers the licensure program, hoping that the warning will lead the miscreant to mend his or her ways. Thus far, forfeitures or suspensions (or, more frequently, voluntary surrenders) of licenses of speech-language pathologists and audiologists have resulted from defrauding governmental third-party payers or from sexual offenses, such as child molesting. In general, then, once licenses are granted, they are only lost under dire circumstances.

It is important to recognize that no action related to denial or revocation of a license is trivial, because of the grave consequences to a professional's ability to earn a living. Accusations must always be proven according to established legal procedures. In the meantime, in conformity with our legal system, the accused is innocent until proven guilty. Such procedures protect professionals against capricious actions based on false accusations. But they also limit the regulatory effectiveness of licensure programs. Consumer advocates frequently damn licensure programs as controlled by the professional groups they presumably regulate and hence as more concerned with self-protection and self-preservation than with consumer interests. Although these charges have some merit, the limited effectiveness of licensure programs is more likely to result from the laggardness of due process and to their usual inability to deal with other than the gravest offenses.

Licensure also merely attests to the qualifications of a holder at the time the license was granted and in no way assures currency in the profession. Several states have responded to this concern by requiring evidence of continuing professional education as one aspect of licensure renewal. Currently—in part because of the lack of evidence that continuing education requirements have achieved their purpose and in part because of the overall de-emphasis on governmental regulation—few new continuing education requirements are being legislated, and some existing requirements have been rescinded.

Recognizing the growing use of support personnel in the delivery of human services, several states have enacted laws and regulations pertaining to the use of paraprofessionals in speech-language pathology and audiology. These laws generally assign the legal responsibility for services carried out by paraprofessionals to the licensed speech-language pathologists and audiologists responsible for their supervision. They may provide for an official registration procedure as well. State education codes may also define the use of aides in school speech, language, and hearing services programs.

ETHICAL CONSTRAINTS

ASHA's Code of Ethics addresses issues related to professional qualifications in several different ways. Basic provider qualifications are defined by the following principle:

> Individuals engaging in clinical practice shall possess appropriate qualifications which are provided by the Association's program for certification of clinical competence.

Recognizing that the ASHA certificates define only minimal levels of competence, this principle is amplified and extended through the following proscription:

> Individuals must neither provide services nor supervision of services for which they have not been properly prepared, nor permit services to be provided by any of their staff who are not properly prepared.

This proscription clearly implies that every professional must not only possess minimal competencies, but must also offer expertise in the specific areas of practice in which he or she engages. It affords the potential for more discrete consumer protection than can ever be afforded by legal regulation. In the final analysis, however, it is a subjective standard which professionals impose on themselves.

ASHA's Code of Ethics also addresses the need for maintaining professional currency in this principle:

> Individuals shall continue their professional development throughout their careers.

To implement this concept, ASHA announced, several years ago, its intention to institute a program for the renewal of clinical certification on the basis of completion of a required program of continuing professional education. This practice has been adopted by many human services professions in their certification programs. After considerable study, revealing that the effectiveness of mandatory continuing education programs is questionable and that such programs create serious practical and financial problems to many professionals—particularly to professionals outside of urban centers—ASHA reversed its earlier position and developed, instead, a voluntary continuing education program.

The Code of Ethics also defines professionals' responsibilities for support personnel and for other people who have not completed full professional preparation for the delivery of clinical services:

> Individuals must not delegate any service requiring the professional competence of a certified clinician to anyone unqualified.
>
> Individuals must not offer clinical services by supportive personnel for whom they do not provide appropriate supervision and assume full responsibility.
>
> Individuals must not require anyone under their supervision to engage in any practice that is in violation of the Code of Ethics.

ASHA's Code of Ethics clearly assigns to speech-language pathologists and audiologists the responsibility to assess their professional competencies and to continually upgrade those competencies. It also broadly defines professionals' responsibilities for the people they supervise. It further offers some general standards for peer evaluation. If taken seriously by professionals, then, the Code affords the potential for more effective assurance that consumers are served by qualified individuals than can ever be offered by legal regulation.

Informed Consent

Concepts of informed consent rest on two basic precepts: Every responsible citizen in a free society has the right to accept or reject whatever services are proposed. Furthermore, he or she must be given sufficient information to make reasoned choices among whatever options are available. These notions may seem so unequivocal that they do not even merit discussion. Yet, they have only recently been regarded seriously in many segments of the human services delivery system, particularly in the health care system. That concern has intensified in the wake of numerous legal actions related to informed consent.

LEGAL CONSTRAINTS

Understandably, most legal concerns about informed consent have thus far focused on medical practice, particularly on issues relating to treatments that hold risks of death, permanent disability, or disfigurement. When such treatments are recommended, the law has repeatedly held that an individual must have the opportunity to make an informed choice, weighing the likely benefits against the risks.

Thus far most court cases centering on informed consent have related to grave consequences of medical treatment (Annas et al., 1981, p. 75):

> When one looks at the informed consent decisions, one sees that the cases do not deal with trivial side effects. They involve risks of paralysis, sterilization, death, deafness, disfigurement, and other serious complications.

According to Annas et al., from a medical-legal standpoint, the doctrine of informed consent is based on four postulates (p. 73):

1. Patients are unlearned in the medical sciences.
2. A person of adult years and sound mind has the right to determine whether or not to submit to medical treatment.
3. The patient's consent, to be effective, must be informed consent.
4. The patient is in abject dependence upon his physician for the information upon which he relies in reaching his decision.

The increasing proclivity of our citizenry to litigation has caused concern in other possibly sensitive areas. Psychotherapists, for example, are scrutinizing their practices to identify areas of risk. When treatments involving drug therapy or electroconvulsive therapy are involved, the same risks obtain as in any area of medical practice. But when behavioral therapy or other psychotherapeutic approaches are at issue, few precedents are available; the potential risks of treatment are more difficult to define. Furthermore, among clients with serious psychological and behavioral problems, it may be problematic to ascertain whether a client fully comprehends those risks and is capable of making an informed choice.

Halleck (1980, p. 93) addressed these concerns:

> The issue of how much understanding the patient needs to provide an informed consent remains murky. So far the courts have focused on the transmission of information rather than on its reception and assimilation. If the information transmitted is such that a reasonable person would have received and assimilated it, consent decision is valid. Problems could certainly arise if the patient were unable to receive and assimilate information as a reasonable person would. Theoretically, this could happen if the patient's sensorium were clouded by illness or medication, if the patient had a hearing or language problem, or if the patient had a mental illness. The issue of mental illness brings us right back to the question of competency. A mentally ill patient who cannot receive and assimilate information relative to treatment is not competent to make a reasonable decision regarding treatment. Faulty comprehension of information regarding treatment can lead to an incompetent acceptance or an incompetent refusal of treatment.

So long as legal concerns regarding informed consent are restricted to grave consequences, it seems unlikely that speech-language pathologists and audiologists are likely to be at considerable risk. It would be difficult to imagine a situation in which serious physical consequences would attend any of our usual evaluative or therapeutic procedures. One can, however, imagine not-too-far-fetched eventualities in which clients might charge that they ultimately suffered because a member of our profession failed to specify clearly the possible negative consequences of refusing treatment. Consider these hypothetical situations:

> A high school junior who stutters refuses to accept a program of speech therapy recommended by the school speech, language, and hearing specialist. Following graduation, he discovers that his stuttering seriously interferes with his ability to find employment. He sues the school specialist, alleging that the possible negative vocational consequences of refusing therapy were not explained to him.
>
> A woman who uses her voice professionally is referred to a speech-language pathologist for voice therapy. Following the initial evaluation she refuses to return for further therapy. Eventually a surgical procedure is carried out to strip the vocal folds, and permanent changes in voice quality occur. She sues the speech-language pathologist, alleging that the negative consequences of refusing therapy were not mentioned.

These examples are fictional, but they are far from inconceivable.

We have probably reached the point in our development as a profession at which we must consider whether the risks of submitting to, or refusing to submit to, the services we provide are sufficient to require the kind of written statements now secured by physicians and other health care providers. Conceivably, the special nature of such procedures as auditory brainstem response testing (which entails sedation), electronystagmography (if administered by audiologists), and the fitting of speech appliances to laryngectomees following tracheoesophageal puncture may prudently require written consent from the client or responsible agent. Otherwise, for the present at least, securing written consent for each service we provide may be unnecessary, although such written consent may be a standard requirement of all departments in some settings where speech-language pathologists and audiologists are employed. Furthermore, individual professionals or departments may opt for routine written consent statements, recognizing that these may be useful even when litigation is not involved, particularly when disputes arise over the recommendations that are made or about the likely outcomes of those recommendations, and especially about matters relating to financial liability.

Whether written consent is secured or not, it is probably always advisable to note in client records the precise procedures that were carried out, that the nature of the procedures was explained and results interpreted, that recommendations were discussed, and that the possible consequences of following or not following those recommendations were outlined. Records should also probably show clinicians' impressions as to clients' understanding of what has transpired.

A further possible involvement of speech-language pathologists and audiologists in questions regarding informed consent can be surmised from Halleck's (1980) earlier-quoted discussion of the question of determination as to whether clients with hearing and language impairments comprehend physician interpretations of treatment risks. Again, I know of no actual instance of such an involvement in litigation, but it is certainly conceivable.

When a client is judged not competent to give fully informed consent, the consent of a family member is usually considered sufficient. In the strictest sense, however, authorization to make legally binding decisions for another individual occurs only after a judicial determination of incompetency, and then only to a parent of a minor child or a legally appointed guardian. Generally, parents must participate when informed consent is required in matters involving minors, except when that minor is "emancipated" (i.e., no longer under the care, custody, and control of the parents). Some states have defined what constitutes "emancipated" in more precise terms. In recent years, various laws and regulations have specified other instances in which parental involvement need not occur, particularly with reference to counseling about contraception and in the prescription of contraceptive devices. Several states also limit parental authority in effecting voluntary commitments of minors to psychiatric hospitals.

Concerns for informed consent recur in several provisions of PL 94-142. Written parental consent must be secured before the child is assessed for placement in a special education program. If parents fail to respond to requests for their consent, they may be compelled to respond through due process hearings or court actions, the assessment may go forward without consent, or any educational placement may be denied until consent is obtained. Parents must be informed of any assessments that are conducted subsequent to the preplacement evaluation, but written permission is not required. Written parental consent must also be obtained for initial placement in a special education program. Following that initial placement, changes may be effected after informing the parents, but do not require formal consent. All communications with parents in connection with assessments and placements must employ the language spoken by the parent and must inform them of the procedures they may pursue should they disagree with the proposed plan. Dublinske and Healey (1978) discussed these and other provisions of PL 94-142 in considerable detail.

ETHICAL CONSTRAINTS

Concern for the importance of informed consent is evident in this principle from ASHA's Code of Ethics:

> Individuals shall fully inform persons served of the nature and possible effects of services.

One issue that must be considered in elucidating the possible effects of services, however, is our frequent inability to predict what will occur. Particularly with respect to the outcomes of therapy programs, we do not have the kinds of data that are often required to make such predictions with any real confidence. Clearly, these kinds of data are sorely needed. In the meantime, however, we must strike some sort of compromise between offering clients the information necessary for their informed consent and overreaching the state of our art and science in making claims that are purely conjectures. This problem is addressed in one of the proscriptions that follow the ethical principle just cited:

> Individuals must not guarantee the results of any therapeutic procedures, directly or by implication. A reasonable statement of prognosis may be made, but caution must be exercised not to mislead persons served professionally to expect results that cannot be predicted from sound evidence.

Confidentiality

The Hippocratic Oath, probably the earliest recorded code of conduct for a group of human services professionals, includes these words:

> Whatever things I see or hear concerning the life of man, in any attendance on the sick or even apart therefrom which ought not to be noised about, I will keep silent thereon, counting such things to be professional secrets.

Concern for the sanctity of information disclosed in the course of relationships between professionals and their clients is evident in all professional codes of ethics and is buttressed by laws regulating professional conduct.

LEGAL CONSTRAINTS

Most federal and state statutes relating to the confidentiality of personal information deal with two principles: (1) except under certain overriding circumstances, such information should be released only with the specific permission of the subject of the information, or of his or her legal agent; (2) the subject, or his or her legal agent, should have the right to review any records containing that information to ascertain its accuracy and to correct inaccuracies. Although the first principle has guided human services providers for many years, the second has been considered only recently, and then often only sporadically.

Consent to disclose confidential information may be in three different forms. First, under *implied consent*, it may be assumed that when a client seeks services from a facility, all staff members who are participating in those services, and all support personnel, may have access to any and all information without the client's specific authorization.

Second, *written consent* is required for the release of information to all individuals outside of that facility. Clients maintain the right to determine what information may be released from clinical records and to whom the information may be released. There have been attempts to classify data in clinical records as confidential and nonconfidential. Nonconfidential data consist of the fact that the client has been seen and the dates of admission and discharge. Confidential data comprise all information concerning the nature of the client's problems, services provided, outcomes of these services, and recommendations proposed. Ostensibly, nonconfidential data may be provided without client consent. Even here, however, some discretion is advisable since clients may be reluctant to have it known that a contact was established with a program providing speech-language pathology and audiology services. In the final analysis, a client is probably within his rights to suppress even the information that he has been seen by a particular agency.

Agencies often employ all-purpose release forms, signed by clients or clients' agents at the time of the initial registration for services. These forms presumably authorize the agency to release any and all information about the client to any concerned professional or to appropriate educational, health, social, or rehabilitation agencies. Such all-purpose releases are highly questionable on both legal and ethical grounds. A person who is unaware of the kinds of information that may accrue during contacts with an agency should not be asked to give advance consent for release of any and all information. Furthermore, that person should not be asked to waive all future rights to determine the individuals or agencies that may receive the information.

Insofar as possible, each release of information should be preceded by a signed document which specifies the kind of information that may be released and the individual or agency to whom it may be sent. For example: "I authorize the release of the results of the hearing evaluations conducted on May 16, 1975 and September 22, 1978 and October 28, 1978, respectively, to Floyd G. Everhart, M.D."; or "I authorize the release of the following information about my son Joseph Anderson: the report of the speech and language evaluation conducted on March 19, 1979 and a summary report on the speech and language therapy program in which he was enrolled from June 28, 1979 to August 16, 1979 to Ms. Susan Kushner, Language, Speech, and Hearing Specialist, Brookville Unified School District."

Under no circumstances, in the absence of subpoena, should information be released that was not acquired directly by the individual speech-language pathologist or audiologist providing the information or by a member of the staff when the report is prepared by an agency. Information supplied by other professionals and agencies during the course of evaluation or treatment should never be released. Those professionals or agencies maintain the right to determine the appropriate recipients of their information and the right to know when such information is provided. Furthermore, the client maintains the right to determine whether he wishes that information to be disseminated.

The third form of consent is *consent inherent in the private interests* of the client, an essentially intangible concept which can also be equivocal. This form covers disclosures by professionals that are deemed essential to the client's best interests. Typically, these disclosures are made to spouses and other family members, without the client's consent, when the professional believes the client will benefit.

State laws also specify conditions and situations under which confidential information may be released without consent. These fall under four headings. *Public reporting statutes* may require professionals to supply information for birth and death certificates; report certain infections and contagious or communicable diseases; report instances of suspected child abuse; and report injuries that may have been caused by a firearm or other weapon. Laws may require the release of information in connection with *judicial processes*, i.e., professionals may be required, usually through subpoena, to release all information that may be related to some legal action. *Statutes concerning cost and quality control* may permit access to confidential records in connection with such procedures as peer review, utilization review, audits of services covered by public third-party payment programs, and to licensing and accrediting agencies. Finally, confidential information may be released in *instances of known danger to a third party*; typically, this statute is invoked in instances in which clients being treated by mental health professionals threaten harm to other individuals or in which physicians diagnose infections, such as tuberculosis or venereal disease, that may threaten a patient's family or other associates.

Three of these statutory areas may directly concern speech-language pathologists and audiologists. Two, judicial processes and statutes concerning cost and quality control, are discussed in Chapters 10 and 12. The third, public reporting, particularly as the statutes apply to suspected child abuse, must be of grave concern to all human services professionals working with children.

In 1973, Congress enacted into law the Child Abuse and Treatment Act, which required all states to enact laws that met certain standards with respect to establishing programs for the prevention and reporting of child abuse. Subsequently, all states have developed appropriate laws and regulations. These laws and regulations vary as to the specification of age ranges and in definitions of what constitutes child abuse. Nevertheless, all mandate reporting by concerned professionals, specify the social, welfare, or law enforcement agency to receive these reports, and grant immunity from suit to persons reporting, in good faith, instances of suspected child abuse. Speech-language pathologists and audiologists would almost certainly be included among the professionals required to file reports. Virtually all of the educational, health, and community agencies that employ members of our profession have established procedures that must be followed; it only remains for each professional to become familiar with those procedures. Private practitioners and employees of facilities with no established procedures should determine what is prescribed by local regulations and policies. It is important to remember that most child abuse laws assign reporting responsibilities to individual professionals, not just to the agencies and institutions that employ those professionals.

Another issue related to confidentiality deserves consideration. Although specifically discussing psychotherapy, Halleck (1980, p. 190) raises a point that merits the attention of speech-language pathologists and audiologists:

> There are no legal precedents regarding control of information in group therapy. This does not mean that psychiatrists have been unaware of serious ethical questions regarding confidentiality in groups and do not fear future litigation. Many group therapists feel that they are sitting on a legal and ethical volcano. Obviously, patients in group therapy might gossip about each other and there is little that can be done to control this. Conceivably the patient could be damaged by this breach of confidentiality and might have a cause of action against other group members or the therapist. Thus far, however, there has been no litigation involving breach of confidentiality in groups. Nor is there any litigation which raises the question of whether information generated in the group is privileged.

Clearly this is one more area which remains undefined, yet bears consideration by anyone who treats clients through group therapy.

ETHICAL CONSTRAINTS

Concern for confidentiality is expressed in all professional codes of ethics. It figured as a dominant consideration in the very earliest discussions of ethical matters by the founders of our profession. In its present version, ASHA's Code of Ethics contains the following proscription:

> Individuals must not reveal to unauthorized persons any professional or personal information obtained from the person served professionally, unless required by law or unless necessary to protect the welfare of the person or the community.

Negligence and Malpractice

Although it might be wished that all professionals at all times delivered services of exceptional quality, reality falls considerably short of that mark. At times, the shortcomings are so great that those services are clearly unacceptable or even harmful. Even when the overall quality of services is acceptable, misadventures may occur that leave deleterious aftereffects. Both legal and ethical considerations address problems related to protecting consumers against inexpert and injudicious management and against such misadventures.

LEGAL CONSTRAINTS

Courts generally hold individuals to be negligent when they fail to do something a reasonable and prudent person would do, or do something that a reasonable and prudent person would not do, given similar circumstances, and someone is injured as a result of that action or failure to act. When the person is a professional, his or her actions or failures to act are presumably compared to what "reasonable and prudent" members of the same profession would do under similar circumstances.

The concept of malpractice may well include negligence, but it also goes beyond negligence. Its definition adds professional misconduct, unreasonable lack of skill, and immoral conduct to what is usually included within the definition of negligence. As applied to health care providers, malpractice refers to bad, wrong, or injudicious treatment leading to injury, unnecessary suffering, or death which results from ignorance, carelessness, lack of proper professional skill, disregard of established rules and principles, or neglect.

To be valid, claims of malpractice must usually show four elements: *duty*, *breach*, *proximate cause*, and *damages*. Duty is usually defined according to "standard of care," which is, in turn, defined in terms of what a reasonable practitioner would do in similar circumstances. (Standard of care was once defined in terms of the usual practices of members of the same profession in the same community. Increasingly, however, courts disregard this "locality rule" and base comparisons on nationwide standards.) A breach of duty is judged to have occurred when the practitioner's actions or inactions do not conform to that standard of care. Proximate cause denotes a causal relationship between the breach and the alleged damages. Damages, then, refer to the harm or injury sustained and are usually equated with monetary compensation for that injury. (A plaintiff can recover damages only when the malpractice has resulted in harm or injury.)

Malpractice is usually covered under tort law. A tort is defined as a civil wrong, other than a breach of contract, for which a person can seek remedy through damages. Occasionally, however, malpractice claims involving allegations of breach of contract, usually an implied contract, have been successful. A contract may be held to exist when there is a specific offer to accomplish something, a client accepts that offer, and pays or promises to pay a fee for the promised product or service. Annas et al. (1981) relate the case of a surgeon who recommended stapes surgery, allegedly advising the patient that even though surgery might not improve the hearing, it would not be worsened. After three operations, the patient's hearing was indeed worse. The patient successfully sued the surgeon, basing that suit on the breach of an expressed contract.

One aspect of malpractice litigation that has received particular attention recently concerns the duty of professionals to refer to other, usually more specialized, professionals. Courts have held that providers must refer clients when they lack the degree of competence, knowledge, and skill necessary to diagnose or treat the client's problems. In general, the referring provider is relieved of all legal responsibilities once the referral has been made.

Thus far, few malpractice suits have been filed directly against speech-language pathologists and audiologists. It seems virtually inevitable, however, that as all malpractice suits become more prevalent, and more and more professionals besides physicians are included in these suits, our current exclusion from these claims will disappear. Every speech-language pathologist and audiologist, regardless of work setting, is well advised to become familiar with situations that foster malpractice claims and learn to avoid, amicably resolve, or otherwise obviate those situations. Many situations that can lead to claims of malpractice can be avoided by prudent professionals. Furthermore, all members of our profession should be assured they are adequately covered by individual or institutional insurance that will cover the costs of defense against malpractice claims and cover any judgments or settlements that result.

One important aspect of our erstwhile immunity to malpractice claims has been our apparent dependent relationship on physicians in those situations where such claims are most likely to arise. It has often been held that physicians are legally responsible for the activities of allied health professionals working under their supervision. Here again, however, if we wish to claim that we represent a fully independent and responsible profession we must accept direct exposure to malpractice claims.

I recall an instance of the inclusion of an audiologist in a malpractice suit against an otolaryngologist. The client consulted the otolaryngologist because of a monaural hearing impairment. The otolaryngologist referred to the audiologist for confirmation and quantification of the loss. The audiologist defined a moderately severe monaural impairment with profoundly reduced speech discrimination. The otolaryngologist dismissed the patient with no recommendations other than for an annual reevaluation. Several months later, the client developed other symptoms and, following evaluation by a neurologist, an VIIIth nerve tumor was diagnosed. (A more extensive evaluation by a second audiologist was included among the procedures used to establish the diagnosis.) The client eventually sued the otolaryngologist and the audiologist, alleging that competent and prudent professionals could have diagnosed the tumor at the time of the initial evaluation. Regrettably, the attorney defending the audiologist claimed that he was not at fault because the physician had not specifically ordered tests that might assist in identifying a retrocochlear lesion. This clearly defined the audiologist as a subprofessional who bore no responsibility for his actions.

The increasing exposure of speech-language pathologists and audiologists to the risks of malpractice litigation can be attributed to more than the increasing risks facing all human services professionals; it also relates to increasing acceptance as a responsible and independent profession.

Independent profession or not, most malpractice claims involving speech-language pathologists and audiologists also involve members of other professions. No professional should ever protect another professional from the consequences of his or her misdeeds at the expense of a client's welfare. However, professionals should not incite malpractice actions against other professionals unless there is obvious evidence of dereliction. Furthermore, when allegations of malpractice are made against another professional, speech-language pathologists and audiologists must be absolutely certain that whatever evidence they provide is completely objective and scrupulously accurate. The following rules are essential:

1. Never criticize another professional in the presence of a client. When differences of opinion are obvious, they should be clearly identified as differences of opinion, not as reflections on the competence of another professional.
2. When a client seems to be receiving or to have received services that may reflect on the competence of another professional, encourage the client to seek a second opinion from another member of the same profession (enter that recommendation in the client's record). In the final analysis, the competence of any professional is best assessed by a member of the same profession.
3. When a client is distressed about services provided by another professional, inform that professional—preferably through a personal conversation—of the client's discontent. (All of us experience instances in which we are completely unaware of clients who are grossly dissatisfied with our services.) Every professional deserves the opportunity to resolve dissatisfactions when such is possible.
4. When reporting, either orally or in writing, about clients in litigious circumstances, include only factual material and such observations as fall clearly within areas of primary professional expertise. Be particularly wary of attributing causes to observed behaviors unless there is unequivocal evidence of direct cause-effect relationships.
5. Be wary of becoming a client's advocate in instances of alleged malpractice. A professional should be dedicated to ensuring that all salient facts are available that may facilitate a just disposition of whatever is at issue. However, his or her participation must always be as an impartial expert, rather than as an advocate.

Recognizing that malpractice litigation has become an important fact of life in the human services professions, some routine practices may decrease the likelihood of such litigation and, at least equally importantly, facilitate defense against such litigation when it occurs. These practices particularly concern record keeping, as discussed in Chapter 6.

ETHICAL CONSTRAINTS

By definition, negligence and malpractice are legal rather than ethical issues. Nevertheless, some ethical constraints clearly relate to negligence and malpractice or, perhaps more precisely, forestall the conditions under which allegations of negligence and malpractice are most likely to occur.

The issue of negligence is addressed directly in the following principle from ASHA's Code of Ethics:

> Individuals shall take all reasonable precautions to avoid injuring persons in the delivery of professional services.

The following principles and proscriptions point to factors that may both avert allegations of malpractice and, conversely, serve as a basis for defining instances where malpractice has occurred:

Individuals shall use every resource available, including referral to other specialists as needed, to provide the best service possible.

Individuals shall evaluate services rendered to determine effectiveness.

Individuals must not exploit persons in the delivery of professional services, including accepting persons for treatment when benefit cannot reasonably be expected or continuing treatment unnecessarily.

Individuals must not guarantee the results of any therapeutic procedure, directly or by implication. A reasonable statement of prognosis may be made, but caution must be exercised not to mislead persons served professionally to expect results that cannot be predicted from sound evidence.

Use of Clients in Research and Teaching

It seems virtually inconceivable that until relatively recent years scientists employed human subjects in about any way their consciences permitted. Prison convicts and residents of institutions for the mentally retarded were injected with live viruses to test the efficacy of vaccines. In the infamous "Tuskegee Study," a group of uneducated residents of a rural community who contracted syphilis were left untreated to permit studies of the natural history of the disease. During the 1960's, more than 20,000 patients (residents of the United States as well as American servicemen and their dependents serving overseas) were administered thalidomide, an experimental drug that produced severe fetal malformations.

The first major document to delineate principles governing human experimentation was the Nuremberg Code, drafted subsequent to the trials of 23 Nazi physicians for crimes against humanity committed during experiments involving concentration camp internees. The first principle of that Code states (Annas et al., 1981, p. 131):

The voluntary consent of the human subject is absolutely essential. This means that the person involved should have legal capacity to give consent; should be so situated as to be able to exercise free power of choice, without the intervention of any element of force, fraud, deceit, duress, overreaching, or other ulterior form of constraint or coercion; and should have sufficient knowledge and comprehension of the elements of the subject matter involved as to enable him to make an understanding and enlightened decision. This latter element requires that before the acceptance of an affirmative decision by the experimental subject there should be made known to him the nature, duration, and purpose of the experiment; the method and means by which it is to be conducted; all inconveniences and hazards reasonably to be expected; and the effects upon his health or person which may possibly come from his participation in the experiment.

The duty and responsibility for ascertaining the quality of the consent rests upon each individual who initiates, directs, or engages in the experiment. It is a personal duty and responsibility which may not be delegated to another with impunity.

The concepts enunciated in the Nuremberg Code have subsequently been expanded in federal and state statutes. They are also reflected in the codes of ethics of all human services professions. Although originally deriving from concerns about medical and biologic research, the use of human subjects in behavioral research is now also addressed in laws and regulations and in codes of ethics.

LEGAL CONSTRAINTS

In 1966, the United States Department of Health, Education, and Welfare published regulations requiring peer group approval of all federally funded research involving human subjects. These provisions were extended in 1974 when Congress enacted PL 93-384, the National Research Act, which created the National Commission for the Protection of Human Subjects of Biomedical and Behavioral Research. This law also encouraged the development of local Institutional Research Boards to review and approve specific research proposals.

Regardless of funding source and whether or not a formal institutional review mechanism is in place, every researcher is well advised to follow the procedures defined for federally funded research before embarking on any project involving human subjects. The essential areas for consideration are: first, that voluntary participation by subjects, indicated by free and informed consent, is assured; and second, that an appropriate balance exists between potential benefits of the research to the subject and to society and the risks assumed by the subject. Since few studies conducted by speech-language pathologists and audiologists entail significant physical, or even psychological, risks, regulations concerning informed consent are more likely to be important. Such regulations generally require:

1. A statement that the procedures involving the subject are being carried out for research, explaining the purposes and expected duration of the research, and describing the procedures to be followed, identifying which, if any, are experimental in nature.
2. Description of any forseeable risks or discomforts.
3. Description of possible benefits to the subjects or to others.
4. Disclosure of available alternative procedures or courses of treatment that might benefit the subject.
5. A statement regarding the confidentiality of experimental records and the approaches to be employed to safeguard confidentiality.
6. Identification of the person to be contacted for immediate answers to whatever questions may arise during the course of the subject's participation.
7. A statement that participation is voluntary and that refusal to participate will involve no penalty or loss of benefits, and that the subject may withdraw at any time without prejudice.

Institutional research boards sometimes waive the requirement of informed consent when the research involves only those procedures normally carried out in the evaluation or treatment of clients in similar circumstances. Furthermore, most boards have developed expedited review procedures for research that could be considered to be educational, research that merely involves interviewing (except in certain highly sensitive or "personal" areas), research that entails observation of subjects in common social interactions, or research involving recorded speech samples.

Even when research involves retrieval of data from clinical records, with no direct involvement of clients, it may be necessary, or at least advisable, to follow formal consent guidelines. Occasionally, agencies—particularly agencies affiliated with colleges and universities—include the possibility of the use of records for research in the blanket consent forms signed by clients. It is dubious whether such forms really constitute informed consent, and consequently they would not be likely to suffice if questions arose about the use of a client's records in a research project.

Apparently, there have been few specific legal definitions of matters related to the use of clients in teaching programs. Nevertheless, one could reasonably anticipate two areas for concern. First, an informed consent procedure patterned after the one followed for human experimentation should probably be employed whenever clients are used for student observation or clinical practice. Second, it seems virtually certain that all legal responsibilities rest with the supervisor should questions of liability arise. Some state licensure laws and regulations specifically address issues related to students in training. In permitting unlicensed students to deliver professional services, states may assign legal responsibility to the students' supervisors (who must be licensed) and may also require the clear designation of students as trainees or interns to the clients served and to all other concerned parties.

Questions may also arise relative to the use of client records in teaching programs. These questions may relate to access to records and to authorization to enter material in records. In the first instance, students should be allowed access to records only after thorough orientation regarding confidentiality. General accessibility to records by any student who is observing evaluations or therapy, or by any student who is engaged in some sort of class project, is probably best avoided. Some programs that accommodate students file particularly sensitive material separately from the records used for daily clinic functions. In any event, it is essential that it be recorded, in writing, that clients are aware that their records are available to students and that they have consented to this.

Because all records are legal documents, some controls are essential in every teaching program to ensure that all entries into those records could withstand scrutiny as a part of some legal procedure. Many university speech and hearing clinics file anything written by any student about a client in that client's record, with no verification of the accuracy of information. This practice could prove to be regrettable. All entries by students into records should be reviewed and countersigned by their supervisors. This practice might well extend to the record entries of all uncertified or unlicensed clinicians, including those engaged in the clinical fellowship year. (Such a practice may be required by regulations supporting state licensure laws.)

Many college and university speech and hearing clinics consider the education of students to be their major function. So long as clients are served, the welfare of those clients, not the education of students, becomes the overriding consideration. This principle would almost certainly guide any court should questions arise regarding the management of a client in a college or university clinic.

ETHICAL CONSTRAINTS

As have most human services professional organizations, ASHA has included reference to the use of clients in research and teaching in its Code of Ethics. The following proscription is included:

> Individuals must not use persons for teaching or research in a manner that constitutes invasion of privacy or fails to afford informed free choice to participate.

Fees and Other Financial Arrangements

Both legal and ethical constraints relating to the financial aspects of the delivery of human services seem to demonstrate fundamental incongruities. On the one hand is the essential notion that professionals should be constrained from profiteering on ailments and misfortunes. On the other hand is the precept that citizens of a free society should be able to pursue economic success with the fewest possible restrictions. The incompatibility of these attitudes is often evident when financial matters are addressed by laws and regulations and by professional codes of ethics.

LEGAL CONSTRAINTS

Except for instances in which professionals' financial transactions constitute outright fraud, the law has tended to remain silent with respect to professional fees. For example, charging excessive fees is not usually included among the offenses defined as unprofessional conduct in licensure laws and regulations. So long as misrepresentation or a breach of contract has not occurred, the investigative and disciplinary arms of most state professional licensure boards will not examine allegations of exorbitant fees.

Furthermore, the federal government, through the Federal Trade Commission (FTC), has restrained attempts at professional self-regulation of fees as illegal, holding that this represents price fixing. Whether valid or not, the FTC has held that consumers' interests are best served when price competition is encouraged, presumably resulting in lower fees. At this writing, Congress is under considerable pressure from certain professional organizations, in particular the American Medical Association, to remove the authority to regulate professions from the FTC. Nevertheless, many states still have laws and regulations that negate fee regulation by professional associations.

While actively opposing attempts to regulate fees, governmental agencies have simultaneously exerted vigorous indirect influence on fee setting through regulations governing the payment of fees under public third-party programs. As more and more beneficiaries have been included in these programs, the greater the influence on setting all professional fees. Herein lies another paradox. The current era of deregulation, manifested in such efforts as to exclude the FTC from concerns for professional fees, is also an era of efforts to control the costs of human services through exercising controls over the fees paid for those services.

Legal scrutiny of fee payments is most likely to occur in instances of disputes between clients and providers and in instances where clients fail to pay for the services they have received. Fees disputes are viewed legally from the standpoint of whether an enforceable contract exists between the client and the provider. There are two types of contracts: express and implied. Express contracts exist when terms and conditions are specifically stated and understood by the concerned parties. Implied contracts may be inferred when four factors can be demonstrated: (1) a service has been rendered; (2) the provider reasonably expected payment for that service; (3) the client should have reasonably known that the provider would expect payment; and (4) the client had the opportunity to reject the service but failed to do so. Usually, actions to recover fees must be based on demonstrating the existence of an implied contract. Sometimes, however, speech-language pathologists and audiologists, and agencies providing speech, language, and hearing services, execute signed agreements with clients, particularly before embarking on an extended therapy program. Audiologists also often execute such agreements in conjunction with hearing aid dispensing programs. Even though an agency or private practitioner may never pursue legal redress for lost fees, these agreements may afford clarification of likely financial responsibility before substantial indebtedness occurs, thus forestalling future disputes. It may also be important to clarify the client's financial responsibility in instances in which only a portion of the professional fee is covered by insurance and the client will be liable for the remainder.

When fees disputes lead to legal action, such disputes usually center on whether the fees charged are fair in terms of the services provided. Typically, courts consider the following five factors in making their determinations: (1) the qualifications of the professional; (2) the time expended in delivering the services; (3) the complexity of the services; (4) the customary fees charged by similar professionals for similar services; and (5) the materials and equipment used. Some courts have also included the client's ability to pay the fees among the factors considered, but this practice is not universal.

Despite legalities, professionals may be well advised to weigh all actions referable to fees disputes carefully before initiating legal procedures. First, one must consider whether the amount owed justifies the costs of legal action and whether the client actually has the means to pay whatever judgment might be awarded. Even more important, the professional should determine whether the client is merely dilatory or irresponsible, or whether he or she is actually disgruntled. Litigious clients may express their dissatisfaction merely by failing to pay their bills. If pressed for payment through legal action, they may respond with malpractice suits. The investment of time and money in defending such suits, no matter how unjustified, will almost certainly far exceed whatever is lost in writing off bad debts.

ETHICAL CONSTRAINTS

One of the principles enunciated in ASHA's Code of Ethics is, "Individuals' fees shall be commensurate with services rendered." The Code also contains provisions specifically addressing fees connected with dispensing products. Those provisions are presented later in this discussion.

Advertising and Public Information

Professionals may have two different motivations for disseminating information about their fields of service. On a general level, they may consider their responsibilities to include increased public awareness, both to encourage people to seek the help they need and to lead them to be more understanding of the problems confronted by other people. More specifically, however, professionals may also wish to encourage more people to seek the services they provide. The first motivation is generally regarded as laudatory; the second motivation has been considered suspect by many professional groups. Their negative views have been reflected in laws they have fostered and in their codes of ethics.

LEGAL CONSTRAINTS

Legal proscriptions against advertising have figured prominently as targets for the efforts of consumer interest groups. These proscriptions were usually initiated by professionals, who generally believed that advertising impaired professional dignity in the eyes of the public. Price advertising, i.e., advertising that in any way sought to convince consumers that a particular professional or facility offered economic advantages over another professional or facility, was absolute anathema to virtually all professional groups. As a part of the consumer movement of the 1970's, however, virtually all laws and regulations that restricted professional advertising were struck down. Furthermore, the Federal Trade Commission and various state professional licensure programs have taken vigorous stands against professional groups which attempt to proscribe advertising through their codes of ethics. The essential rationale of these efforts held that restricting advertising limited competition that was ultimately in the best interests of consumers.

Although advertising is generally permissible, some states still impose restrictions on solicitation by professionals. The distinction between advertising and solicitation may be elusive. Annas et al. (1981) offered the following distinction: "... one can think of advertising as messages directed to the general public, whereas solicitation is an attempt to induce a particular consumer to avail himself of a specific provider's products or services." This distinction might be illustrated in an area of audiologic practice. Any agency providing audiology services might advertise a free hearing screening program. However, if the hearing-impaired people identified in the screening program were pressed to seek further services exclusively from that agency, this would constitute solicitation.

With the current growing emphasis on deregulation, and the returning influence of professional associations as opposed to consumer advocates, we may see some reappearance of restrictions on advertising. The return of the once common absolute proscriptions, however, seems unlikely.

Advertising practices in connection with dispensing hearing aids have been extensively scrutinized. Substantial segments of the never-finalized trade regulation rules for the hearing aid industry, proposed by the Federal Trade Commission, were directed at advertising practices. Among the practices to be forbidden were statements that implied that the hearing aid seller was a fully qualified health professional or that his or her place of business was a medical, educational, or research institution; statements that hearing aids can restore normal hearing or prevent further hearing loss; representations that hearing aids can be fitted prescriptively; claims relative to invisibility; and other false claims relative to the likely benefits of hearing aid use. Although the proposed FTC regulations never achieved adoption, regulations adopted by the Food and Drug Administration (FDA) concerning hearing aid dispensing did exert some vague controls over advertising practices. Furthermore, some local jurisdictions have applied laws and regulations, directed at deceptive practices in all advertising, in actions against hearing aid dispensers and manufacturers. Nevertheless, despite claims by the FDA to the effect that its regulations, together with strong state and local licensing laws, would adequately address the abuses in the hearing aid industry, many unfortunate advertising practices continue unchecked.

Public statements, other than advertising, made by professionals are subject to the same legal restrictions as statements by any other citizen. Such statements become matters of legal concern if they are demonstrably deceptive, libelous, or defamatory. The law, therefore, provides little control over this aspect of professional practice.

ETHICAL CONSTRAINTS

As do most professional associations, ASHA directly confronts issues related to advertising and statements to the public in this principle:

> Individuals' statements to persons served professionally and to the public shall provide accurate information about the nature and management of communicative disorders, and about the profession and services rendered by its practitioners.

This principle leads to three proscriptions:

> Individuals must not misrepresent their training or competence.
>
> Individuals' public statements providing information about professional services and products must not contain representations and claims that are false, deceptive, or misleading.
>
> Individuals must not use professional or commercial affiliations in any way that would mislead or limit services to persons served professionally.

Despite the changes that have occurred in official and public attitudes toward advertising by professionals, it would be unrealistic to conclude that only restrictions relative to the accuracy of the advertising apply. Most potential consumers do expect a different pattern of conduct from professionals than from commercial enterprises. They may be wary, therefore, of professionals who use the kind of advertising they associate with Madison Avenue. Furthermore, other professionals may be disinclined to recommend the services provided by members of other professions who seem to pursue vigorous public relations campaigns, either through outright advertising or through other efforts in the popular media. While neither illegal nor frankly unethical, these are matters of professional propriety and are addressed as such in ASHA's Code of Ethics:

> Individuals should announce services in a manner consonant with the highest professional standards in the community.

Dispensing Products

Many human services professions face quandaries with respect to dispensing products related to their areas of practice. Physicians have been concerned about their role in dispensing pharmaceuticals, dentists with their role in dispensing products related to dental hygiene, and physical and occupational therapists with their roles in dispensing various aids and appliances. Some states have enacted laws to regulate these roles, most notably with respect to physician ownership of pharmacies. Most professions address issues related to dispensing products, either directly or indirectly, in their codes of ethics.

There are fundamental differences between dispensing products and all other areas of practice of human services professionals. The public tends to make essential distinctions between professionals and merchants, ascribing different motivations, attitudes, and approaches to carrying out daily affairs. Laws and regulations have tended to reflect these distinctions, and codes of ethics have served to preserve them.

Many distinctions between professionals and merchants derive from assumptions about sources of income. Professionals derive their incomes from fees for services or from salaries that relate, at least to some extent, to the services they provide. Merchants are compensated through profits on the sales of products, profits that represent the difference between the price paid by the consumer and the cost of procuring and delivering the product. Although many merchants provide services in connection with the delivery of their products, those services are usually included within the purchase price of the product.

Popular assumptions have held that

these income source differences between professionals and merchants substantially influence their motivations, that is, professionals base their decisions on the best interests of the consumer since those decisions do not influence income, but merchants are primarily interested in accomplishing the sales from which their incomes exclusively derive. However, these assumptions reflect gross oversimplifications. The decisions and recommendations made by professionals often affect, at least indirectly, their incomes. On the other hand, the merchant who is solely interested in effecting sales, with no regard to the needs of the consumer, is not likely to succeed. Regardless of these realities, when a professional engages in dispensing products, he or she invites new forms of legal and ethical scrutiny.

LEGAL CONSTRAINTS

By most legal definitions, the professional who engages in dispensing products becomes a retailer and is, therefore, subject to whatever laws and regulations states and local communities impose on retailers. Often retail sales licenses are required. Laws governing collection of state and local sales taxes apply. Other laws may apply to retailing by nonprofit agencies or by agencies incorporated under particular statutes. Still others may refer to the name or names used by the professional or agency when engaging in retail sales.

Hearing aids are obviously the products most likely to be dispensed by members of our profession. The specific legal constraints that we are most likely to confront, therefore, are laws and regulations related to hearing aid sales. Currently, most states require hearing aid dispensers to be licensed. Some states exempt licensed or certified audiologists, either partially or completely, from hearing aid licensure requirements, but others do not. Some laws make special provisions for institution-based dispensing programs, but others do not. Most state licensure laws, in addition to establishing minimal requirements for dispensers, contain provisions that regulate their sales practices.

The federal government has launched several forays into the arena of regulating hearing aid sales practices. Early investigative efforts, first led by Senator Kefauver and later by Senator Church, resulted in news releases and other reports that alerted the public to prevalent problems but did little to prevent or control those problems. During the mid-1970's the Federal Trade Commission initiated a massive effort to develop a set of trade regulations to apply to the sale of hearing aids. The results of their investigations and their recommended regulations were published in 1978. Their recommendations as related to advertising have already been mentioned. Other provisions included restrictions on in-home sales, the marketing of used hearing aids, the use of testing programs to identify potential customers, and, most importantly (and most vigorously contested), a "buyer's right to cancel." This latter provision specified that a hearing aid purchaser or renter maintained the right to cancel the sale or rental within 30 days and to receive a refund. Primarily because of vocal opposition from hearing aid manufacturers and sellers and, regrettably, even from some physician organizations, the FTC rules were never adopted.

Almost simultaneously with the FTC efforts, the Food and Drug Administration carried out its own development of regulations under its program of regulating medical devices. The fundamental purpose of the FDA effort was quite different from the FTC program. The FDA was solely charged with the consideration of the "safety and effectiveness" of hearing aids as medical devices, not with sales practices per se. Since they were much less restrictive than the FTC rules, the FDA regulations met considerably less opposition and they were adopted, becoming effective in August 1977. Since these regulations were at odds with the laws and regulations of several states, those states applied for exemption from pre-emption by the new federal rules.

The FDA reviewed these applications and published their final decisions in 1978, granting some exemptions and denying many others.

The salient features of the FDA hearing aid regulations relate to labeling and to conditions of sale. Labeling requirements specify that the hearing aid must show the name of the manufacturer or distributor, the model name or number, serial number, year of manufacture, and an indication of the correct battery position. Those requirements also specify essential information that must be contained in an instructional brochure, to be provided with the aid, which illustrates and describes the operation, use, and care of the aid; sources of repair and maintenance; and a statement to the effect that the use of a hearing aid may be only part of a rehabilitative program that may also involve speech reading or auditory training. (This latter statement has been about as effective in motivating new hearing aid users to seek rehabilitative services as has the Surgeon General's warning on cigarette packages in leading people to give up smoking.) The regulations also require a fully disclosed warning to dispensers and to purchasers that under certain circumstances medical advice should always precede hearing aid purchase. These circumstances include: (1) visible congenital or traumatic deformity of the ear; (2) history of active drainage from the ear within the previous 90 days; (3) history of sudden or rapidly progressive hearing loss within the previous 90 days; (4) acute or chronic dizziness; (5) unilateral hearing loss of sudden onset or rapidly progressive unilateral loss within the previous 90 days; (6) audiometric air-bone gap equal to or greater than 15 dB at 500 Hz, 1,000 Hz, and 2,000 Hz; and (7) pain or discomfort in the ear. The warning also cautions dispensers to exercise special care in fitting aids with maximum power output exceeding 132 dB because of the potential for further damage to the residual hearing.

The FDA conditions for sale require that a client must, prior to delivery of the hearing aid, present to the dispenser a written statement from a licensed physician, dated within the previous 6 months, certifying that the hearing loss has been medically evaluated and that the client may be a candidate for a hearing aid. However, if the client is 18 years of age or older, he or she may sign a waiver to the medical evaluation. The conditions for sale also specify that the client has the right to review the instructional brochure prior to purchase, and that the medical clearance form or the medical waiver must be retained by the dispenser for 3 years following sale of the aid.

Other direct legal restrictions on hearing aid dispensing may be in the form of regulations governing public third-party payment for hearing aids (primarily through Medicaid, departments of rehabilitation, or Crippled Children Services). In 1978, the Health Care Financing Administration proposed regulations governing dispensing of hearing aids under Medicaid, but those regulations were never adopted. Nevertheless, most states that include hearing aids among the benefits of their Medicaid programs have adopted regulations specifying the conditions under which hearing aids may be purchased, the procedures to be followed in selecting appropriate candidates, the amount of payment allowed, and the procedures to be followed in obtaining that payment. With the growing efforts to control all expenditures of funds for human services, it seems inevitable that increasingly stringent regulations will be imposed on the purchase of hearing aids by public agencies.

As more and more audiologists become involved in dispensing of hearing aids, it is possible that their activities may fall within the purview of regulations intended for other purposes. A fundamental concept in certain state regulations holds that, in the field of health care, consumer interests are served when the professional recommending or prescribing a product is a different individual from the dispenser of that product. This concept is most frequently applied with respect to physicians and pharmaceuticals. Specifically, states may constrain physicians from directly or indirectly engaging in the sale of pharmaceuticals. Similar concerns have been studied with respect to the prescription and sale of prostheses, including eyeglasses. To my knowledge, no legal questions have been raised as yet with respect to audiologists both recommending and dispensing hearing aids (although the matter was considered in the course of the Health Care Financing Administration's development of its proposed Medicaid hearing aid regulations). Nevertheless, there may well be increasing scrutiny of their practices as more audiologists engage in hearing aid dispensing.

ETHICAL CONSTRAINTS

Our profession's concerns for ethical issues related to product dispensing have thus far focused on audiology services. Although most discussions have centered on dispensing hearing aids, matters related to dispensing products connected with industrial hearing conservation programs have also been considered. Except for occasional questions about the sale of clinician-prepared materials to clients, speech-language pathologists have been essentially exempt from concerns about product dispensing. As more speech prostheses become available, particularly nonoral communication devices, speech-language pathologists may also come under increased scrutiny related to sales practices.

For many years, the leaders of our profession and its association adopted a hard line toward product dispensing. That position was enforced through ASHA's Code of Ethics, which carried the following proscription:

> He must not accept compensation in any form from a manufacturer or a dealer in prosthetic or other devices for recommending any particular product. . . . He must not perform clinical services or promotional activity for any profit-making organization that is engaged in the retail sales of equipment. . . .

In the last major revision of the Code there was a substantial change in the expressed attitude toward dispensing practices. Currently it espouses the following principles and practices:

> Individuals who dispense products to persons served professionally shall observe the following standards:
>
> 1. Products associated with professional practice must be dispensed to the person served as a part of a program of comprehensive habilitative care.
> 2. Fees established for professional services must be independent of whether a product is dispensed.
> 3. Persons served must be provided freedom of choice for the source of services and products.
> 4. Price information about professional services rendered and products dispensed must be discussed by providing to or posting for persons served a complete schedule of fees and charges in advance of rendering services, which schedule differentiates between fees for professional services and charges for products dispensed.
> 5. Products dispensed to the person served must be evaluated to determine effectiveness.

The specificity of several of these statements—in comparison to the broader provisions of most other segments of the Code—offers further evidence that dispensing products is still regarded as inherently different from other professional services. Although some of these attitudes are likely to remain, their influence will probably wane in the face of increasing evidence that the involvement of our profession in dispensing products may well have substantially served the best interests of our clients.

Nondiscrimination and the Right to Receive Services

The civil rights movement has impacted on virtually every aspect of American life. Appropriately, all human services professions have been permanently influenced by many consequences of that movement. Two major principles have emerged. The first specifies that services must be available to the people who need them regardless of race, sex, age, economic circumstances, or disabilities. The second specifies that all qualified individuals must be afforded equal opportunity to prepare themselves for a chosen profession and to enter that profession once preparation has been completed. These principles are elaborated in both legal and ethical standards.

LEGAL CONSTRAINTS

The Civil Rights Act of 1964, with its subsequent amendments, invoked broad proscriptions against discrimination on the basis of race, color, national origin, religion, sex, age, or handicap. Although the major issues it addressed related to employment, other manifestations of discrimination were also considered. Particular attention was paid to nondiscrimination in institutions and agencies receiving federal funds, either directly or indirectly, which includes the majority of programs providing human services.

Subsequently, even stronger measures were invoked that went beyond the maintenance of policies of passive nondiscrimination. These measures required institutions and agencies to take positive, "result-oriented" steps toward the elimination of barriers (again primarily employment barriers) affecting minorities and women. The efforts initiated by these requirements are usually referred to as affirmative action programs.

Most speech, language, and hearing services are provided in institutions espousing affirmative action programs. Usually, the programs have defined specific procedures that must be followed in the recruitment and employment of both professional and support staff. Often, there are specified affirmative action goals that go beyond assuring equal employment opportunities to applicants and actually strive for staff compositions that truly reflect the community as a whole.

Affirmative action efforts toward increasing the number of traditionally underrepresented groups in the professional work force have extended beyond employment practices. There have also been vigorous, but variably effective, efforts toward increasing their representation in the student bodies of professional education programs. These efforts have been encouraged by the provisions of various federal funding programs for professional education.

One further important outgrowth of the civil rights movement was recognition, for the first time, that handicapped people also comprise a group that, historically, has been deprived of rights supposedly assured to all citizens. Efforts to remedy this situation were codified into Section 504 of the Rehabilitation Act of 1973, entitled "Nondiscrimination on the Basis of Handicap," which became law in 1977. The regulations supporting Section 504 specified that "no otherwise qualified handicapped individual in the United States shall, solely by reason of his handicap, be excluded from participation in, be denied the benefits of, or be subjected to discrimination under any program receiving federal financial assistance."

The provisions of Section 504 extended well beyond issues related to employment. Most importantly to providers of human services, all programs that were direct or indirect recipients of federal funds were mandated to become accessible to handicapped people and, in all other respects as well, to be operated in a nondiscriminatory manner. Two particular areas were of concern to speech-language pathologists and audiologists. Their clinical facilities had to be made accessible to clients with limitations in ambulation, and those facilities serving hearing-handicapped clients had to be equipped with telecommunication devices and prepared to accommodate clients who use sign language. Furthermore, as in all higher education programs, departments of speech-language pathology and audiology were confronted with the need to ensure that no artificial obstacles were created for the entry of disabled individuals into our profession.

The influences of the civil rights movement and the other efforts toward social reform that characterized the three decades following World War II were also readily apparent in struggles to overcome deliberate and de facto discrimination throughout the realm of human services. Although efforts to overcome discrimination in education probably received the greatest attention, similar efforts were directed to such other human services as health care.

One of the federal government's earliest efforts at improvement of the availability of private sector health care was the Hill-Burton Act, ratified by the legislature in the late 1940's. This act authorized funds for the construction of new health care facilities, primarily hospitals. One of its conditions, unfortunately often ignored, was that all facilities built with these federal funds were to provide some free and below-cost care.

Medicaid represented the most vigorous governmental effort to improve the availability of medical care. The Department of Health, Education, and Welfare included these optimistic words in the handbook of policies prepared for the state agencies that were to administer the Medicaid program (United States Department of Health, Education and Welfare, 1966, Section D-540, Supplement D.):

> The passage of Title XIX (i.e., the Medicaid law) marks the beginning of a new era in medical care for low-income families. The potential of this new title can hardly be overestimated, as its ultimate goal is the assurance of complete, continuous, family-centered medical care of high quality to persons who are unable to pay for it themselves. The law aims much higher than the mere paying of medical bills, and states, in order to achieve its high purposes, will need to assume the responsibility for planning and establishing systems of high quality medical care, comprehensive in scope and wide in coverage.

The Medicaid program not only aspired to make health care available to everyone, it also aspired to offer its beneficiaries freedom of access to the same health care systems that serve all other citizens. To reinforce further the objectives of the Medicaid legislation, Congress addressed improved access to health care in the Comprehensive Health Planning and Health Services Amendments of 1966 as well, announcing these goals (Section 2(a) PL 89-749):

> The Congress declares that fulfillment of our national purpose depends on promoting and assuring the highest level of health attainable for every person, in an environment which contributes positively to healthful individual and family living; that attainment depends on an effective partnership, involving close intergovernmental collaboration, official and voluntary efforts, and participation of individuals and organizations; that Federal financial assistance must be directed to support the marshaling of all health services—national, state, and local—to assure comprehensive health services of high quality for every person but without interference with existing patterns of private professional practice of medicine, dentistry, and related healing arts.

These various federal programs did not stop with mere attempts to remove barriers to the procurement of health care. They also contained affirmative action provisions which encouraged, or even required, efforts to actively seek clients from groups that were historically underserved by America's health care system.

All of these efforts, however, stopped short of declarations that health care constitutes a legal right. In Sparer's (1976, pp. 39–40) excellent discussion of the legal right to health care, he observed:

> A "legal right to medical care" may be said to exist when two conditions are met: (1) there exists a definable duty on the part of ascertainable medical care providers to give medical care to particular persons (or persons in general); (2) the persons who are the beneficiaries of the duty have a legal remedy which they can use to enforce the performance of the duty, or collect damages for failure to perform. Without these conditions, one may request medical care. One may offer to purchase it. One may always claim that a moral obligation on the part of a provider to give care exists. But one does not have the legal right to medical care.
>
> There is no legal right to medical care in the United States. For those who have purchased them, there are legal rights created under private contract. For others, there are rights to limited medical care under some circumstances. The precise circumstances are often elusive. For many, there are no legal rights to medical care whatsoever.

With regard to the legal rights to care under such statutory programs as Medicaid and Medicare, Sparer wrote (p. 42):

> Neither program creates a "right" to medical care as such. Like private insurance, they create rights to payment for care if the applicant is eligible for the program.

Despite their apparent pessimism, Sparer's observations were made at a time when vestiges of the social reform efforts of the Great Society era remained. Subsequently, however, the combined influences of escalating health care costs and efforts to restrict federal expenditures for human services make even more unlikely any declaration that health care is a fundamental right of the citizens of our nation.

In the entire realm of laws concerning human services, the most vigorous enunciation of rights may be found in PL 94-142, which declares that *all handicapped children have a legally enforceable claim to a free, appropriate education in the least restrictive environment.* Several aspects of PL 94-142 requirements, such as the contents of the Individualized Education Program (IEP) and the mandated opportunities for parent participation in the development and implementation of that plan, have been discussed in previous chapters. The law's provisions go substantially farther in assuring individual rights by specifying due processes that parents may follow in the event of dissatisfaction with the IEP or with its implementation.

After receiving notification of the plans that have been formulated for a handicapped child's education, the parent or guardian may present complaints with respect to any matter relating to the identification, evaluation, or educational placement of the child or the provision of a free, appropriate public education for such a child. In the earliest stages of due process, most school districts strive for an informal and amicable resolution of complaints. Often, misunderstandings can be resolved and mutually satisfactory solutions reached. If these efforts fail, formal procedures that are defined in the law begin (Section 615 b 2):

> Whenever a complaint has been received, the parents or guardian shall have an opportunity for an impartial due process hearing which shall be conducted by the state education agency or by the local education agency or intermediate educational unit, as determined by state law or by the state educational agency. No hearing conducted pursuant to the requirements of this paragraph shall be conducted by an employee of such agency or unit involved in the education or care of the child.

Due process hearings constitute an adversarial proceeding between the school and the family, presided over by a presumably impartial hearing officer. Downey (1980a, p. 256) characterized these hearings:

> The nature of an adversarial process is one of confrontation—witnesses are called and examined by each side, facts or conclusions are challenged; each party wants to win acceptance of their view, not achieve a compromise ... The initial and ultimate goal will be to have the hearing officer agree with either party on what the child's identification, evaluation or placement should be. A secondary goal may be to compile a sufficient record based on statements of witnesses and evidence to change a procedure or policy that will ultimately be resolved by the state education agency or the courts.

PL 94-142 further prescribes that if the hearing does not lead to a solution that is satisfactory to the parents they may forward an appeal to the state education agency. That agency must then conduct an impartial review of the hearing, reviewing the entire record to determine whether all procedures were consistent with due process requirements. The state reviewing officer may seek further evidence and solicit further oral and written arguments from the adversaries. The officer then renders an independent decision and sends a copy of that decision to the two parties.

If the parents or, in unusual circumstances, the school district are dissatisfied with the outcome of the appeal to the state education agency, they may initiate civil action through the courts. Such court action, however, is usually limited to scrutiny of procedures to determine that due process occurred. Conceivably, the court could find that the conclusions of the reviewing officer were unfounded and either order a new hearing or define the educational placement that must be effected.

At this writing, there is considerable question as to whether the present due process provisions of PL 94-142 will remain in place. Nevertheless, although they may well be modified, it seems highly unlikely that they will be eliminated entirely.

ETHICAL CONSTRAINTS

Most professional association codes of ethics now include statements that address nondiscrimination directly. The following proscription occurs in ASHA's Code of Ethics:

> Individuals must not discriminate in the delivery of professional services on any basis that is unjustifiable or irrelevant to the need for and potential benefit from such services, such as race, sex or religion.

The profession's concern for discrimination has gone well beyond the terms of this proscription. There have been recurrent efforts toward the recruitment of members of minority groups into the profession and toward improving the opportunities of these individuals after they have completed their professional education. As with similar efforts in other professions, the results have probably been less impressive than were the efforts, but unquestionably some minority groups are better represented in the profession today than 20 years ago.

The issue of sex discrimination has also been the focus of widespread concern. Since most estimates suggest that approximately 85% of the members of our profession are women, it can scarcely be charged that, in contrast to many professions, barriers exist to the entry of women into the profession. However, it is readily apparent that women are not proportionately represented in leadership positions in our profession. This has been evident in the composition of senior faculty members in colleges and universities, in administrative positions in agencies and clinics, and in positions of responsibility in our national professional organization.

The relative position of women in our profession is also expressed in economic terms. In 1979, Perrin reported comparisons between the mean salaries of male and female members of ASHA. Even among the speech-language pathologists and audiologists in the youngest age group, the males reported mean salaries 11% higher than the females. By the 51 to 55 age group, that difference rose to 33%. In the older age groups, the mean salaries of males were 40% higher in hospital clinics, 43% higher in colleges and universities, and 63% higher in federal and state agencies. Perhaps, as the result of various affirmative action programs, more recent studies will show some improvement in this situation. Unquestionably, however, many manifestations of sex discrimination in our profession remain.

Intraprofessional and Interprofessional Relationships

Two salient characteristics of all professions are their concerns for self-regulation and their espousal of the free sharing of information with other members of the same profession. Traditionally, these two characteristics figured prominently in professional codes of ethics but were essentially outside of legal purviews. However, intraprofessional relationships are no longer immune from legal scrutiny.

The same situation has obtained with respect to interprofessional relationships. With occasional exceptions, regulatory bodies have left such matters to the concerned professions, but recent years have seen promulgation of more and more regulations that at least indirectly define interprofessional relationships.

LEGAL CONSTRAINTS

The essential incongruities in legal positions with reference to self-monitoring by professions can be seen in the following quotations. The first is from a paper by Grimm (1972, p. I-14) published as a part of a report on the Study of Accreditation of Selected Health Educational Programs:

> In many respects, national accreditation has served state licensing agencies well. The accredit-

> ing programs of health professional associations have relieved most state licensing boards of the responsibility for evaluating educational programs and the expense of mounting their own full-scale accrediting programs. Whereas the incorporation of specific course work requirements into licensing statutes may ossify educational standards and inhibit necessary and desirable educational innovation, the requirement for national accreditation provides a built-in mechanism by which educational prerequisites for licensure may be kept automatically abreast of changing educational needs and requirements. Moreover, there is little doubt that interstate mobility has been greatly facilitated by the existence of national educational standards and norms. By providing state boards a readily usable yardstick for evaluating licensure candidates, national professional accreditation has, in effect, established national baseline standards for selected categories of health personnel.

The second quotation is from a booklet entitled *Deceptive Packaging* (Schulman and Geesman, 1974, p. 68) published by a consumer action group. Their use of the terms "trades" and "occupations" definitely includes professions:

> The most controversial aspect of licensing, as it relates to the public interest, lies in the fact that the trades and occupations are not merely regulated but self-regulated as well. The instances found in most statutes that board members be actively engaged in the trade they regulate pose some obvious problems. The main criticism here is that, as a result of this requirement, board members are often faced with a conflict of interest when considering matters that inevitably affect their private livelihood. In short, the problem with asking a man to wear two hats is that . . . at one time he may not take off the right hat.

Clearly the situation is paradoxical. On the one hand, governmental regulatory bodies have openly lauded professions' efforts to improve standards through self-regulation. On the other hand, it has been charged that these efforts are self-serving and not in the public interest.

During the 1970's, several federal agencies became increasingly involved in the direct and indirect regulation of professional practices. Most evident were the activities of the Federal Trade Commission in addressing issues related to professional self-regulation that they considered to restrain "free trade," particularly in such fields as medicine and dentistry. They considered practices that raised professional standards to result in artificial shortages of professional personnel, which in turn reduced competition among professionals and resulted in increased costs to consumers. These efforts by federal agencies seem to be waning in the 1980's, however, which may result in the restoration of greater freedom of self-regulation by professional groups.

Two major moves away from self-regulation were also apparent at state levels. Several states established requirements for public representation on licensure boards; that is, professional licensure boards were required to include one or more lay people in their membership who were to participate in the establishment and monitoring of licensure standards. Furthermore, several states removed disciplinary authority from their licensure boards, assigning the responsibility for receiving and investigating complaints and for recommending disciplinary actions to bodies that were not, like the licensure boards, primarily constituted of members of the same profession as the alleged miscreants. Despite the apparent reversal of trends at federal levels, thus far no substantial movements seem to be under way at state levels to restore these responsibilities to profession-dominated groups.

The law has shown little concern for the second-mentioned aspect of intraprofessional relationships, that is, the free interchange of information. Nevertheless, concerns do arise about the propriety of professionals using legal mechanisms to protect their interests in their discoveries and developments. The law provides, through copyrights and patents, means of restricting the use of another's work; or, more specifically, it requires that a royalty be paid to the holder of the copyright or patent. Although patents and copyrights are taken for granted in business and industry, this has long been an area of controversy in the scientific community. At the present time, however, with the growing limitations of governmental research funds, scientists are increasingly turning to industry for research support. Those industries obviously assume that any resultant developments will be secured by copyrights and patents that may ultimately return a profit to the holders. This situation has precipitated even more heated controversies in the scientific community.

Speech-language pathologists and audiologists have always assumed that their published works and the testing and therapy materials they develop will be protected by copyright. Occasional patents have been granted on equipment designed by members of our profession. Some professionals have questioned whether these practices are entirely consonant with the free exchange of information, but little real concern has been voiced. It remains to be seen whether the growing controversies among other scientists will extend to researchers in our field.

Some aspects of interprofessional relationships are defined directly in law. These are usually on the basis of a "master-servant" principle, in which a professional must direct the activities of, and hence assume legal responsibilities for, another professional or technical specialist. In some states this describes the legal relationship between physicians and physical and occupational therapists, between ophthalmologists and opticians, and between dentists and dental hygienists. There have been isolated and abortive efforts to define, legally, similar master-servant relationships between physicians and speech-language pathologists and audiologists, but none has achieved even fragmentary success.

Legal definitions of interprofessional relationships are more likely to be accomplished indirectly. These occur most frequently in regulations for public programs. The most obvious examples are found in regluations for public third-party payment programs, which inevitably require that speech-language pathology and audiology services may be provided only when recommended by physicians. Regulations and policies of school programs may also assign authority to representatives of particular professions in such a way as to effectively define interprofessional relationships.

ETHICAL CONSTRAINTS

ASHA's Code of Ethics addresses both intra- and interprofessional relationships. With regard to intraprofessional relationships, the Code states:

> Individuals should strive to increase knowledge within the profession.

The fundamental ethical responsibility of professional self-regulation is reflected in these statements:

> Individuals shall inform the Ethical Practices Board of violations of the Code of Ethics.
>
> Individuals shall cooperate fully with the Ethical Practices Board inquiries into matters of professional conduct related to this Code of Ethics.

Statements referring to both intra- and interprofessional relationships are found in many different sections of the Code. Among these are:

> Individuals should establish harmonious relations with colleagues and members of other professions, and endeavor to inform members of related professions of services provided by speech-language pathologists and audiologists, as well as seek information from them.
>
> Individuals shall identify competent referral sources for persons served professionally.
>
> Individuals should present products they have developed to their colleagues in a manner consistent with the highest professional standards.
>
> Individuals should assign credit to those who have contributed to a publication in proportion to their contribution.

A specific and forthright statement about interprofessional relationships may well be one of the most important provisions of the Code since it clearly enunciates the role of speech-language pathology and audiology as an independent and fully responsible profession:

> Individuals must not provide clinical services by prescription of anyone who does not hold the Certificate of Clinical Competence.

This statement has been the focus of widespread discussion in the light of prevalent requirements by third-party payers for physician approval of speech-language pathology and audiology services. It is important to remember, however, that such policies do not state that speech-language pathology and audiology services can only be provided when ordered by a physician. Rather, they hold that our services can only be *covered* when ordered by a physician. In many instances, this may amount to the same thing since, in some settings, speech-language pathologists and audiologists may be permitted to provide only those services for which someone is willing to pay. Nevertheless, such requirements for physician approval do not define the kind of master-servant legal relationship described earlier. All manner of institutional policies influence the services we provide, including policies related to authorization for payment. However, these policies are quite different from mandates by members of other professions, which require particular services to be provided—perhaps even specifying the way in which the service is to be carried out—or which stipulate that a needed service may not be provided, without regard for the judgment of the professional who is directly concerned. A speech-language pathologist or audiologist who accedes to the latter situation is indeed in violation of ASHA's Code of Ethics.

SPEECH-LANGUAGE PATHOLOGISTS AND AUDIOLOGISTS AS EXPERT WITNESSES

One direct consequence of the increasing recognition granted to our profession is the growing use of our services as expert witnesses. This role can be onerous, but it can also be gratifying. There are few greater challenges to one's professionalism. Seldom do situations occur which hold more opportunities either to establish the prestige of our profession or to appear completely ridiculous.

Downey (1980b, p. 333) defined the role of an expert witness:

> There is a difference between a witness and an expert witness. A witness is a person who has direct sensory experience of an event and who is competent to testify as to what took place . . . An expert witness is an exception to the rule of law that prohibits taking of evidence from persons who do not have direct sensory knowledge and who are competent to testify. An expert witness is one who does *not* have direct knowledge of the issue at hand but whose expertise (via education, research or experience) is such that the court finds that the witness can help resolve particular issues. Expert testimony is offered where special knowledge is necessary, and there is a qualified expert who can testify.

The roles of expert witnesses differ somewhat, depending upon the legal processes and procedures that are under way. Speech-language pathologists and audiologists are most likely to serve in five different types of proceedings: litigation, hearings to determine testamentary capacity, actions related to disability determination, fair hearings under the provisions of PL 94-142, and legislative hearings.

Litigation

The following are actual incidents that have occured in the past several years:

> An 8-year-old was struck by an automobile while walking home from school. She apparently suffered only surface contusions and abrasions. However, after she returned to school, she seemed to show some behavioral changes. According to her parents, her speech also became hesitant and she showed difficulty in finding words.

> A 32-year-old sales representative sustained a unilateral vocal fold paralysis during thyroid surgery. He alleged that his vocational future was seriously impaired by this surgical misadventure.

> A 2-year-old with the multiple handicaps of visual impairment and a congenital heart defect was seen in an audiology clinic because she did not respond to sound. The mother probably contracted rubella during the first trimester of pregnancy. She sued the clinic where she received prenatal care, alleging that she was not told of the possible consequences of the rubella and offered the option of terminating the pregnancy.

> A 10-year-old girl sustained serious injuries while playing with some other children at a building con-

struction site. While hospitalized she developed an osteomyelitis that was eventually treated with streptomycin. During the course of that treatment, she lost virtually all of her hearing.

Each of these incidents has a common element. During the attendant legal proceedings, speech-language pathologists or audiologists were called as expert witnesses.

Although local practices differ, there may be four stages at which expert witnesses may be involved in litigations. The first two stages, records subpoena and deposition, comprise what is usually referred to as the discovery phase, that is, the phase during which the attorneys are determining what the issues of the case are, what evidence is available, what witnesses are available, and what additional information should be obtained before a settlement is sought or the case proceeds to trial. The next two stages are the pretrial attorney-witness conferences and the trial itself. Although settlements may occur at any time before the end of the trial, these two stages are usually not pursued unless it appears that matters can only be settled through a trial.

RECORDS SUBPOENA

A subpoena is issued by a court, usually at the request of attorneys seeking evidence to be used in litigation. The agency that has compiled the records has no control over their use, i.e., whether they are used in a client's behalf, whether they will be used against the client, or whether they will be used both to support and refute allegations. States also differ in laws regarding the form for acceptable clinical records. Some permit submission of complete and certified photocopies. Others require submission of the original record. (Always make a copy before turning over the original; courts have been known to "mislay" records—sometimes forever.)

When records are subpoenaed, it need not follow that they will be received in evidence by the court. Their admissability is governed by rules of evidence; records may or may not be admissable on the basis of the circumstances of the case and the laws relating to those circumstances. Rejecting as evidence an entire record or any portion of a record need not imply a reflection on the accuracy or completeness of the record; it may merely be considered inadmissable in, or irrelevant to, the particular action.

Most professionals are dismayed on the first occasion of service of a subpoena. Inevitably, a review of the subpoenaed record reveals oversights, omissions, and regrettable statements. As we gain experience in such matters, however, we learn to accept subpoenas as a simple fact of professional life. Furthermore, subpoenas can sharpen one's meticulosity in keeping clinical records.

DEPOSITION

Depositions generally serve two purposes. They amplify and add new information to whatever records and reports have been subpoenaed, and they also offer the attorneys the opportunity to "audition" potential witnesses, to determine what they will be able to contribute, and to surmise how they are likely to perform on the witness stand.

Depositions are formal procedures, conducted under strict legal regulation. A witness may be summoned to appear at an attorney's office, or, in some instances, the attorneys will come to the witness's office. During a deposition, each attorney has the opportunity to examine the witness under oath. A court reporter is present who prepares a verbatim transcript.

The following should be kept in mind during a deposition:

1. Depositions can be deceptive. Sometimes they are characterized by an informal joviality that can encourage the witness to make offhand speculations and ill considered remarks that can lead to grave embarrassment if the case goes to trial.
2. Make no statements during a deposition that you would not readily repeat on the witness stand in a courtroom. Be certain that you clearly understand the attorney's question before answering it. Define any technical terms clearly.

Explain how you reached any conclusions, but never defend yourself or your conclusions.

3. Never criticize another professional. If your conclusions differ and you can account for the differences objectively, it is proper to do so. If you cannot account for them objectively, do not speculate.
4. Do not answer questions that fall outside your areas of expertise and the scope appropriate to speech-language pathologists and audiologists, even if you know the answer. If the question falls outside those boundaries, say so. Even though a question does fall within the area of your expertise, if you do not know or are uncertain of the answer, say so.
5. Never speculate about the causes of whatever conditions are in question unless you are absolutely certain of the cause.
6. Avoid using such words as "diagnosis" and other terminology popularly ascribed to physicians unless quoting physician statements already in the record. Although speech-language pathologists and audiologists may properly use these terms in most situations, they may set you up for challenges of your qualifications that have nothing to do with the substance of your testimony.
7. Take as much time as you wish to be certain that you understand questions, to frame your responses, and to answer as completely as you believe necessary (albeit keeping answers as cogent as possible). Remember, the purpose of the deposition is to seek whatever information you, as an expert, can provide. Do not permit yourself to be rushed.
8. Admit freely the limitations of whatever procedures you have used to arrive at your conclusions, noting when findings are equivocal or when there may be reasonable differences of professional opinion in interpreting the same set of findings.
9. Remember that your responses during a deposition not only give the attorneys a view of what you can contribute as a witness, they also expose your areas of vulnerability under cross-examination. This is a further reason for keeping responses clear, succinct, factual, and strictly focused on answering precisely the question that was asked.
10. *Always* insist on receiving a copy of the transcript of your deposition for your review (unless specifically precluded by the laws of your state). Make the request at the end of the deposition so that it appears in the transcript together with the attorneys' consent. Most states require that deposition transcripts be sent to the witness on his or her request and permit the witness to correct any errors within a stated time interval. In order to cut costs, attorneys sometimes imply that a witness must go to their offices or to the court reporter's office to conduct this review. Since you can conduct a more thorough review if provided with a copy, insist that it be sent to you. Remember: *you will be held accountable for all statements attributed to you in the final deposition transcript whether they are accurate or not.* Therefore, make all corrections immediately, retaining a copy of those corrections for your records. Within some limits, you may correct errors or omissions that are not just transcription errors. For example, if on review you note statements that might be misinterpreted, poorly chosen words, or even minor omissions, include these among your corrections.

In most instances, an expert witness is paid for the time involved in giving a deposition. If the fee is at your discretion and not determined by your employer, it should fairly represent the time spent in preparing for the deposition, traveling to and from the deposition, giving the deposition, and reviewing the transcript. A reasonable amount can usually be set on the basis of lost income to the witness or to his or her employer for the time required.

Because of crowded court calendars, growing trial costs, and the increasing proclivity of juries to award settlements in instances of dubious merit, more and more cases are settled on the basis of depositions, before going to trial. Often, even if the case does go to trial, some deposed witnesses are not called to testify. This need not imply criticism of the witness or of his or her testimony. The attorneys may simply conclude that the testimony does not contribute to the specifics of the case they are trying to put forward.

PRETRIAL ATTORNEY-WITNESS CONFERENCE

Despite depositions, most attorneys schedule conferences with the expert witnesses they are calling before a trial begins. Such conferences usually serve two purposes. They provide an opportunity for the attorney to orient the witness to the role of the expert witness and to describe the procedures to be followed. They also lead to preparation for the line of questioning that will be pursued.

During the pretrial conference, an expert

witness should determine the specific points the attorney will attempt to establish during the testimony. If those points lie outside the expertise of the witness, or if they are inconsistent with the witness's findings and conclusions, these matters should be clarified during the pretrial conference. Many attorneys permit a witness to draft a script that presents verbatim the questions and answers that are most likely to establish the salient features of the witness's potential testimony. Although the attorney may deviate from that script during the actual trial, it can be helpful both to the attorney and to the witness. The attorney will be provided with clear and readily answerable questions, and the witness will have the opportunity to prepare in advance the best answers to those questions. Furthermore, the attorney may be able to identify for the witness the points that are most likely to be targeted in cross-examination.

Witnesses should also use the conference to orient the attorney as to the nature and limits of their expertise. Since courts and juries are often unfamiliar with our profession, the attorney should be provided with statements about our profession, its appropriate scope of practice, and the preparation of its practitioners. Witnesses who practice in a state offering licensure should provide the attorney with a copy of the licensure law, which will legally define the profession and its scope of practice.

The witness should also ensure that the attorney has some basic understanding of any tests that were administered, of the essential nature of the client's communicative disorders, and of the basis for any recommendations for management.

The purpose of the pretrial conference, then, is to obviate any surprises—for either the attorney or the witness—during the direct examination (i.e., the examination of the witness by the attorney calling that witness).

Expert witnesses may also claim payment for participation in a pretrial conference. Usually, charges covering the conference itself and the preparation for the conference are included in the billing for the expert witness fee that is rendered following the trial.

THE TRIAL

Most of what the average speech-language pathologist or audiologist knows about the conduct of trials comes from movies and television. This is a most inadequate orientation.

The role of an expert witness in litigation is clearly and simply defined: *An expert witness is called to assist a jury to understand the facts of a case and to reach a just decision based on those facts.* The major task of the witness, then, is to communicate clearly to the jury. The witness may be assisted or impeded in this task by the line of questioning pursued by the attorneys, but the failure of an expert witness to accomplish this purpose can never be excused on the basis of the inadequacy of the questions that are posed. In other words, the witness must use whatever direction of inquiry is pursued to somehow communicate the essential information.

Procedurally, the first interrogation of an expert witness is conducted by the attorney who has called that witness. At the outset of that interrogation, the opposing attorney may, with the consent of the judge, interject questions that are intended to impeach the witness's expertise before he or she offers testimony. Thereafter, the opposing attorney may, and usually does, raise objections both to the questions that may be asked and to the answers given, once again usually based on the witness's competence to answer whatever question has been posed. When objections are raised, the judge rules as to whether the question or the answer may stand, or should be rephrased, or is to be ignored by the jury. Following the direct examination, the opposing attorney cross-examines the witness; cross-examination may then be followed by rebuttal, led by the other attorney. Many of the suggestions offered for testifying during depositions also apply to trial testimony. These additional suggestions may be helpful:

1. Throughout the entire testimony, talk directly to the jury, in the same way you would talk to any group of lay people. Maintain eye contact with as many jurors as possible. Be alert for signs of confusion or disinterest. If you perceive general confusion, adjust your level of language usage or clarify your answers. If you perceive disinterest, try to make your answers more succinct. Since the attorneys are asking the questions, you will be tempted to look at them while answering. Instead, look at the attorney when listening to and clarifying the question, then face the jury to respond to the question. Be particularly careful to continue to talk to the jury during cross-examination.
2. Usually, your testimony as an expert witness begins with a review of your qualifications. Here, you should strike a delicate balance between excessive modesty and self-aggrandizement. The review should include a summary of your professional education, specification of certification and licensure, previous and present employment, and areas of special professional interest. If you have published material relating to those areas, this should be mentioned. Because lay people are often unfamiliar with our profession, it is wise to define briefly the scope of practice of speech-language pathology or audiology. If you work in a state offering licensure, that definition is best accomplished by paraphrasing the scope-of-practice statement in the licensure law. It is also advisable to emphasize that speech-language pathologists and audiologists are not physicians.
3. Always be certain that you understand a question before attempting to answer. Do not, however, clarify questions by restating them or saying something like "Do you mean . . .?" Simply say, "Would you repeat the question, please?", or "I don't understand your question, would you rephrase it, please?"
4. If you cannot answer a question because it is based on false assumptions, or because the answer lies outside of the scope of your professional practice or of your expertise, do not attempt to answer the question. Simply say, "I can't answer that question." (If the question is unanswerable because of a false premise, you may point this out, if you can do so without appearing argumentative.) Or state, "I can't answer that question because it is outside my area of expertise."
5. Never bluff. Never guess at an answer. Never make any statements unless you are completely certain of their accuracy. Even though you feel that you should know the answer, and that your ignorance reflects on your expertise, do not take any chances; simply say, "I don't know the answer to that question." Although the opposing attorney may use this to disparage your expertise, an admission of ignorance on a particular point is much less damaging than the identification of inaccuracies in your testimony. If even one or two factual errors are identified during cross-examination, your entire testimony may be negated.
6. If objections are raised to a question or to the substance of your testimony, sit calmly until the matter is resolved by the judge's ruling. If the judge overrules an objection to a question, ask that it be repeated before answering it. (Even if you have not forgotten the original question, the jury probably has.) If the objection is sustained and the question is restated, wait for a comment before beginning your answer because an objection may be raised against the restated question.
7. If permitted by the court, bring all of your records concerning the matters at issue with you to the witness stand. If your participation in the case involved any kind of test administration, have the manuals for the tests at hand. If you have been deposed, you should also have the deposition transcript immediately available. When asked questions based on these materials, you should have the specific item in front of you when answering the question. You may always take whatever time is required to find the statements that are being questioned and to read those statements before answering the question.
8. If, in asking a question, an attorney reads an excerpt from the report of another professional, from a test manual, from a textbook, or from any other source, always ask to read the material yourself before answering any questions. Attorneys have been known to misread statements or to take them out of context.
9. Try to anticipate in advance where the substance of your testimony may conflict with the testimony of other witnesses and to analyze the likely bases of these differences of opinion. (The attorney who calls you as a witness will either have, or can obtain, reports of all other evaluations.) This may guide you in framing your responses. For example, if different conclusions can be attributed to differences in the tests that were administered, this can often be introduced early in your testimony by means of a statement such as, "To assess Ricky's language, I administered the Sequenced Inventory of Communicative Development, among other tests. Although many clinicians use the Illinois Test of Psycholinguistic Abilities for this purpose, I prefer the SICD because. . . ." Or, "Neurologists often conclude that a patient does not have any problem understanding language on the basis of

informal conversations, where they seem to respond appropriately. However, in the tests I administered, Mr. Locke was asked to respond to much more complex language, and under these circumstances it was obvious that he does, indeed, have problems understanding language." When conflicting professional opinions exist, the role of an expert witness is not to win a debate or even to win the jury over to his or her opinion. Instead, the witness should assist the jury to understand the possible bases for the disagreements, so that they can make an informed choice among the opinions.

10. Prepare yourself psychologically for the cross-examination. It is the job of the attorney who is conducting the cross to negate your testimony in the minds of the jury. He or she may use several devices to accomplish this. The attorney may seek to establish that you are unqualified to offer opinions that should be taken seriously. The attorney may attempt to demonstrate that your testimony is biased. The attorney may try to point out errors in your testimony by highlighting conflicts with other expert opinions or by citing references in the literature that disagree with statements you have made. The attorney may attempt to identify conflicting statements or other inconsistencies in your testimony—inconsistencies between your testimony and your deposition or between your testimony and statements in your records and reports on the case under litigation. In conducting cross-examinations, attorneys may be abusive, contemptuous, patronizing, and rude. The best defense against these tactics is to be unflappable, dignified, gracious, confident, and suitably modest in return. The moment an expert witness becomes defensive, the cross-examiner has succeeded.
11. No matter how strongly you feel about the clients or circumstances involved in litigation, never become an advocate for one or another possible outcome. Once you become an advocate, you forfeit your value as an expert witness, since it will inevitably be reflected in what you say or do not say. To reiterate: your role is to provide the jury with the information they will need to make an informed decision. It is not your role to lead the jury to make what you consider to be the "right decision."
12. Always remember, when you are an expert witness, *you are not on trial.* Furthermore, *your profession is not on trial.* Adopt the point of view that you are on the witness stand because you have something valuable to contribute. As in every area of your professional practice, the consumers of your services (in this instance the jury) may disregard your opinions and conclusions. But if those opinions and conclusions derive from your best efforts and most considered judgments, and if you have done your best to communicate them clearly, you have played your role successfully.

Hirsch et al. (1979, p. 218) concluded their chapter on service as an expert witness with this admonition:

> Remember the jurors are anxious to understand and very conscientiously trying to do the right thing by both sides and by justice. Theirs is no easy task, nor do they take their responsibilities lightly. In other words, be as good a member of the justice team as you can. Never forget that you are a part of that team—an important part—and that justice, in the end, is every citizen's responsibility.

Due Process Hearings

I earlier outlined some of the provisions of PL 94-142 with respect to due process, including the fact that parents are granted the right to demand reconsideration of the results of assessments or the provisions of IEP's. As noted, one step in this procedure is a fair hearing. Any speech-language pathologist or audiologist who has seen a child, whether as a school employee or in connection with services provided in some out-of-school facility, may be called as an expert witness. Occasionally, speech-language pathologists with acknowledged expertise in a field may be called, even if they have never seen the child who is the subject of the hearing.

The procedure followed in fair hearings usually resembles closely the procedure of court trials. A hearing officer's role is similar to the role of a judge in a court proceeding that does not involve a jury. The parents may represent themselves or be represented by an attorney or other advocate. If they are represented by an attorney, the school district is usually also represented by an attorney. Each party presents its case, calling witnesses to support its position. After a witness is examined, the opposing side may cross-examine the witness. The hearing officer may also ask questions. After all witnesses have been examined, each party makes closing statements, summarizing the merits of its position.

Downey (1980b, p. 333) outlined typical

questions asked of expert witnesses during fair hearings:

1. What is your name, address, occupation and current position?
2. What is your educational background?
3. What previous positions have you held?
4. Have you written in this field?
5. Have you held positions with the government or professional associations?
6. Have you had occasion to evaluate children suspected of having X condition?
7. How many?
8. Did you evaluate the child in question?
9. By what methods?
10. Are those methods commonly used in your field to make judgments on identification, evaluation and placement?
11. Are they reliable?
12. What were the results of your tests?
13. Given your expertise in this area, what is your opinion of the test results?
14. Given your expertise, do you have an opinion as to the identification, assessment or placement contained in this IEP?

Again, as when serving as expert witnesses in court actions, professionals must remember they are there to share expertise, not to serve as advocates. This may be particularly difficult when the professional is an employee of the school district that is being challenged, or even more difficult when the professional's own recommendations are challenged. Yet, it is still the professional's responsibility to provide all relevant information to assist the person who must reach a decision—in this instance the hearing officer—rather than to defend any particular points of view or set of recommendations.

Fair hearings may also focus on sharp differences of opinion between school clinicians and clinicians employed in out-of-school settings. Unless a clinician from an out-of-school setting has objective evidence, he or she should never attempt to evaluate the quality of services provided within school programs. Statements should be restricted to such facts as the length and frequency of special services that can be provided, the number of children being served within the special classes or programs that are under consideration, and the nature and extent of the problems presented by other children in those classes or programs. The qualifications of the specialist conducting an assessment or a special program should be at issue only when they do not meet the qualifications specified by the authors of whatever tests have been administered or fall short of the qualifications established by the state education department.

Because they have recommended placement in their facilities under the options for nonpublic facility placement within PL 94-142, speech-language pathologists and audiologists from out-of-school settings often have vested interests in the outcome of these hearings. Although such a clinician may recommend nonpublic facility placement as an expert witness, he or she should also specify all options that may exist. It is possible to express the opinion that the agency the witness represents offers the most suitable program, but it is not appropriate to advocate that placement.

Disability Determination

For practical purposes, disabilities are usually differentiated as short-term disabilities and long-term disabilities. The former assume that after a reasonable period of recovery, the client will be able to return to independent productivity. The latter assume that the client will not be able to achieve independent productivity during the forseeable future, if ever.

Operationally, short- and long-term disabilities may be managed quite differently. As noted in an earlier chapter, provisions for short-term disability are usually in the form of insurance that may be supplied by an employer, purchased privately by a client, or shared jointly by the employer and the client. Provisions for long-term disability, however, are covered through Social Security. In either instance, final decisions regarding eligibility for disability coverage must be made by physicians. But when the disabilities include communicative disorders, physicians may depend wholly or partially on information provided by speech-language pathologists and audiologists in making their determination. Because of the variety of provisions for short-term disability, it is impossible to specify the procedures to be followed. In general, however, when an opinion is sought from a speech-language pathologist or audiologist the question to be answered is "When can the client return to work?," or, occasionally, "When will it be possible to determine whether the client is permanently disabled?" Speech-language pathologists are most often consulted when language is disrupted as the result of trauma or cerebrovascular accidents or when major structural changes have been effected through trauma or such surgical procedures as laryngectomy or glossectomy. Occasionally, less devastating conditions, such as vocal nodules, may be under consideration for clients who place heavy demands on their voices to pursue their occupations. Audiologists may be consulted to offer opinions as to when optimal benefits will be achieved from aural rehabilitation or regarding problems in vocational readjustment that are likely when a hearing loss has been incurred. Speech-language pathologists and audiologists may often confront these questions with little dependable objective information. Yet, however uncertain their opinions, those opinions are likely to be more authoritative than can be offered by members of any other profession.

Provisions for long-term disability may be covered either under Title II of the Social Security Act or under the more recent Title XVI that added the Supplemental Security Income (SSI) program. Under Title II, there are three basic categories of beneficiaries. *Disabled workers under age 65* may qualify when they have been employed for sufficient lengths of time in positions covered by Social Security. *Persons continuously disabled since childhood* may qualify when one parent who is covered by Social Security retires, becomes disabled, or dies. *Disabled widows or widowers*, age 50 or older, may qualify if the deceased spouse was covered by Social Security. Under Title XVI, disabled adults and children may qualify for SSI support even though they do not meet Title II criteria with respect to previous coverage under Social Security for themselves, their spouses, or their parents.

Once again, the responsibility for determination of disability is assigned to physicians, working with local or regional Disability Determination Units. These physicians review reports from physicians and other specialists and, when needed, secure additional evaluations to reach their decisions. According to the law, they must certify that the client is unable "to engage in *any* substantial gainful activity by reason of a medically determinable physical or mental impairment which can be expected to result in death or has lasted or can be expected to last for a continuous period of not less than 12 months. . ." (Social Security Administration, 1979, p. 1). Medically determinable impairments are defined as manifesting themselves through signs or laboratory findings apart from symptoms (i.e., the claimant's own perception of his or her own physical or mental impairments). Signs are defined as "anatomical, physiological, or psychological abnormalities which can be observed through the use of medically acceptable clinical techniques." Laboratory findings are "manifestations of anatomical, physiological phenomena demonstrable by replacing or extending the perceptiveness of the observer's senses and include chemical, electrophysical, roentgenological, or psychological tests." In the instance of communicative disorders, data provided by speech-language pathologists and audiologists may be used to verify observed signs or treated as laboratory findings.

In classifying disabilities involving communicative disorders, hearing loss is included in Section 2.00 of the *Listing of Impairments*, entitled Special Senses and Speech, under a subsection entitled Otolaryngology (pp. 18–19). That section specifies:

> *Hearing impairment.* Hearing ability should be

evaluated in terms of the person's ability to hear and distinguish speech.

Loss of hearing can be quantitatively determined by an audiometer which meets the standards of the American National Standards Institute (ANSI) for air and bone conducted stimuli (i.e., ANSI 3.6-1969 and ANSI 3.13-1972, or subsequent comparable revisions) and performing all hearing measurements in an environment which meets the ANSI standard for maximum permissible background sound (ANSI 3.1-1977).

Hearing tests should be preceded by an otolaryngologic examination and should be performed by or under the supervision of an otolaryngologist or audiologist qualified to perform such tests.

In order to establish an independent medical judgment as to the level of severity in a claimant alleging deafness, the following examinations should be reported: Otolaryngologic examination, pure tone air and bone audiometry, speech reception thresholds (SRT), and speech discrimination testing. A copy of reports of medical examination and audiologic evaluation must be submitted.

Cases of alleged "deaf mutism" should be documented by a hearing evaluation. Records obtained from a speech and hearing rehabilitation center or a special school for the deaf may be acceptable, but if those reports are not available, or are found to be inadequate, a current hearing evaluation should be submitted as outlined in the preceding paragraph.

Organic loss of speech. Glossectomy or laryngectomy or cicatricial laryngeal stenosis due to injury or infection results in loss of voice production by normal means. In evaluating organic loss of speech, ability to produce speech by any means includes the use of mechanical or electronic devices.

Speech disorders are also included in the section on Neurological Disorders. These include "central nervous system vascular accident" with "sensory or motor aphasia" resulting in impaired communication more than 3 months following the vascular accident, and cerebral palsy with "significant interference in communication due to speech, hearing, or visual defect."

Hearing impairment may qualify a client for long-term disability coverage when it is "not restorable by a hearing aid" and is "manifested by average hearing threshold sensitivity for air conduction of 90 decibels or greater, and for bone conduction to corresponding maximal levels, in the better ear, determined by the simple average of hearing threshold levels at 500, 1000, and 2000 Hz; or speech discrimination scores of 40 percent or less in the better ear." Organic loss of speech qualifies clients for long-term disability coverage when characterized by "inability to produce by any means speech which can be heard, understood, and sustained."

Although devoted to coverage of long-term disability, Social Security and SSI coverage need not be lifelong. When impairments may reasonably be expected to improve, clients are re-evaluated periodically. If the impairment is no longer sufficiently severe to obviate gainful employment, benefits may terminate after a 3-month "adjustment period." Under certain circumstances, clients may engage in a period of "trial work" without termination of coverage. Disabled clients covered by Title II and Title XVI may qualify for vocational rehabilitation services, and most are also covered either by Medicare or Medicaid or both.

Hearings on Testamentary Capacity

Occasionally speech-language pathologists are called as expert witnesses to testify in actions inquiring into the validity of a will. Virtually always, these actions concern decedents who had language impairments resulting from cerebrovascular accidents or some other traumatic encephalopathy. When these individuals execute wills after they acquire their communicative disorders, questions may arise about their competency at the time the will was executed. Usually these inquiries are carried out through hearings; however, challenges can ultimately lead to trials.

In most states, testamentary capacity is based on three factors: (1) the person must understand that he or she is making a will; (2) the person must know, without prompting, who his or her natural heirs are; and (3) the person must know, without prompting, the nature and extent of his or her property. Expert witnesses, then, are consulted to determine whether these factors obtained at the time the will was executed.

A speech-language pathologist is often in an unenviable position when called as a witness in proceedings regarding testamentary capacity. If a client clearly showed completely intact language comprehension, and, perhaps with some lapses in word finding, had essentially intact language production, it may be possible to offer useful evidence. It may also be possible to give an unqualified opinion if the client showed massive deficits in all aspects of language comprehension and production, with likely attendant cognitive impairments. For most clients, however, whose impairments lay somewhere between these extremes, clear-cut testimony is virtually impossible.

It is usually possible to present some evidence about the client's orientation to his or her surroundings, awareness of events, and other evidence of his or her purposeful and rational behavior. A speech-language pathologist may also be able to testify as to the client's ability to recognize and name members of his or her family or the other people who are named as heirs. A speech-language pathologist may even be able to describe instances that demonstrate presence or absence of awareness of property and other aspects of financial affairs.

The role of speech-language pathologists in testamentary hearings can be stated succinctly: They may offer information that will assist the court in making determinations about testamentary capacity; they should not, however, ever presume to state definitively that a client did or did not have testamentary capacity.

Governmental Hearings

I have reiterated the contention that one consequence of asserting our professional independence is our increasing involvement with current laws and regulations. But an even more significant hallmark of professional maturity is active participation in the formulation of new laws and regulations. One step in drafting those laws and regulations involves hearings at which concerned citizens provide input for the consideration of legislative and regulatory bodies. In the strictest sense, the role of testifier at a governmental hearing differs from the usual role of expert witness, but there are many essential similarities.

Both federal and state governments hold hearings as a part of the legislative process. These hearings may occur at three different times. Fact-finding hearings may occur before any specific legislation is contemplated. Legislative committees and their staff members, or other governmental agencies, may conduct hearings to identify problems, leading ultimately to the formulation of legislation to remedy those problems. When proposed laws are drafted and introduced, the committees that review—and usually amend—those laws prior to congressional or state legislative action also hold hearings. These hearings ostensibly offer advice about the implications of the proposed legislation. Once laws are enacted, regulations are written to specify further the provisions of the laws. Regulations are usually drafted immediately after a law is enacted, but they may be revised and expanded at any time after the law's enactment. In most instances, the task of writing regulations is assigned to the governmental agency responsible for carrying out the provisions of the law (e.g., departments of education or health, licensure boards, the Food and Drug Administration, or the Federal Trade Commission). Once again, hearings are conducted in conjunction with the drafting of regulations.

Although hearings are an important part of all legislative processes, it would be naïve to claim that they are the most important component of that process. Efforts that rely entirely upon testimony at hearings to influence substantially the drafting of new laws and regulations are seldom successful. As in every aspect of our increasingly complex society, to be successful, those efforts must usually be coordinated by legislative advocates who are professionals in their field, i.e., in legislative advocacy. Although the testimony of a member of our profession at a hearing dealing with an area of our concern may sometimes be crucial, it usually comprises only one facet of successful legislative advocacy. Increasingly, success in influencing legislation entails the retention of experienced legislative advocates, who may know little about our profession or its concerns, but who know a lot about influencing legislative processes.

The most important suggestion that can be offered to speech-language pathologists and audiologists who are contemplating testimony at governmental hearings, therefore, is to plan that testimony as one part of a total effort—an effort thoroughly orchestrated by a professional legislative advocate.

Some other suggestions are:

1. Unless there are clearly opposing views among members of the profession, it is best to designate a single official spokesperson, chosen by a group representing the profession. If irreconcilable views exist, the points on which professionals have agreed to disagree should be delineated, specifying the bases for the disagreements. (However understandable, this situation is always regrettable because it assigns to lay people the responsibility for resolving intraprofessional disagreements.) Equally to be avoided are situations in which endless reiterations of similar views are presented by an uncoordinated succession of members of the same profession.
2. Most governmental hearings accept both oral and written testimony. It is usually most effective to present a clear, brief, cogent, and lively oral statement, supported by more detailed written testimony. The oral testimony may pique the interest of the committee, staff, hearing officer, or hearing panel. The written testimony will offer the details that can be studied later and applied in making decisions. Even the written testimony, however, should be as concise as possible.
3. Sometimes, consumers may provide helpful support to professional testimony. However, their participation should be well planned, clarifying the precise objectives to be accomplished. The consumers should be selected for their ability to present viewpoints clearly and to answer whatever questions may be asked following the testimony. The use of clients solely for eliciting sympathy or other emotional reactions should generally be avoided.
4. Confrontational "Mau-Mauing" tactics have been so overused that they have lost much of their effectiveness. They seldom serve to accomplish a profession's objectives at governmental hearings.
5. Testimony at governmental hearings should always stress service to the public welfare. A testifier should emphasize why provisions of laws or regulations are or are not in the consumers' interests, never why they are or are not in the interests of a profession.

Unlike other situations in which speech-language pathologists and audiologists participate as expert witnesses, in governmental hearings they are indeed advocates for a point of view. Although their purpose remains that of enabling those who listen to their testimony to make informed choices, they usually have a substantial personal interest in the choices that are made.

SUMMARY

Consumer protection is the principal goal of both legal and ethical regulation of human services professions. Legal controls, having the force of law, would seem the more effective. Yet, they generally define only the outer limits of acceptable practice. Ethical controls, on the other hand, represent efforts toward professional self-regulation. Although carrying less stringent penalties, codes of ethics offer more detailed definitions of acceptable standards of professional practice.

As we have entered the mainstream of health services professions, speech-language pathology and audiology are increasingly concerned with legal and ethical issues. Those concerns, however, are the inevitable consequences of enjoying the privilege of independent professional practice.

References

Annas GJ, Glantz LH, Katz BF: *The Rights of Doctors, Nurses and Allied Health Professionals.* Cambridge, MA, Ballinger, 1981.

Beresford HR: *Legal Aspects of Neurologic Practice.* Philadelphia, FA Davis, 1975.

Bernzweig EP: *The Nurse's Liability for Malpractice.* New York, McGraw Hill, 1981.

Christoffel T: *Health and the Law.* New York, The Free Press, 1982.

Downey M: Due process hearings and PL 94-142. *ASHA* 22:255–257, 1980a.

Downey M: Conduct of the due process hearing. *ASHA* 22:332–334, 1980b.

Dublinske S: PL 94-142 due process decisions. *ASHA* 22:335–338, 1980.

Dublinske S, Healey W: PL 94-142: questions and answers for the speech-language pathologist and audiologist. *ASHA* 20:188–205, 1978.

Grimm KL: The relationship of accreditation to voluntary certification and state licensure. In *Study of Accreditation of Selected Health Professions, Staff Working Papers.* Washington DC, Study of Accreditation of Selected Health Professions, 1972.

Halleck SL: *Law in the Practice of Psychiatry.* New York, Plenum, 1980.

Hirsch CS, Morris RC, Moritz AR: *Handbook of Legal Medicine.* St. Louis, CV Mosby, 1979.

Hofling CK: *Law and Ethics in the Practice of Psychiatry.* New York, Brunner/Mazel, 1981.

Perrin K: Personal incomes in the speech-language-hearing profession. *ASHA* 21:522–525, 1979.

Schulman M, Geesman J: *Deceptive Packaging.* San Francisco, San Francisco Consumer Action, 1974.

Social Security Administration: *Disability Evaluation under Social Security: A Handbook for Physicians.* Washington DC, United States Department of Health and Human Services, 1979.

Sparer EV: The legal right to health care: public policy and equal access. *Hastings Center Report* 6:39–47, 1976.

United States Department of Health, Education, and Welfare: *Handbook of Public Assistance.* Washington DC, United States Department of Health, Education, and Welfare, 1966.

CHAPTER TWELVE

Assuring the Quality of Clinical Services

Even if institutional and individual providers of speech, language, and hearing services scrupulously adhere to all relevant laws and legal regulations and to all provisions of ASHA's Code of Ethics—or at least to the letter of the Code—they may still deliver less than optimal, or even inferior, services. Therefore, consumer protection must extend beyond the topics discussed in Chapter 11. This chapter is concerned with other types of quality assurance procedures and programs that seek even more effective means for protecting the consumers of our professional services.

ACCREDITATION

Chapter 2 contained the definition of accreditation formulated by the National Commission on Accrediting:

> Accreditation is the process by which an agency or organization evaluates and recognizes a program of study or an institution as meeting certain predetermined qualifications or standards. It shall apply only to institutions and their programs of study or their services.

As defined, accreditation is primarily carried out by nongovernmental agencies and organizations, in contrast to licensure where a governmental body grants to an institution the legal right to provide services. For example, in many states, hospitals must be licensed before they may provide any health care services, or some state education agencies require licensure of nonpublic schools as a qualification for payment for children served under the provisions of PL 94-142. Accreditation, on the other hand, is ostensibly voluntary; an agency or institution may legally provide services whether it is accredited or not. As will be discussed in greater detail, in practice this differentiation is not so precise. When effective accreditation programs are in place, they are used by governmental agencies to define qualified providers of services. Consequently, many accreditation programs have acquired what is, in effect, a quasi-legal status.

There are several groups that carry out accreditation programs for educational institutions. They exist to protect the consumers who are students in or who employ graduates from those institutions. Within our field, ASHA's Education and Training Board is concerned with the accreditation of graduate education programs in speech-language pathology and audiology. This discussion, however, will consider only the accreditation programs that are concerned with the quality of clinical services that include those available to people with communicative disorders, i.e., the programs offered by ASHA's Professional Services Board, by the Joint Commission on Accreditation of Hospitals, and by the Commission on Accreditation of Rehabilitation Facilities.

ASHA's Professional Services Board (PSB)

The Professional Services Board is the one accrediting agency that is exclusively concerned with assuring the quality of speech, language, and hearing services. The American Speech-Language-Hearing Association established its accreditation program in 1959 with the founding of the American Boards of Examiners in Speech Pathology and Audiology (ABESPA). Among the tasks assigned to those boards was the obligation to establish and maintain boards responsible for the formulation of standards, to arrange and conduct examinations to determine the qualifications of individuals, organizations, and institutions, and to furnish proper persons and agencies with lists of individuals, organizations, and institutions that had been certified or accredited by ABESPA. From the outset, ABESPA announced the intention to offer "certification"—later properly changed to "accreditation"—of two types of programs. Educational programs in speech pathology and audiology were to be accredited by the Education and Training Board, and clinical services were to be accredited by the Clinical Services Board. By the time ABESPA announced its readiness to begin the accreditation of clinical services, the name of the responsible body had been changed to the Professional Services Board.

In its initial announcement, PSB invited agencies providing speech, language, and hearing services to apply for accreditation. PSB would then survey the agency to determine whether it met specified standards (which had been developed by PSB and approved by the ABESPA Board of Directors). These standards primarily addressed the qualifications of personnel, clinical practices and procedures, professional interrelationships, and physical facilities and equipment.

With the complete reorganization of ASHA's standards program in 1979, there developed a clearer differentiation between standards setting functions and standards interpretation and administration functions. This separation carried out a pattern under way in most professional standards programs, a pattern established in the belief that placing all of these functions in the same hands created confusions of roles and possible conflicts of interests. In particular, many consumer advocates contend that the bodies that establish standards should not also interpret and enforce those standards. At that time, therefore, all of ASHA's standards setting functions—including setting standards for accreditation of clinical services programs—were assigned to the newly established Council on Professional Standards in Speech-Language Pathology and Audiology. Insofar as accreditation of clinical services was concerned, the interpretive and administrative functions remained with PSB.

Current PSB procedures essentially resemble those announced at the inception of the program. A detailed application is prepared, usually following an extensive self-study procedure by the applicant agency. If preliminary review of the application reveals that the agency meets general requirements for accreditation, a site visit occurs. Site visitors are appropriately certified members of the staffs of agencies that have been accredited by PSB. The site visit team studies the agency for first-hand evidence that it meets the criteria specified for accreditation. In the course of their review they meet with the individual or individuals who are administratively responsible, interview members of the professional staff, review sample client records, observe diagnostic and therapeutic sessions, examine facilities and equipment, and meet with representatives of other agencies or other professionals in the community. After their visit, the team renders a report to PSB. Based on the information provided in the original application, the report of the site visit team, and whatever supplemental information may be requested, PSB then decides whether to award or withhold accreditation.

In its latest revision (1983, pp. 52–58) PSB defines 25 standards, which are further elaborated by the definition of indicators that offer evidence as to whether those standards are met. These standards are:

1. The program shall have established goals which are directed toward achieving the maximum communication competence of individuals with communicative disorders and which are achieved through the provision of comprehensive evaluation, consultation, treatment, and referral services.
2. The development, review, revision and evaluation of program goals shall be the responsibility of the program administrative personnel, utilizing procedures for ongoing recommendations from the speech-language pathology and audiology staff and consumers.
3. Administrative policies and procedures must be effective and appropriate to the program's

goals. Although the program director may not be a speech-language pathologist or audiologist, policies and procedure relating to clinical activities in communicative disorders shall be made by an individual who meets the requirements for the appropriate ASHA Certificate of Clinical Competence.

4. Administrative policies and procedures shall provide fiscal stability and responsibility.
5. The program shall not discriminate on the basis of sex, age, race, religion, national origin, or handicapping condition in providing services to the public or in employment practices.
6. Services provided shall be accurately identified and described to the public.
7. The program shall establish and follow appropriate client admission, discharge, and follow-up policies and procedures.
8. The program shall establish and follow policies and procedures for the evaluation of the communicative disorders of its clients. Speech-language evaluations shall include hearing screening to determine whether the client should be referred for hearing evaluation. Hearing evaluations shall include observations to determine whether the client should be referred for speech-language evaluation.
9. The program shall establish and follow treatment policies and procedures consistent with the program's stated goals and appropriate to the client's communication needs as identified during evaluation.
10. The program shall provide resources for counseling services consistent with the program's stated goals and appropriate to the client's needs.
11. The program shall establish and maintain referral policies consistent with the program's stated goals and appropriate to the client's needs.
12. The program shall establish and maintain appropriate policies for the preparation of written reports.
13. The professional staff of the program shall be qualified and of a size sufficient to provide services essential to the achievement of the program's goals.
14. Speech-language pathologists and audiologists who assume independent responsibility for provision of clinical services shall meet the ASHA CCC requirements in the area(s) in which they provide services. Service providers under contract to the program shall meet the same requirements as salaried personnel.
15. Program staff members from other professional disciplines, including consultants and service providers under contract, shall be credentialed or licensed in their particular specialties.
16. The administrator shall ensure that assignments of staff members are commensurate with the professional qualifications and special skills of these individuals. The program shall ensure that professional staff are allowed time to conduct aspects of their assignments not involving direct client contact.
17. The program shall provide for staff growth and development.
18. Speech-language pathologists and/or audiologists who supervise clinical activities must meet the requirements for the ASHA CCC in the appropriate area, and, in addition, provide evidence of competence in clinical supervision.
19. A speech-language pathologist or audiologist who meets the requirements for the ASHA CCC in the appropriate area shall be responsible for all client services provided in these areas by persons not meeting the ASHA CCC requirements (i.e., clinicians, clinical fellows, and supportive personnel). Individuals who do not meet the ASHA CCC requirements shall be identified as such to the client and shall be appropriately supervised.
20. Supervision of students in clinical practicum shall be sufficiently frequent to ensure provision of quality services to the client at all times. The minimum schedules of direct supervision provided by the program shall be: a) at least 50% of each evaluation; b) at least 25% of treatment sessions.
21. Accurate, complete records shall be prepared and maintained for each client. Records shall be accessible to appropriate personnel and systematically organized to facilitate storage and retrieval.
22. The program shall establish and follow policies and procedures ensuring that all client records are adequately retained and protected with respect to confidentiality, destruction, and loss.
23. The physical plant shall be barrier free, in compliance with all applicable safety and health codes, and suitable for the conduct of those activities required to meet the objectives of the program.
24. The program shall provide and maintain an environment with equipment, materials, and calibration procedures appropriate to its stated goals.
25. The program shall evaluate the efficiency and effectiveness of the various components of its operations, including personnel, budget, equipment, facilities, and needs of the population served. This evaluation shall be accomplished by means of regular reviews of these components. Such reviews shall include for-

mal evaluation of individual client management.

PSB may award accreditation in either speech-language pathology or audiology or in both speech-language pathology and audiology, depending upon the scope of services provided by the program. Accreditation has been awarded to programs in all settings: schools, medical centers, colleges and universities, community centers, and rehabilitation facilities, and to private practitioners. Unquestionably, of the available accreditation mechanisms, it offers the most exhaustive review of speech-language pathology and audiology services. As such, it affords a higher level of quality assurance within our field than do the other two possible clinical services accreditation programs.

Joint Commission on Accreditation of Hospitals (JCAH)

In 1918, the American College of Surgeons instituted a Hospital Standardization Program which sought to encourage the adoption of a uniform medical record format to facilitate more accurate recording of the treatment accorded to hospital patients. This soon led to recognition that this program might also offer a means of identifying institutions that provided quality care. The scope of the program grew steadily until it overreached the resources of the parent organization. Four other organizations responded to pleas for joint sponsorship of the program, resulting, in 1951, in the establishment of a sponsoring coalition comprised, in addition to the American College of Surgeons, of the American College of Physicians, the American Hospital Association, the American Medical Association, and the Canadian Medical Association. At the same time, the program was renamed, becoming the Joint Commission on Accreditation of Hospitals (JCAH). The Canadian Medical Association withdrew its sponsorship in 1959 with the establishment of the Canadian Council on Hospital Accreditation. The American Dental Association became a member of JCAH in 1979.

At its inception, JCAH adopted the standards developed by the Hospital Standardization Program. The first revision of standards was published in 1953, and revisions have continued during the ensuing years. New editions of the JCAH manuals are published annually, with each containing some revisions of previous standards.

JCAH achieved its first legal recognition from the federal government with the enactment of the Medicare law in 1965. The law specified that hospitals participating in the Medicare program must maintain the level of patient care called for in JCAH standards. Thus, JCAH-accredited hospitals were automatically deemed to comply with Medicare standards of care. Subsequently, most public and private third-party payment programs have given similar status to JCAH accreditation.

With respect to accreditation, the announced purposes of JCAH are (p. ix):

1. to establish standards for the operation of hospitals and other health-related facilities and services.
2. to conduct survey and accreditation programs that will encourage members of the health professions, hospitals, and other health-related facilities and services voluntarily:
   a. to promote high quality care in all aspects in order to give patients the optimum benefits that medical science has to offer.
   b. to apply certain basic principles of physical plant safety and maintenance, and of organization and administration of function for efficient care of the patient, and
   c. to maintain the essential services in the facilities through coordinated effort of the organized staffs and governing bodies of the facilities.
3. to recognize compliance with standards by issuance of certificates of accreditation.

At the present time, JCAH has established standards for and offers accreditation to four different types of institutions: (1) acute care general hospitals, including hospital-sponsored ambulatory health care services; (2) long-term care facilities; (3) facilities and programs providing services to psychiatric and substance-abuse patients, including community mental health programs; and (4) ambulatory health care organizations, excluding hospital-sponsored ambulatory health care services.

The JCAH accreditation process is initiated by an institution filing an Application for Survey. The items included in the survey are detailed in the *Hospital Survey Profile* which is available both as a self-study document and as a means of providing information for accreditation surveys. This profile amplifies each accreditation standard through checklists to be completed by personnel at the applicant institution. On completion of the application procedure, a team of JCAH surveyors visits for on-site observations to confirm the information provided by the institution. In addition to visits to various departments, "public information interviews" must be held, during which consumers or other members of the general public, and any members of the staff or other personnel from the institution, may appear to express their concerns. At the conclusion of the on-site survey, the team must hold a summation conference with representatives of the hospital's governing body, administration, and medical staff. During this conference, the surveyors present their findings and the hospital representatives may comment on those findings.

Following completion of the survey, the team's findings are reviewed by JCAH staff, who, in turn, recommend to the Accreditation Committee of the Board of Commissioners whether accreditation should be awarded or denied. When an institution is deemed substantially in compliance with relevant standards, it is granted accreditation for 3 years; however, an interim study (using the *Hospital Survey Profile*) must be conducted approximately midway through that accreditation period. At the end of 3 years, the hospital must go through the same survey procedure in order to renew its accreditation. An accredited institution may, however, be surveyed at any time at the discretion of JCAH.

One group of JCAH standards applies to the institution as a whole, considering such factors as administration and governance, building and grounds, emergency services, functional safety and sanitation, infection control, and medical records services. In addition, however, they have established standards applicable to individual departments and programs.

Speech-language pathology and audiology services are considered within the standards for rehabilitation services. The basic principle underlying these standards is: "Rehabilitation programs or services shall be regularly and conveniently available to meet the needs of the patients." The first standard addresses the fundamental organization of all rehabilitation services (p. 151):

> Organized rehabilitation programs or services within the hospital shall be provided by an adequate, qualified staff that receives competent medical direction, as required, and is provided with adequate physical resources.

Standard IV in the section on rehabilitation programs and services specifies: "Speech pathology and audiology services shall be provided as required." That standard is elaborated with the following interpretation (p. 167):

> Speech pathology and/or audiology services provided within the hospital from either hospital or community resources shall meet the requirements contained in Standard I of Rehabilitation Programs/Services. When provided from hospital resources, the speech pathology and audiology program/service may be organized as a separate hospital unit or subsumed under the overall rehabilitation program/service organizational structure.
>
> Overall administration and supervision of the speech pathology and/or audiology program/service shall be provided by a qualified speech-language pathologist or qualified audiologist. This individual, as well as all staff speech-language pathologists and audiologists with independent responsibilities, shall hold the Certificate of Clinical Competence or a Statement of Equivalence in either speech pathology or audiology issued by the American Speech-Language-Hearing Association, or have a documented equivalent training and/or experience; shall meet any current legal requirements of licensure or registration; and shall be currently competent in the field.
>
> Support personnel, such as speech pathology assistants and communication aides, shall be qualified by training and/or experience for the level of work performed, and shall be appropri-

ately supervised by a staff speech-language pathologist or audiologist.

Properly credentialed personnel, educational institutions, health care agencies, or other recognized educational or social organizations may be authorized to refer ambulatory care patients for speech pathology and audiology services.

All speech and language evaluations shall be conducted by a qualified speech-language pathologist. All audiometric testing and evaluation procedures beyond routine pure tone testing shall ordinarily be carried out by, or under the direct supervision of, a qualified audiologist.

Criteria for services, including hearing aid evaluations, and norms for specialized testing techniques and methods used in evaluation shall be established. These shall be designed to assure quality goals consistent with those of the criteria and norms recommended by the American Speech-Language-Hearing Association (Standards, Professional Services Board, American Boards of Examiners in Speech Pathology and Audiology, 1979).

Audiometers shall be calibrated at least quarterly, and when relocated. Standards for the performance of calibration and maintenance shall be established. These shall be designed to assure quality goals consistent with those of the standards recommended by recognized national standards organizations. When audiological services are offered, a specially constructed, sound-treated test area shall be available that meets accepted criteria for the attenuation of outside noise.

Without question, JCAH is the single most important program for the accreditation of clinical services. Although its standards are far less detailed than the standards administered by PSB, they clearly demonstrate concern for the quality of our professional services. Obviously, however, no single survey team could contain representatives of all professions considered by JCAH standards. Therefore, the ultimate impact of JCAH accreditation on assuring the quality of speech, language, and hearing services is limited both by the generality of its standards and by the lack of specific expertise of its surveyors.

Commission on Accreditation of Rehabilitation Facilities (CARF)

Although hospital-based rehabilitation services fall within the purview of JCAH accreditation, its view of rehabilitation is somewhat narrower than the view taken by many institutions primarily devoted to the delivery of rehabilitation services. The Commission on Accreditation of Rehabilitation Facilities was established, therefore, in response to expressed needs for an agency exclusively devoted to the establishment of standards for rehabilitation agencies and to the accreditation of institutions and agencies that meet those standards.

Institutions and agencies falling within the purview of CARF are characterized in the first four criteria for eligibility for accreditation. According to these criteria, a facility must: (1) be involved in evaluating and/or minimizing the effects of handicapping conditions of those it serves; (2) be involved in a process of maximizing the individual's functioning, either within the facility or by linkages with other agencies; (3) provide services designed to enhance the independence, self-sufficiency, and productivity of those served; and (4) be involved in a process of goal-oriented, comprehensive, interdisciplinary and coordinated services, either within the facility or by linkages with other agencies. As these criteria suggest, CARF accreditation can be applied to a wide spectrum of models for services delivery. More specifically, however, they cite 12 different types of programs or services that fall within their purview: (1) hospital-based rehabilitation; (2) outpatient medical rehabilitation; (3) infant and early childhood development programs; (4) vocational evaluation; (5) work adjustment; (6) occupational skill training; (7) job placement; (8) work services (i.e., programs providing direct remunerative work to disabled people); (9) activity services (i.e., programs of therapeutic services toward maximizing clients' independent functioning); (10) residential services; (11) independent living programs; and (12) psychosocial programs. Conceivably, speech-language pathologists could be employed, at least on consultative bases, in programs of any of these types; however, they are most likely to be found in the first three types of programs.

The procedure followed for CARF accreditation essentially resembles all accreditation processes. A facility first conducts a self-study, usually employing a questionnaire CARF has prepared. If the facility deems itself ready for accreditation, it completes the application and requests a site survey. A survey-consultation team is appointed to conduct the study and to report its findings to the Commission. Ultimately, the Commission informs the facility of its decision and sends a written report summarizing perceived strengths and weaknesses and making recommendations for program improvement. Three outcomes are possible. If the facility shows "substantial fulfillment of the standards," it is awarded 3-year accreditation. If it has significant deficiencies but shows promise for overcoming those deficiencies, 1-year accreditation is awarded. If major deficits are apparent, accreditation is denied.

CARF standards, like JCAH standards, first address organizational characteristics. Second, they address matters applicable to all programs, including intake and orientation procedures; assessment and evaluation procedures; case coordination and management; and referral, discharge, and follow-up. Finally, there are more specific standards for each of the 12 different programs or services cited above.

Although many of the standards cited by CARF are directly applicable to the delivery of speech-language pathology and audiology services, there are only cursory references to those services, actually even fewer references than in JCAH standards. However, CARF representatives frequently cite PSB standards when detailed information about our professional services is needed. In general, then, speech-language pathologists and audiologists who are employed by facilities accredited or seeking accreditation by CARF may be held accountable according to standards addressing some of the general aspects of organization and client management. But CARF accreditation procedures will not usually address the features that uniquely characterize speech-language pathology and audiology services.

SUPERVISION

Supervision may well be the oldest, most traditional approach to quality assurance. Even in ancient and primitive societies, it has been assumed that the quality of human services will be ensured by placing younger and less experienced providers under the surveillance of masters of the arts and crafts of their fields of service. Furthermore, it has been assumed that the members of some occupational groups concerned with human services require supervision throughout their careers. Until recent years, supervision probably represented the entire quality assurance efforts of most human services programs.

Our profession's greatest concerns have focused on the supervision of students engaged in the clinical practice that comprises one part of professional education, and of beginning professionals who are in the early months of employment (often completing the clinical fellowship year requirement for ASHA certification). Standards specifying the amount of supervision that must be provided to these individuals and the qualifications of their supervisors are addressed in the requirements for the certificates and in standards for accreditation by ASHA's Education and Training Board and Professional Services Board. The emphasis on supervision of apprentice professionals and new professionals is readily apparent in our literature. Culatta and Helmick (1980, 1981) published an exemplary review of the literature on supervision in speech-language pathology and audiology.

Approaches to Supervision

In discussing supervision, many writers characterize supervisory "styles," i.e., the approaches supervisors use in attempting to improve the proficiencies of the students or professionals under their charge. (Gouran, 1980, offered a succinct summary of supervisory styles.) It may be more accurate, however, to view supervisory practices on a continuum from unilateral to bilateral. Unilateral practices involve establishment of standards by the supervisor (or by the supervisor's employer) and holding the supervisee accountable according to those standards. Bilateral practices involve joint development, by supervisor and supervisee, of standards, and joint determination of whether or not those standards were met.

In practice, good supervision is seldom consistently at one end of this continuum or the other. Even when standards are established unilaterally, some degree of self-assessment by the supervisee usually occurs. On the other hand, good supervision is seldom completely bilateral. Unless the supervisor is providing greater input in the establishment of standards and in evaluating the supervisee's success in meeting those standards, there is really no supervision.

Supervisory practices will also vary according to circumstances. When a supervisee is engaging in practices that are worthless, erroneous, or even harmful, a good supervisor will intervene directly and immediately. Practices will also differ substantially depending on the capabilities of the supervisee. A good supervisor will use very different approaches in working with a student or beginning clinical fellow than in working with an experienced professional seeking skills in a new area of clinical endeavor.

When supervisees are evaluated according to a predetermined set of standards, those standards should be clear from the outset. Many programs prepare evaluation protocols or use protocols devised by other institutions. One of the more fully developed and researched evaluation instruments is the Wisconsin Procedure for Appraisal of Clinical Competence (W-PACC) (Shriberg et al., 1974, 1975). This instrument employs a 38-item Clinician Appraisal Form which is divided into two scales. One scale assesses interpersonal skills, including such items as, "Conveys to the client in a nonthreatening manner what the standards of behavior and performance are." The other scale assesses professional-technical skills and is divided into four subscales: developing and planning, teaching, assessment, and reporting. It includes such items as, "Sequences teaching tasks to implement designated program objectives." A supplementary 10-item scale is also included to summarize such personal qualities as appearance and punctuality. The supervisor rates supervisees on each item according to a 10-point scale, with four descriptors as guides to that scale, ranging from the lowest—"Specific direction from supervisor does not alter unsatisfactory performance and inability to make changes"—to the highest—"Demonstrates independence by taking initiative, makes changes when appropriate, and is effective." Based on these ratings, a percentage score is derived for the interpersonal and the professional-technical scales. The *W-PACC Applications Manual* further offers data to permit comparison of the ratings of a particular supervisee with others of comparable training and experience.

Many bilateral approaches to supervision derive from such systems as Management by Objectives (MBO) (Odiorne, 1969). MBO was originally proposed to facilitate planning and decision making in business and corporate enterprises. Many subsequent variations of the essential design of MBO have been proposed, but their similarities generally outnumber their differences. MBO and its various derivatives have been widely used in planning human services programs. Dublinske and Grimes (1979) formulated an approach to program planning evaluation that was specifically applied to speech, language, and hearing services programs.

Although MBO and its offshoots emphasize overall program development, supervision is often an important element of that development. Furthermore, its basic precepts can be applied to supervisory practices even in those instances where no program innovations are contemplated. It can be applied to supervision at all levels, from the supervision of clinical practice by inexperienced clinicians to supervision of the most senior staff members.

Essentially, MBO entails the clear definition of objectives through the participation of all parties responsible for accomplishing those objectives and the assessment of success in terms of progress toward meeting those objectives. Odiorne described three classes of objectives. *Regular* or *routine objectives* are concerned with the daily, ordinary requirements necessary for survival of the program. *Problem-solving objectives* address areas of deficit performance, particularly where matters tend to get worse if left alone. *Innovative* or *improvement objectives* seek to effect changes in current modes of operation toward achieving improved quality of performance. To apply these to supervision in our field, regular or routine objectives relate to the daily routines of providing services within the context of the particular agency or institution. Problem-solving objectives would address specific deficits in a clinician's performance or areas of limited competence in dealing with particular clinical problems. Innovative or improvement objectives would be concerned with assisting a clinician to develop innovative approaches and practices that could improve the quality or efficiency of services of the entire program.

Dublinske and Grimes (1979) proposed six components which must be considered in stating objectives. They must specify: (1) what is to be accomplished; (2) when it is to be accomplished; (3) who is to do it (to be valid, an objective must always be controllable by the person assigned the responsibility); (4) to whom the activity is to be directed; (5) the criteria according to which the outcomes are to be assessed; and (6) how the outcomes are to be evaluated. The fifth and sixth components illustrate a fundamental tenet of MBO: all objectives must be measurable. This recalls discussions at other points in this text about problems in accountability in our field resulting from the as yet unquantifiable complexities of many of the behaviors that concern us. Nevertheless, in discussing problems in measuring achievement toward objectives, Odiorne (1969) suggested five possible levels. (All levels apply to results rather than to the activities pursued to achieve those results.) The best measurements involve real-time or raw data (dollars of sales, tons of output, number of home runs hit). Next best are ratios—batting averages, percents, fractions, etc. Third best are rating scales employing check lists of items that may be rated numerically, or as to worth (excellent, good, fair), or according to some other qualifiers. Fourth are verbal scales where specific actions ("directs," "checks," "reports," etc.) are identified. Least reliable are general descriptions that compare current conditions with conditions as they should be.

As applied to supervisory practices in our field, an MBO-derived approach would require the supervisor and supervisee jointly to target aspects of clinical practice where changes should occur. Objectives would then be developed, including the six components cited above (the "who" is always the supervisee). During subsequent conferences, each objective would be reviewed, determining, through mutual discussions, the supervisee's progress toward its achievement. When the specified final date is reached, the supervisee would then be held accountable, through comparisons of actual outcomes to the original objectives. This approach is best suited to the assessment of clinician performance as it is reflected in accuracy in administering and interpreting diagnostic procedures, in effecting measurable changes in communicative behaviors, in achieving improved client attendance, in reducing instances of disruptive behaviors, and in working toward other objectives that lend themselves to quantification. As noted by Odiorne, however, when objectives preclude quantitative assessment, descriptive assessment can be employed.

Supervision as an Interpersonal Process

Ultimately, all supervision is an interpersonal process with two participants: the supervisor and supervisee. Its fundamental effectiveness as an approach to quality assurance, therefore, depends on those participants, or, more specifically, on the supervisor's own proficiencies as a clinician and his or her skill in guiding another person in the mastery of those proficiencies, and on the supervisee's willingness and capacity to grow and change.

Our literature holds abundant discussions of the critical qualities for good supervisors and good supervision. Those discussions were well summarized in the Culatta and Helmick (1980, 1981) articles cited earlier. Recently (1982), ASHA's Committee on Supervision in Speech-Language Pathology and Audiology published suggested competencies for effective clinical supervision. These competencies are manifested in 12 different tasks involved in clinicial supervision (p. 1021):

1. establishment and maintenance of an effective working relationship with supervisees.
2. assistance of supervisees in developing goals and objectives.
3. assistance of supervisees in evaluation and case management.
4. observation of supervisee-conducted evaluation and treatment sessions.
5. evaluation of supervisee performance.
6. conduct of supervisory conferences.
7. demonstration of clinical procedures.
8. instruction in ethical, legal, and regulatory aspects of the profession.
9. instruction in report writing and editing.
10. maintenance of client records.
11. instruction in the use and maintenance of clinical equipment.
12. exemplification of professional conduct.

A most provocative discussion of the roles of supervisees in the supervisory process was written by Kandushin (1968), using the then-popular idiom, in discussions of human relationships, of "games people play." Although he was discussing supervision of social workers, several of his formulations apply, with equal aptness, to supervision of speech-language pathologists and audiologists. Kandushin defined games as "a scheme, or artfulness, utilized in the pursuit of some objective or purpose" and added: "The purpose of engaging in the game, of using the maneuvers, snares, gimmicks and ploys that are, in essence, the art of gamesmanship, lies in the payoff. One party to the game chooses a strategy to maximize his payoff and minimize his penalties."

Several of Kandushin's games are familiar to experienced speech-language pathologists and audiologists. For example, he described a series of games designed to manipulate the level of demands made by supervisors. One he entitled "Two Against the Agency" or "Seducing for Subversion." In this game the supervisee explores the theme that there is a fundamental conflict between a bureaucratic orientation, which is concerned with records, filling out forms, writing reports, and with such details as when a staff member appears for work and goes home, and a professional orientation, which is concerned with direct work with clients. The supervisee declares a commitment to a professional orientation. This game can be effective because most supervisors can identify with the supervisee's professed primary concern for serving clients and may also share resentment for bureaucratic demands. Thus the supervisee may win in the game and be able to do his or her "own thing" in the guise of being more "professional."

Another game, in which human services professionals are particularly vulnerable, involves recasting the relationship from supervisor-supervisee to therapist-client. Kandushin called this game "Protect the Sick and Infirm" or "Treat Me, Don't Beat Me." In this game the supervisee confides personal problems that affect his or her job performance, seeking to engage the supervisor in a concern for these problems. Once the shift in roles to therapist-client is accomplished, the supervisee achieves reduced demands in the work situation since therapists are accustomed to expect less of clients than supervisors expect of student clinicians or employees.

Role changes can also be effected through the games "Evaluation Is Not For Friends" and "Maximum Feasible Participation." In the former game, the supervisee achieves a social relationship with the supervisor, thus mitigating the judgmental aspects of the supervisor-supervisee relationship. The latter game involves a shift in roles to peer-peer. This game capitalizes on the earlier characterized bilateral approach to supervision that conceives of the process as one of shared responsibilities. In it, supervisees express the attitude that they know best what they need and want to learn and should, therefore, determine their own agendas. Supervisors may be vulnerable to this game because it involves the appearance of supervisees showing initiative and responsibility for improving their skills. But this game may also result in diversion from areas where improvement is most urgently needed.

An intriguing game with obvious parallel versions in our field is one Kandushin calls "If You Knew Dostoevsky Like I Know Dostoevsky." To illustrate: in supervisory conference, "the supervisee makes a casual allusion to the fact that the client's behavior reminds him of that of Raskolnikov in *Crime and Punishment*, which is, after all, somewhat different in etiology from the pathology that plagued Prince Myshkin in *The Idiot.*" The ploy comes when the supervisee says, "You remember, don't you?" When, as usually occurs when the game is well planned, the supervisor does not remember, the supervisee proceeds to instruct the supervisor. This game is particularly effective when the supervisor has been in the profession for several years and may not be completely current in all of the areas the supervisee has recently studied. In any field of abounding new information—and changing fashions—like speech-language pathology and audiology, this can be a particularly effective game since it can quite successfully neutralize a supervisor.

A related game is called "So What Do You Know About It?" This game involves identifying areas in which the experience of the supervisee surpasses that of the supervisor. It can work well in our field when the supervisee has come from another field, such as teaching in the public schools, is nearer to the age of the client than is the supervisor, or has personal experiences with a communicative disorder.

Three of Kandushin's games involve supervisees seizing control, particularly in supervisory conferences. The first, called "I Have a Little List," involves the supervisee arriving with a series of questions about his or her work. The skilled player will arrange these questions to tap areas of the supervisor's special interests. The conference, then, becomes a lecture delivered by the supervisor, usually with great satisfaction, and never gets around to discussions of the supervisee's shortcomings. The second control game, called "Heading Them Off At The Pass," involves a supervisee avoiding critical analyses by beginning conferences with free admissions of all of the mistakes that have been made. Under these circumstances, in the face of such overwhelming self-derogation, the supervisor will almost inevitably become sympathetic and reassuring. The third control game is "I Did It Like You Told Me." Here, the supervisee seeks specific prescriptions for case management and slavishly follows those prescriptions. The real responsibility for the client is thus transferred to the supervisor from the supervisee, who is merely dutifully carrying out instructions.

It would be unfair to consider only games played by supervisees; supervisors, too, can be accomplished game players. Kandushin makes passing reference to one or two supervisor games but by no means explores them in equal detail. Most supervisor games seek one of two prizes. Some seek relief from the authoritarian role that is an inevitable part of supervision—many human services professionals have problems appearing authoritarian. Others seek concealment of inadequate information, particularly in situations where a supervisor has no helpful suggestions for a struggling supervisee.

Supervisors may have their own version of Kandushin's "Evaluation is Not for Friends," which might be called "What Say? Let's Be Buddies." In this game, the supervisor can avoid both the unpleasant aspects of evaluating the supervisee and the responsibility of offering needed assistance by effecting a peer level relationship, so that the supervisee expects neither evaluation nor assistance.

Two effective games for forestalling exposure of areas of supervisor ignorance might be called "Let's Hear It For Carl Rogers" and "How Do You Feel When You Say That?" These games can be particularly successful in the hands of supervisors who find reassurance in such catch phrases as "helping the whole person" and "creating an atmosphere for growth." The former game involves a perversion of nondirective approaches, in which the supervisor responds to every question with a question (e.g., Supervisee: "How can I help Tommy produce an /r/?" Supervisor: "You don't know how to help Tommy produce an /r/?" Or, even better, "Tommy won't produce an /r/ for you?") When confronted with this endless return of every question, the supervisee will usually stop asking questions entirely, and the supervisor wins the game. The latter game involves the supervisor exploring the motivations of an "emotional tone" underlying every question asked by the supervisee. Or, even better, it can be played by the supervisor making such observations, as "I noticed that Tommy's mother didn't stop to talk to you at the end of the therapy session today. How did you feel about that?" This game can also protect the supervisor from expectations of any real assistance because it casts all problems as manifestations of the supervisee's hangups. In acknowledging problems in the conduct of his or her clinical responsibilities, therefore, the supervisee also confesses to deeper personal problems.

"Yes, But" is a game that succeeds in keeping the supervisee constantly off balance. It involves seeking a flaw in every activity carried out by the supervisee. It is most effective in situations where many responsibilities assigned to the supervisee lie outside the expertise of the supervisor. Once a flaw is identified, attention can be shifted from the core of the clinical session to something that is within the supervisor's ken.

Finally, "Those Were The Good Old Days" can be a useful game to supervisors who have failed to keep up with current professional practices. (Its essential dynamics are akin to Kandushin's "If You Knew Dostoevsky Like I Know Dostoevsky.") This game involves frequent citation by the supervisor of the contributions of two decades or more ago, which are unlikely to be known by the supervisee. A particularly effective gambit entails reducing a current approach to a feeble reincarnation of an earlier school of thought (e.g., "The whole field of pragmatics is nothing but a new version of general semantics."). The prize in this game is protection of the supervisor from accountability for any current information because anything that is current is merely a new version of older ideas or something that pales by comparison with conventional wisdom.

With respect to supervisee games, Kandushin concludes his paper with a discussion of possible responses by the supervisor (p. 32):

> . . .another approach is to share honestly with the supervisee one's awareness of what he is attempting to do but to focus the discussion neither on the dynamics of his behavior nor on one's reaction to it, but on the disadvantages for him in playing games. These games have decided drawbacks for the supervisee in that they deny him the possibility of effectively fulfilling one of the essential, principal purposes of supervision—helping him grow professionally. The games frustrate the achievement of this outcome. In playing games the supervisee loses by winning.

Presumably, antidotes to supervisor games should be essentially similar. The supervisor, however, has a distinct edge since few supervisees can confront their supervisor "honestly, with an awareness of what he is attempting to do." The effect of supervisor games can, however, be at least as deleterious as supervisee games since they provide formidable interference to professional growth for both parties in the relationship. Once again, when a supervisor wins a game, he or she also loses by winning.

Although probably the oldest means of

quality assurance, supervision still retains the potential for being one of the most effective. Regardless of how many other quality assurance efforts are pursued by any agency or institution, some supervision will always be necessary.

PEER REVIEW

The essential concept underlying peer review holds that the quality of services delivered by a professional is best assessed by his or her peers in the same profession. As a rule this concept is quite valid. When several professionals work together on the same staff, they usually make accurate assessments of the competencies of the other members of that staff. Professionals who practice in the same community can usually identify colleagues with particular competencies and, on the other hand, colleagues with limited proficiencies. The few deceptions that occur are usually short-lived.

Although applied informally throughout the history of all human services professions, peer review has been increasingly formalized as an approach to quality assurance. It figures to some extent in most accreditation programs. It is one of the basic tenets of utilization review. It is commonly used as one facet of claims reviews by third-party carriers, or at least in reviews engendered by appeals of denied claims.

In many instances, so-called peer review processes are spurious. Typically, in multiservice accreditation reviews and claims reviews, although the services of some professionals are indeed reviewed by members of the same profession, other professionals' services are reviewed differently. This is typified by some peer review activities in the health care system in which physician services are reviewed exclusively by physicians, but the services of other professionals are reviewed, not by their peers, but by physicians or by a token member of another health profession, often a nurse. (Currently, in my community, a major third-party carrier assigns review of claims for audiologic services to a physician consultant who is certified in obstetrics and gynecology.) Peer review is usually less formalized in the educational system, but essentially similar perversions of the process can occur when review responsibilities are assigned to general and special education personnel who may have little knowledge of the specialized services they are reviewing. These practices bring to mind the famous proclamation in Orwell's *Animal Farm*, "All animals are created equal, but some animals are more equal than others," which might be paraphrased "All professionals should be reviewed by their peers, but some professions are more peer than others."

In the health care system, peer review passed from a concept to an institution in 1972 with the enactment of Public Law 92-603, which amended the Social Security Act. This legislation was engendered to some extent by concerns for the quality of health care provided through such federal programs as Medicare, Medicaid, and Maternal and Child Health Care. However, even stronger motivation probably arose from the growing alarm over the escalation of expenditures for those programs. In response to these dual concerns for quality and costs, the new law mandated the establishment of a nationwide network of Peer Standards Review Organizations (PSRO), to be charged with the responsibility of reviewing the institutional care (i.e., care in hospitals, nursing homes, and other institutions) provided to beneficiaries of these federally funded public programs. Initially, the PSRO's had no jurisdiction over care delivered in physicians' offices, clinics, and other ambulatory care facilities unless reviews were specifically requested by local physicians. Many proponents of the PSRO program, however, aspired to the ultimate inclusion of ambulatory care services within their purview. Hare (1981) described some early efforts in ambulatory care review such as the experimental statewide programs carried out in New Mexico and Utah.

Fundamental to the PSRO was the concept that not only should review be in the hands of peers, it should also be based at the community level, that is, it should recognize local conditions and practices. The legislation, then, specified standards for local organizations and described the procedures for their establishment. The ultimate responsibility for standards setting, nevertheless, was assigned to the local organizations. Ultimately, approximately 200 PSRO's were recognized throughout the nation. These organizations were established on a nonprofit basis and were principally comprised of doctors of medicine or osteopathy, with occasional members of other professions, such as dentistry, who also had independent hospital admitting privileges. As will be discussed later, some limited participation of other health professionals was also permitted.

Local PSRO's were not required to assume direct responsibility for all reviews conducted within their assigned territories. They were permitted to delegate responsibilities to those hospitals that demonstrated the capability to carry out review according to the requirements established by each PSRO.

PSRO Procedures

A fundamental responsibility assigned to each PSRO was the development, again presumably at local levels, of norms, criteria, and standards according to which reviews were to be conducted. These terms, as defined by the National Peer Standards Review Council, were quoted by Nelson (1981, p. 27) in his discussion of the influence of that Council on PSRO:

> *Norms.* Medical care appraisal norms are numerical or statistical measures of usual observed performance.
>
> *Criteria.* Medical care criteria are predetermined elements against which aspects of the quality of medical service may be compared. They are developed by professionals relying on professional expertise and on professional literature.
>
> *Standards.* Standards are professionally developed expressions of the range of acceptable variation from a norm or criterion.

Local PSRO's (or hospitals to which review privileges have been designated) carry out their responsibilities through three different types of review: *concurrent review*, *medical care evaluation study*, and *profile analysis*.

CONCURRENT REVIEW

This is a process under which a PSRO certifies the necessity, appropriateness, and quality of services provided during a hospital stay. Such reviews are customarily conducted by coordinators who are not themselves physicians (often they are nurses), but who carry out their responsibilities under medical supervision. These coordinators first check each new hospital admission to ascertain its necessity—usually inquiring whether the diagnostic or treatment procedures to be accomplished during the hospitalization could as well be carried out on an outpatient basis. Next, based on defined norms for similar hospitalizations, a checkpoint is established at the end of the typical length of stay. When that checkpoint arrives, the coordinator determines whether the patient is still hospitalized. If so, the reason for exceeding the normal stay is ascertained. If a reasonable basis is not apparent, the case is referred to a physician advisor for investigation. If an extended stay is justified, a new checkpoint is established and the same procedure repeated when that checkpoint is reached. Inevitably, concurrent reviews consider not only the length of stay, but the necessity of whatever diagnostic procedures may prolong the stay, the quality of treatment provided, and any other factors that might account for longer hospitalization than is normal for patients with similar diagnoses.

MEDICAL CARE EVALUATION (MCE) STUDY

MCE studies are carried out on the basis of records reviews. Such studies closely resemble records audit procedures, discussed in another section of this chapter. According to Oestreicher and Smits (1981, pp. 172–173) there are eight basic steps that are essential for a valid study. (Their definitions of these steps were abstracted from a detailed discussion by Goran et al., 1975.)

1. *Determine the objective of the study.* The topic should be one that occurs with reasonable frequency, one in which medical care makes a difference and one in which some problem is at least suspected.
2. *Establish criteria.* One of the utilization review committee's most interesting and challenging jobs is to set the criteria for "standard" medical care. These criteria may be elaborate, complex, and involve branching logic, as in the case of criteria for treatment of myocardial infarction. They may also be extremely simple; one PSRO conducted an audit of the use of blood in which the only criterion for identifying charts for physician review was transfusion of a single unit of blood.
3. *Design the study.* The utilization review committee must decide on the conduct of the study; will all charts be examined or only a sample; how long will the work take; is any extra training of review coordinators needed:
4. *Collection of data.* Information is usually collected from patients' charts by review coordinators or medical records personnel by means of a form designed by the utilization review committee.
5. *Develop reports.* The results of data collection are aggregated and displayed for committee consideration.
6. *Analyze results and identify deficiencies.* The committee must determine if variances from the criteria are justified; they must decide how serious any deficiencies are and how best to correct them.
7. *Develop a corrective plan.* Development of such a plan usually involves work with specialty departments as well as with physicians who appear at fault. Seminars, grand rounds, and special hospital bulletins may all be used to notify staff of problems.
8. *Restudy.* After the corrective plans have been implemented, restudy after a reasonable period of time should ensure that the problems have been corrected.

PROFILE ANALYSIS

This third type of review has thus far seldom been used by PSRO's. This approach involves examination of aggregate health care data, considering such issues as death rates and infection rates—usually analyzed by procedure—for particular hospitals; the frequency with which particular surgeons carry out certain operative procedures; or the frequency with which a particular physician prescribes narcotic drugs. These data are then compared to profiles of other physicians in the community. Because it demands consistent data management, profile analysis may gain increasing use as more and more complex automatic data storage and retrieval systems become available in health care institutions.

PSRO and Other Health Care Practitioners

PL 92-603 required that services provided by health care practitioners other than physicians (not surprisingly, referred to as HCPOTP in governmentese) were to be included within the aegis of PSRO's, and, further, that these practitioners were to be included in some way in the review of the services they provided. The PSRO advisory group rules and regulations published in the July 12, 1976 *Federal Register* defined HCPOTP as follows:

> Health care practitioners other than physicians are those health professionals who (a) do not hold a doctor of medicine or doctor of osteopathy degree, (b) meet all applicable State and Federal requirements for practice of their profession, and (c) are actively involved in the delivery of patient care or services which may be paid for, directly or indirectly, under Titles V, XVIII, and/or XIX of the Social Security Act.

Within those titles are specified 15 "generic disciplines" that provide such health care services. Speech-language pathology and audiology is included among those disciplines.

Transmittal No. 44 of the Bureau of Quality Assurance of the Health Services Administration, issued on January 25, 1977 and entitled *Policies Applicable to PSRO's Involving HCPOTP in Peer Review in Short Stay Hospitals*, addressed questions related to the circumstances under which HCPOTP might be involved in PSRO activities:

1. Where health care practitioners other than physicians are accorded active staff privileges

and have responsibilities for hospital admission, continued stay and discharge, review for admission certification and continued stay should involve such practitioners.

2. Participation of health care practitioners other than physicians in MCEs and profile analysis shall be similar to that of physicians when care provided by other practitioners is being reviewed. This policy applies to all categories of health care practitioners other than physicians who are authorized to perform review under the act and to conduct any MCE study or profile analysis that includes the review of patient care or services provided by peer practitioners.
3. Criteria, standards, and norms are an integral part of the peer review system, and must be developed by peer practitioners for their specific areas of practice.

In their discussion of the roles of nonphysicians in the PSRO program, Ellis and Sadin (1981) proposed several illustrations of instances in which the participation of other professionals would be essential for the justification of certain hospital admissions and surgical procedures. Among the illustrations was "...before a pharyngeal flap procedure to achieve appropriate speech and voice quality should be performed, there should be confirmation by a speech-language pathologist that there is a speech or voice problem requiring surgical correction."

Despite the provisions for inclusion of nonphysicians in PSRO activities, their participation has probably been sporadic at best. In occasional instances, voting membership in local PSRO's and membership on state PSRO councils has been extended to nonphysicians, usually dentists or nurses. Rarely, PSRO boards and councils have designated one token slot for a representative allied health professional who might be a speech-language pathologist or audiologist. However, the major involvement of nonphysician professionals has occurred in peer review activities in individual institutions. Within these institutional programs, many speech-language pathologists and audiologists have been active participants in review procedures. Often, when a speech-language pathology and audiology department has an ongoing quality assurance program, such as routine patient care audits, institutions will accede to those programs as comprising one facet of the peer review process.

Iowa Quality Assurance Program

The Iowa Quality Assurance Program can be cited as a model statewide peer review program in the field of speech-language pathology and audiology. This program, first called the Iowa Peer Review Program, was initiated in 1974 by the Iowa Speech and Hearing Association. The mission of this quality assurance program, as described in their manual (1977), was broader than usual peer review activities, aiming at the development of "a method for looking at groups of records to determine trends in service delivery" toward the primary goal of "improved care—not practitioner critiquing." Nevertheless, they asserted (p. 2):

> Our statewide activities to date have put us in a favorable position to serve in an advisory capacity to the Iowa Foundation for Medical Care, our PSRO. This will assure that professional services we provide are being reviewed according to standards set by speech-language pathologists and audiologists, rather than by persons outside our profession.

Several facets of the Iowa program deserve careful study. Their diagnostic taxonomy was presented in Chapter 8 of this text. Even more noteworthy is their effort to establish standards of care and to set down client management criteria for each of the communicative disorders included in that taxonomy. The concept that professions should define standards and criteria of care is inherent in the peer review process. This concept has been accepted as feasible by most health care professionals. As a result of apathy, or even overt resistance—usually based on contentions that our profession lacks the data required for such definitions—speech-language pathologists and audiologists have generally been unwilling to participate in efforts to define standards of care. Regrettably, this has often resulted in abdication of that responsibility to the members of other professions, and the resultant standards and criteria range between woeful inadequacy and complete intolerability.

Many members of our profession—undoubtedly including many members who practice in Iowa—would question specific points in the Iowa Quality Assurance Program Standards. Nevertheless, they are exemplary in terms of the willingness of a group of professionals to commit themselves to some reasonable standards. By way of illustration, Table 12.1 reproduces the Standards of Care defined for malignant neoplasms of the larynx. Table 12.2 reproduces the audit criteria for the same condition.

The Future of PSRO

It is impossible to estimate the national impact of PSRO's on the delivery of health care services, either in terms of improving the quality of care or in terms of cost containment. The enthusiasm that attended the institution of the program is evident in an article published in *ASHA* by Schoeni (1974), who was a member of the public affairs staff of the Office of Professional Standards Review during the early days of

Table 12.1.
Iowa Quality Assurance Program: Standards of Care—Malignant Neoplasm of Larynx

Communication Disorder: Aphonia Due to Total Laryngectomy

1. The initial evaluation may include:
   A. Case history
   B. Presurgical examination of oral mechanism
   C. Presurgical hearing screening
   D. Presurgical counseling
   E. Presurgical estimate of habitual communication pattern
   F. Postsurgical examination of oral mechanism
   G. Postsurgical hearing screening
   H. Postsurgical estimate of habitual communication pattern
   I. Estimate of potential for producing esophageal sound
   J. Observation of client's and/or significant others' attitudes which may affect diagnosis and/or treatment
2. Consultations may include:
   A. Another speech pathologist
   B. Audiologist
   C. Physician
   D. Psychologist
   E. Nurse
   F. Social worker
   G. Employer
   H. Vocational rehabilitation counselor
   I. Chaplain
3. Long-term goals should be set which reflect the client's rehabilitation potential and are feasible to attain considering the client's current status.
4. Rationale for long-term goals should include any or all of the following: mastery of esophageal speech and/or mastery or communication with adaptive equipment (artificial larynx, language board); enhancement of communication through writing and/or gestures; determination of appropriate subsequent management.
5. Termination should occur only if the long-term goals have been met, or no progress is documented within 24 visits or 2 months (unless complicating circumstances affect the client's status), or the client requests termination.
6. Termination should occur within 200 client visits.
7. At termination of treatment, the client (and if desirable, the client's significant others) should be counseled regarding the client's current status and future needs.

Table 12.2.
Iowa Quality Assurance Program: Audit

Audit topic: Aphonia due to total laryngectomy resulting from malignant neoplasm of the larynx.
Audit objective: To improve service to clients with this communication disorder.
Case sample: X clients discharged from evaluation or treatment for this diagnosis.

Criteria	Expected Compliance %
1. The initial evaluation included:	
A. Case history	99
B. Examination of oral mechanism	95
C. Hearing screening	95
D. Estimate of habitual communication pattern	95
2. Following the evaluation the client and/or significant others were counseled regarding the client's problem, current status, and future needs.	99
3. Long-term goals were set.	95
4. Rationale for long-term goals included at least one of the following: mastery of esophageal speech and/or mastery of communication with adaptive equipment (artificial larynx, language board); enhancement of communication through writing and/or gestures; determination of appropriate subsequent management.	95
5. Termination occurred only if the long-term goals were met, or no progress was documented within 24 visits or 2 months (unless complicating circumstances affected the client's status), or the client requested termination.	99
6. Termination occurred within 200 client visits.	99
7. At termination of treatment, the client (and if desirable, the client's significant others) were counseled regarding the client's current status and future needs.	95

the program. She wrote (p. 680):

> ...PSRO may be potentially the most important health program ever enacted here or any place in the world in terms of its possible beneficial impact on health and the health care system in this country. The PSRO may represent medicine's last chance to monitor and discipline itself and to remain a proud and independent profession, since it offers unlimited opportunity for the medical profession to bring some order in areas where serious problems now exist and to improve the quality of medical care.

Even with due allowance for expected public affairs staff hyperbole, it must be recognized that PSRO has fallen far short of these aspirations. The future of the program seems uncertain at best. At this writing, the Reagan administration has recommended the phasing out of all PSRO's. This position probably derives both from the questionable effectiveness of the program and from an overall withdrawal from governmental regulation of free enterprise, including physician and hospital free enterprise. Thus far, however, many members of Congress persist in their support of the PSRO concept, particularly because of their concerns for health care costs. Therefore, although PSRO's may remain, it seems virtually certain that their number will be reduced by consolidation.

There seem, nevertheless, to be sufficient salutary benefits from programs related to the PSRO movement to assure that, whether PSRO's survive or not, some influences will remain. Furthermore, numerous activities developed through PSRO's are now required by many private third-party carriers. Most health professionals have come to accept the concept that they do not deserve immunity from all scrutiny, and furthermore, that they themselves must participate in that scrutiny. Similarly, although health care costs have continued to escalate during the PSRO era, most public and private third-party payers will continue to demand some protection against the sovereignty of health care professionals. Insofar as speech-language pathology and audiology is concerned, our situation is well summarized in the July 1981 *Governmental Affairs Review*, published by ASHA:

> Even if PSRO's are reduced or eliminated, some form of quality assurance will probably continue. Speech-language pathologists and audiologists should monitor the status of their PSRO and participate in planning the quality assurance activities that may replace the PSRO if it is eliminated.

Presently, then, the future of peer review is in doubt. Nevertheless, the concept of peer review is likely to remain as an important approach to assessing the quality of clinical services. Although peer review has received the widest attention as an approach to quality assurance in the health services system, it holds equal potential for application in the other settings in which speech-language pathology and audiology services are delivered.

RECORDS AUDITS

Records audits may be carried out by different people for different purposes. Such audits involve reviews of samples of client records to assess conformity to preestablished standards. They may be conducted by external agencies, as in the instance of third-party payers seeking confirmation that claimed services were actually provided, or they may be internal audits conducted by administrators, professional staff review committees, or the clinicians immediately responsible for providing services. This discussion will consider only internal audits carried out as a part of quality assurance programs.

Once again, quality assurance procedures involving records audits have developed primarily in health care programs. Increasingly, however, those procedures are being adapted for application in other settings.

Griffin (1978) defined four major types of records audits used for quality assurance. *Monodisciplinary* or *single disciplinary* audits are conducted by a department or by another group of professionals representing a single discipline. *Parallel* audits occur when a single topic or focus is selected and all departments or programs within an institution conduct single disciplinary audits concurrently, focusing on that topic. The results are then shared among all disciplines. *Multidisciplinary audits* are characterized by the selection of a topic and focus by a committee comprised of representatives of several disciplines. Each member of that committee then consults with his or her professional peers to develop criteria specific to their shared discipline. The audit committee applies these criteria in conducting a records audit and utilizes the results of that audit to identify problems and to develop remedial action plans. *Interdisciplinary* audits occur when an audit committee, comprised of representatives of several professions, develops criteria for a given topic and proceeds with the records audit, problem identification, and development of remedial actions. Interdisciplinary audits are usually outcome-oriented because outcomes are generally determined by all members of the team.

Kaplan and Hopkins (1980) summarized a representative sample of approaches to the assessment of quality of care in medical facilities, most dependent to some extent on records audits. Four of those approaches might be applied to quality assurance programs in our field.

Performance Evaluation Procedure for Auditing and Improving Patient Care (PEP) (Joint Commission on Accreditation of Hospitals, 1974) has been widely employed in hospital quality assurance programs. It is described as an outcome-oriented method of retrospective review. Criteria are established to describe key factors in the management of either those patients with a particular diagnosis or those who have been subjected to a particular diagnostic or treatment procedure. PEP criteria usually focus on such issues as validation of diagnoses, justification for hospital admission, justification for surgery or other treatment procedures, discharge outcomes, complications, and length of hospital stay.

The PEP system involves six steps: (1) An audit committee (usually composed of physicians, with occasional representatives from nursing or other health professions) selects an audit study topic and writes criteria. (2) A committee assistant, who may be a health professional or an experienced clerk, retrieves records and screens them to determine whether the criteria were met, then reports the results of that screening to the committee, forwarding those records that did not meet the criteria. (3) The committee analyzes the records that failed to meet the criteria to determine whether they are actually deficient or whether extenuating factors are apparent. (4) The committee analyzes the causes of discovered deficiencies and plans and recommends corrective action. (5) The committee defines critical elements of care that should be monitored and makes plans for follow-up. (6) The committee reports the findings of the audit to the people concerned through appropriate hospital channels.

Although JCAH does not require the use of PEP as a qualification for accreditation, they do require that a well organized quality assurance program be in place. Therefore, since PEP is identified as a system developed by JCAH, many hospitals have chosen it in preference to other options.

Criteria Mapping (Kaplan and Greenfield, 1978) is an intriguing approach that seeks to track practitioner logic in the clinical decision-making process. A diagram, called a decision tree, is developed to represent the sequential decisions that must be made in specific clinical situations. Records are reviewed to determine the degree to which actual diagnostic and treatment procedures adhere to that diagram. This approach recognizes that aggregating all people with the same diagnoses and assuming that the same criteria apply to all of them—the usual practice in criteria-based records audits—has many shortcomings. Criteria mapping concedes that the approach a clinician applies may depend on the individual manifestations of the essential problems rather than on the diagnosis. Quality of care, therefore, is signaled by the action taken by the clinician when those manifestations are encountered and by the outcomes of each step in the diagnostic and treatment process.

Problem Status Index-Outcome (PSI) (Mushlin et al., 1978) involves sending questionnaires to clients at a predetermined time following their contact with a health care provider. The timing of the questionnaire depends upon the clinical problem and the expected outcomes of whatever services were provided. The questionnaires seek to elicit client perceptions about the frequency and severity of symptoms and about whatever limitations the condition imposes. Questionnaires are then compared to records data, particularly those data relating to anticipated outcomes. This approach may be particularly useful in instances where a client must follow a specific regimen in order to control problems or to ensure the continuation of whatever salutary results were achieved during treatment.

CMA/CHA Educational Patient Care Audit (California Medical Association/California Hospital Association, 1975) introduced an important modification to previous medical audit systems: The concerned health care providers would be substantially involved in their own evaluations through active participation in the formulation of criteria and in the definition of standards for care. ASHA's Patient Care Audit system, discussed below in detail, derives from the CMA/CHA approach.

Another approach, too recent to have been included in the Kaplan-Hopkins summary, has been attracting attention in health care facilities. This procedure, called *Quality Circles*, may entail records reviews, but need not be restricted to such reviews. The potential for applying the quality circle concept to speech, language, and hearing services was discussed by Adair (1983). She characterized it as "a system for identifying and solving problems using the creative ideas of the personnel at the grass roots level of the organization." The concept, derived from industry, originated in Japan, where it has been used since their industries began rebuilding following World War II.

Quality circles are comprised of a group of people who work together. In human services programs, circles may either be made up of staff members from the same department or established as multidisciplinary teams. They meet once weekly to identify and seek solutions to problems, with a supervisor usually serving as facilitator.

Quality circles follow an eight-step procedure which is cyclic, that is, when the eighth step is completed, it leads to a new cycle of problem-solving efforts involving the same eight steps. The steps are: (1) select problem, (2) collect baseline data, (3) analyze what is causing the problem, (4) set a goal, (5) develop solutions, (6) implement solutions, (7) evaluate results, and (8) report results. In her characterization of quality circles, Adair observed:

> An important part of the Quality Circle process is the use of very specific group process techniques that assure equal input from all participants. This allows the circle to tap a great deal of creative potential and excellent ideas that previously have been seriously underutilized. It also provides ongoing reinforcement of circle members through seeking the successful resolution of problems they, themselves, were concerned about.

Two records audit procedures, Patient Care Audit and Child Services Review, have been developed by the American Speech-Language-Hearing Association specifically for quality assurance programs in speech, language, and hearing services agencies. The procedures are presented here in some detail because of their singular importance to members of our profession.

Patient Care Audit

According to the ASHA model (Griffin, 1978, p. 22):

> Patient Care Audit is a process for retrospectively monitoring and improving *group performance.* Patient Care Audit is primarily concerned with upgrading patterns of care in a speech-language pathology/audiology program, rather than identifying deviant care provided by an individual speech-language pathologist or audiologist. Audit techniques provide a mechanism both for documenting *appropriate* patterns of care (service and outcomes) and for identifying areas in which improvement is necessary.

The responsibility for the patient care audit program is delegated to a formally organized committee comprised of members of the professional staff of the agency or department. Those staff members must be actually engaged in the delivery of the services under review. In small agencies, the entire staff may comprise the committee. In large agencies, where a broad scope of services is offered, several committees may be appointed, each covering specific areas of service involving special expertise. In all instances where committees involve less than an entire staff, the membership should rotate so that each staff member eventually participates in the audit program. The committee or committees must meet regularly, preferably at least monthly. Among the factors essential to the success of patient care audit programs is the enthusiastic support of the professional staff, as well as the support and cooperation of the agency's administration.

Griffin contends that an effective patient care audit program should be capable of carrying out four major functions: (1) to perform enough retrospective audit studies each year to ascertain whether the patterns of care provided by the agency meet professionally recognized standards; (2) to document the agency's activities, including compilation of statistics, summaries, and analyses; (3) to afford regular written summaries of the audit committee's activities to administration (both to the administration of the speech pathology and audiology department and to the administration of the institution within which that department resides); and (4) to assist in planning continuing education activities through determination of the educational needs of staff members.

Patient care audit, like quality circles, is conceptualized as a cyclic model, with nine steps leading from one to the other, and the final step leading once again to the first step in the next cycle, so that the process is continuous. Figure 12.1 is a graphic representation of that process. The nine steps are delineated as follows:

STEP 1: SELECT AUDIT TOPIC

A topic or "problem" for audit can be a diagnosis (e.g., clients with cleft palate), a symptom (e.g., clients with persistent hoarseness), an abnormal test result (e.g., clients with severely reduced speech discrimination scores), a social-psychological problem (e.g., family support of laryngectomees), or a treatment procedure (e.g., hearing aid selection and orientation). Among the aspects of client care that can be examined are justification of admission to a particular treatment program, accuracy of diagnosis, indications for referral, adequacy and appropriateness of management, and adequacy of short-range outcomes. Griffin proposes five conditions for the selection of a problem as an audit topic: (1) *high frequency*, that is, the problem must be encountered frequently; (2) *problem severity in absence of appropriate diagnosis, treatment, or referral*—there must be significantly adverse consequences to clients if clinicians fail to make appropriate diagnoses, offer appropriate treatment, or make appropriate referrals; (3) *amenability to proper intervention*, i.e., it must have been established that the speech-language pathology and audiology services to be scrutinized may potentially affect the health and well-being of clients; (4) *generally agreed upon methodologies in handling the problem*—areas of significant controversy as to appropriate and effective methodologies for evaluation and treatment do not lend themselves to audits; and (5) *interest*

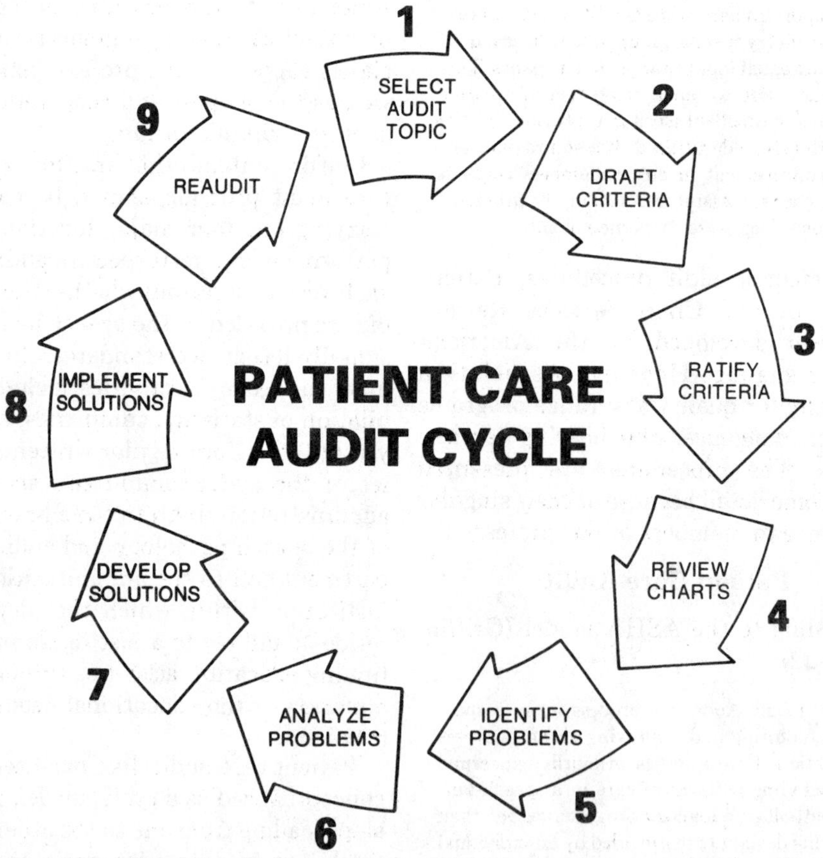

Figure 12.1. Graphic representation of patient care audit cycle. (Reproduced by permission of American Speech-Language-Hearing Association from their *Patient Care Audit Manual*.)

and enthusiasm in doing an audit on a problem—unless all concerned staff members demonstrate active interest in a topic, the audit is not likely to achieve the ultimate goal of improved standards of care; therefore, particularly during the early phases of a new patient care audit program, topics should represent general interests, rather than "pet" interests of audit committee members.

Once a general topic has been identified, the study objective must be formulated. Griffin defined a study objective as a "narrower aspect of care or outcome of care within an audit topic which serves as a focus for developing criteria, identifying problems and planning remedial actions to solve those problems" (p. 35). She elaborated this definition further (p. 35):

> The audit topic identifies a general area of concern for review. Within this general area will be a number of components, some more crucial to patient care than others. By focusing on a single component of the topic, the audit committee is able to examine in detail the quality of care associated with a critical aspect of the topic. Consequently, any remedial actions resulting from the audit can be specifically directed at deficiencies in significant elements of patient care. This is especially necessary in multi-/inter-disciplinary audit, where the relative importance of criteria may vary among the discipline representatives.

Study objectives are usually stated as "to assess. . ." or "to improve. . ." such factors as adequacy of evaluation procedures, accuracy of diagnostic results, criteria for initiating treatment, adequacy of treatment outcomes, and criteria for terminating services.

Next, the client population that is to serve as the focus of the audit is defined. Among the factors that may be considered in that definition are age and sex; type and severity of communicative disorders; diagnosis; and nature, frequency, and duration of services. After defining the client population, the study size is defined, that is, the number of client records to be reviewed during the course of the audit. That sample must be large enough to warrant interpretation of the results and formulation of conclusions, but at the same time sufficiently restricted to enable completion of appropriately detailed studies within a reasonable time interval. Finally, a time period is defined, i.e., the span of time during which the services under study were delivered; this is to ensure that all clients being reviewed were served by current staff according to current practices.

STEP 2: DRAFT CRITERIA

The definition of criteria most often applied to patient care audit resembles that applied to peer review studies, as presented in the earlier discussion of PSRO's. Audit criteria are of two general types. *Process* criteria focus on the professionals providing the services and consider the nature of treatment, sequence of events, and activities pursued in providing care to a client. *Outcome* criteria focus on the client and pertain to the end results of whatever care was provided.

Fundamental to the entire patient care audit procedure is the concept that criteria must be developed by the actual providers of services; they may not be made up of textbook statements or profiles formulated by external professional groups (which is not to say that such profiles have no place in other types of quality assurance activities). Griffin amplified this point (p. 54):

> The advantage of self-developed criteria is the resulting sense of identification and commitment. Any time health care professionals engage in professional dialogue, the patient benefits. The exchange of ideas about patient care, which is an automatic by-product of setting audit criteria, provides a forum for ongoing professional development, particularly in multi-/inter-disciplinary patient care audit.

Audit criteria should demonstrate five essential characteristics: (1) They should be specifically related to the topic and the audit objectives and be effective indicators of the quality of care delivered to the specific client population. (2) They should be understandable, i.e., clear enough so they will be interpreted in the same way by all readers and specific enough so that no confusion will arise. (3) They should be measurable in terms such as elapsed time, or frequency or range of test or treatment data expected. (4) They should be behavioral; that is, they specify expected actions of the clients or professionals involved. (5) They should be achievable in the sense that they are realistic and appropriate to the audit population and to the capabilities of the staff and agency delivering the services.

The *expected level of performance* for all criteria must always be 100% because, by definition, criteria represent elements that are essential to good client care. Nevertheless, there may be instances in which reasonable exceptions may reasonably occur; therefore, a *threshold for action* is defined which may be lower than the expected level of performance. This threshold, also expressed as a percent, represents the minimum number of client records that may meet a criterion and still indicate an acceptable standard of care. When the number of records fails to reach that minimum, remedial action is necessary. In instances where a criterion is absolutely necessary to clients' health and safety or is otherwise unequivocal, the threshold for action may, like the expected level of performance, be 100%. If thresholds for action are set below 75%, it is usually advisable to reconsider whether the criterion is, indeed, an important element of good client care.

STEP 3: RATIFY CRITERIA

In this step, the criteria prepared by the audit committee are presented to a group comprised of all the professionals providing the services under study. Griffin specified the purposes of this ratification process as: (1) to ensure that all concerned professionals will acknowledge the importance of whatever problems are found and support efforts toward their solution; (2) to complement the work of the audit committee with other input and ideas; (3) to define and clarify any criteria drafted by the committee that are ambiguous; (4) to provide staff educational experiences through critical appraisal and discussion of the drafted criteria; and (5) to foster true peer review through ensuring that all professionals whose performance is to be reviewed understand and accept the standards by which they are to be judged and have the opportunity to modify or reject those standards with which they do not agree.

The goal of ratification, then, is to achieve agreement among the concerned professionals that the proposed criteria are, indeed, essential to good client care. Such agreement may be of three types. Ideally, there is unanimous agreement, signifying that all participants concur. Agreement may be by simple majority, indicating that, although some participants disagree, they will abide by the majority decision. (Those opposed to the criteria may request that records of clients they have served be excluded from review according to the disputed criteria.) The third type, consensus, means that, although some participants may not completely agree with a particular criterion, they will consent to inclusion of their client records in the audit and accept the results. When a criterion presented by the audit committee does not receive agreement from the concerned staff members, that criterion is deleted from the audit and referred back to the committee for further consideration.

STEP 4: REVIEW CHARTS

All records in the previously defined sample are reviewed to determine the frequency with which ratified criteria have been met. To achieve these data, client records are reviewed by the audit committee or by their delegate to assess conformity to each of the ratified criteria. The total number of records within that sample that conform to each criterion is expressed as a percentage of the sample. For example, if 20 of a sample of 25 records conform to a particular criterion, the actual level of performance for that criterion would be 80%.

STEP 5: IDENTIFY PROBLEMS

For the purposes of patient care audit, problems are identified on the basis of instances in which the actual level of performance falls below the threshold for action defined in step 2.

Before concluding that a particular performance discrepancy—i.e., a discrepancy between the actual level of performance and the threshold for action—should be pursued further, the committee may wish to verify the study. If the sample constitutes a small segment of the total number of clients in a particular population, the committee may wish to determine whether sampling errors occurred. Criterion statements may also be reviewed to be certain of their clarity and validity. Finally, the committee may consider whether uncontrollable variables are interfering with performance. When problems are attributable to factors beyond the control of the providers of the services under audit, it may be fruitless to pursue those problems further.

Once identified and verified, problems are then ranked for planning remedial action. Ranking is based on such factors as the importance of the criterion to quality care, size of the performance gap, and the susceptibility of the problem to improvement. At the conclusion of this step, therefore, all identified problems are prioritized for remediation.

STEP 6: ANALYZE PROBLEMS

Griffin (1978, p. 88) characterized problem analysis:

> Probably the most neglected, yet the most critical, phase in the audit process is problem analysis. If carefully and properly completed, the criteria setting process and review of failed charts might clearly reveal performance deficiencies. It is true, however, that in most cases the mere revelation of the performance deficiency is not sufficient to alleviate it. Rather, there are a minimal number of steps needed before deciding to commit the resources necessary for effectively alleviating the performance problem. Without this type of effort, the audit experience is reduced to an academic exercise devoid of its potential to effect the needed changes in health care.

Problem analysis is accomplished by means of two maneuvers. First, possible reasons for the problem are identified. These reasons may be due to limitations in the knowledge and skills of staff members, or failure to use their available knowledge and skills, or they may be due to a shortage of equipment and materials, budgetary limitations, and other organizational deficiencies. Second, the probable causes of the problem are verified. Here, the possible bases are reviewed to determine which are most likely to account for performance discrepancies. Again, for the purposes of patient care audit, the identified factors must be amenable to change.

The problem analysis step occurs even when the records audit has revealed no discrepancies. In such an event, ASHA's *Patient Care Audit Manual* (American Speech-Language-Hearing Association, 1978) enjoins its users to re-evaluate the list of criteria and the thresholds for action by asking four questions: (1) Given available knowledge and hunches about potential problems in client care, is each audit objective appropriate? (2) Given the program's capabilities, do the criteria represent the best indicators of client care? (3) Were the thresholds for action too low? (4) Were the criteria clear and specific enough? If the answers to these questions affirm the validity of the audit, the Manual advises, "accept the audit findings with pride, publicize the fact that good patient care is indicated by this set of criteria and go on to the next audit."

STEP 7: DEVELOP SOLUTIONS

This step involves definition of the actions to be taken for the solution of whatever problems have been identified. Possible solutions may involve such management actions as modification of policies and procedures. They may relate to personnel factors such as staff development and inservice and continuing education. They may address the availability of such resources as space, supplies, and equipment. In weighing any potential solutions, it is usually wise to consider such factors as the relative simplicity of each solution, its cost, the degree to which its effectiveness can be measured, and other factors that determine ease of implementation.

Once potential solutions are identified and their relative merits appraised, the apparently optimal solutions are selected and a *remedial plan for action* formulated. That plan involves five stages: (1) statement of desired action to improve quality of care; (2) identification of the person or persons responsible for each action; (3) specification of the date by which the actions are to be completed; (4) development of procedures for documenting changes; and (5) specification of the date for reaudit. When the remedial plan for action is developed by the audit committee, it is ratified by the staff, following essentially the same procedure used for ratification of audit criteria.

STEP 8: IMPLEMENT SOLUTIONS

This step consists of carrying out the remedial plan for action. Since a properly developed plan has basic monitoring mechanisms, the amount of progress toward implementation of solutions should always be immediately apparent. Furthermore, the evaluation of the ultimate effectiveness of the solutions is foreordained by establishing the date for reaudit within the plan.

STEP 9: REAUDIT

This step involves repetition of the same audit procedure on a sample of records representing the same population defined for the first audit, except that it considers clients served since the completion of the remedial action plan. The reaudit uses the same criteria and thresholds for action defined for the original study.

Four reaudit outcomes are possible. First, the new actual performance levels may exceed the earlier performance levels and meet the thresholds for action. This would demonstrate that the remedial actions were effective and should be continued, and that no further remedies are currently needed. Second, although the new performance levels might exceed the previous levels, they may still fall below the thresholds for action. In this event, although the remedial actions may have effected some improvement, they were still insufficient; additional solutions may be required. Third, the performance levels may remain unchanged. This outcome suggests that the remedial actions were ineffective and that a new plan is needed with a subsequent reaudit. Fourth, the new performance levels may fall below the previous performance levels, indicating that the remedial actions were actually detrimental and that significant reorientation is in order.

If the initial audit revealed actual performance levels that reached or exceeded thresholds for action, or if the reaudit shows that the remedial plan has produced satisfactory results, the cycle is completed. However, as Figure 12.1 demonstrates, the patient care audit process is continuous; when one audit cycle reaches satisfactory conclusion a new audit cycle begins, addressing a new topic to ascertain whether acceptable standards of care are practiced in another area of service.

Example of Patient Care Audit

The following fictitious example is constructed to illustrate the steps in the patient care audit cycle.

The audiology staff of a large speech and hearing center became concerned about the quality of their diagnostic services for preschoolers. This concern was precipitated by a series of incidents in which school-age children, who had previously been seen as preschoolers, returned for re-evaluation. Reviews of the records of their earlier evaluations showed serious deficiencies in information and, more importantly, instances where misevaluations seemed likely. Discussions of these concerns for the adequacy of audiologic services for preschoolers led the staff to select this topic for their next patient care audit and to refer it to the three staff members who comprised the patient care audit committee.

At their next meeting, the audit committee agreed that the topic for the audit would be best identified as "Preschoolers with Hearing Impairment." The objective was identified as "To improve hearing evaluation procedures for preschool children." They decided that an effective audit could be best conducted by delineating further the age range of the population to be studied. They concluded that clearer criteria could be defined, and hence a more discriminating audit could be conducted, if they focused on only one segment of the preschool population and examined other segments in future audits. They agreed, therefore, to identify the audit population as children in the age range of 3 years to 4 years 11 months seen for initial basic hearing evaluations. Because the staff had remained constant for the previous year and no major procedural changes, or changes in available equipment, had occurred during the previous year, they agreed to select the audit sample from clients seen during that interval. A review of the summary of all audiologic services provided during that year suggested that approximately 100 children had been seen who were within the defined population. The committee concluded that a sample of 25 records should suffice for the audit; therefore, they proposed a review of the records of every fourth client from the specified population.

The committee proceeded to draft the following criteria:

1. A history (covering prenatal, birth, and neonatal course; general developmental milestones; speech and language development; development of auditory behavior; and medical, educational, and social factors) was obtained.
2. Pure-tone thresholds at 250 to 4,000 Hz were obtained under ear phones and by bone conduction (when AC thresholds were 20 dB or poorer), with masking levels noted.
3. Speech reception thresholds were obtained under earphones and recorded, noting the method of testing.
4. Speech discrimination scores, or estimates of speech discrimination, were reported and the method of testing specified.
5. Impedance testing was conducted.
6. Observations of the intelligibility of the child's speech were recorded.
7. A plan was stated, including recommendations for follow-up, and was interpreted to the family.
8. Reports were sent to the referral source and to other agencies as requested by the referral source or family.

In discussing thresholds for action, the committee agreed that only in rare instances, such as when a family spoke no English and no interpreter was available, or when the child was accompanied by an older sibling or foster parent with little information about the child, should it be impossible to complete a case history. They also foresaw few instances in which reports should not be sent to the referral source. Therefore, thresholds for action of each of these criteria were set at 95%. They agreed that multiple factors might interfere with the achievement of criteria concerning testing procedures, yet, because of the importance of these criteria, the committee concluded that minimally acceptable thresholds for action were 90%. Although they believed that some observations of the children's speech patterns were important, they concluded that many children were so apprehensive during hearing evaluations that such observations would be difficult. Consequently, they established a threshold for action for this criterion at 75%.

After the committee completed their draft, they presented it to the entire audiology staff, seeking ratification of the proposed criteria and thresholds for action. Although the staff was generally supportive of the criteria statements, they expressed some concerns. They contended that, although bone conduction thresholds could be successfully obtained in some children in the specified age range, it was unrealistic to expect such success in all children, particularly because of masking problems. They proposed that, for this age group, the information achieved through impedance measurement would be more reliable in many instances. Therefore, they recommended deletion of the reference to bone conduction in the second criterion, revising it to read, "Pure-tone thresholds were obtained at 250 to 4,000 Hz under earphones." The third criterion, concerning speech reception testing, was acceptable as presented.

The staff questioned the inclusion of the fourth criterion. They contended that the tests available for the assessment of speech discrimination for children of this age were difficult to interpret at best. Furthermore, the majority of children in this population had conductive hearing impairments, making the interpretation of those tests even more problematic. They concluded that a future audit, specifically dealing with children with sensorineural impairments, might well include a criterion related to speech discrimination, but they agreed that the criterion should be deleted from this audit.

The staff further observed that several children seen for hearing evaluations had ventilating tubes in place, as well as other conditions that precluded impedance testing. Consequently, they suggested an addition to the fifth criterion so that it read, "Results of impedance testing were reported, or, when extenuating factors were noted, C[1] volumes were reported."

Finally, although they concurred that it was often difficult to draw conclusions about childrens' speech during hearing evaluations, they believed that some helpful observations could usually be made about their overall communication, including their apparent understanding of spoken language. They proposed a revision of the sixth criterion to, "Observations of the child's overall communication were reported," and proposed changing the threshold for action on that criterion to 85%. After this final change was effected, the amended criteria and thresholds as shown in Table 12.3 were ratified by the staff.

Next, the audit committee proceeded to review the records of the client sample they had specified. The results of their review are summarized in the column headed "Actual Level of Performance" in Table 12.3. It was immediately apparent that on five of the seven criteria the actual level of performance fell below the threshold for action, suggesting that remedies were obviously needed. The results of the audit were distributed to the entire staff.

Following further discussions with staff

Table 12.3.
Patient Care Audit

Audit topic: Preschool children with hearing impairment.
Objective: To improve hearing evaluation procedures for preschool children.
Population: Children in the age range of 3 years to 4 years 11 months seen for initial basic hearing evaluations.
Time period: January 1, 1982 through December 30, 1982.

Criteria	Expected Level of Performance	Threshold for Action	Actual Level of Performance
	%	%	%
1. A history (covering prenatal, birth, and neonatal course; general developmental milestones; speech and language development; development of auditory behavior; and medical, educational, and social factors) was obtained.	100	95	72
2. Pure-tone thresholds were obtained at 250 to 4,000 Hz under earphones.	100	90	84
3. Speech reception thresholds were obtained under earphones and the method of testing specified.	100	90	84
4. Results of impedance testing were reported, or, when extenuating factors were noted, C[1] volumes were reported.	100	90	80
5. Observations of the child's overall communicative abilities were reported.	100	85	68
6. A plan was stated, including recommendations for follow-up, and reported to the family.	100	95	96
7. Reports were sent to the referral source and to other agencies as requested by referral source or family.	100	95	96

members, and utilizing the findings of the records review, the audit committee analyzed each of the problems revealed by the audit. Deficits with respect to the first criterion seemed to relate to difficulties in determining whether missing information revealed oversights by the audiologist taking the history or merely indicated that the audiologist had not recorded anything because no potentially significant information was revealed in that segment of the case history. When the matter was discussed with staff members, it was readily apparent that opinions differed as to the proper approach to reporting history data.

Deficiencies in reporting pure-tone and speech reception thresholds were chiefly attributable to the specification in those criteria that thresholds must be obtained under earphones. Apparently, when a child refused to wear earphones some audiologists conducted sound field tests; if a significant hearing impairment seemed unlikely, they recommended re-evaluation 6 months or so in the future.

Two problems seemed to account for the failure to meet criteria for impedance testing. In some instances it was mentioned that ventilating tubes precluded complete testing, but C^1 volumes were not recorded. More frequently, however, tympanometry was reported, but there was no mention of acoustic reflex measures. Further discussion of this omission revealed that the only equipment that permitted full impedance testing was located in a heavily used hearing test suite. On the other hand, a portable unit that only provided for tympanometry was generally available. When time was limited, therefore, the latter unit was likely to be used.

The most serious discrepancy between actual performance and threshold for action occurred on the criterion regarding observations of the child's overall communicative abilities. Typically, information directly related to auditory responses was noted, but there was no information about other aspects of communication.

After discussions with other staff members, the audit committee concluded that first priority should be assigned to overcoming problems related to actual hearing testing. The second priority was assigned to the observed deficiencies in impedance testing. Next in order was the problem in reporting overall communicative behaviors and, finally, the deficiencies in case history reporting.

In developing a plan to ameliorate shortcomings in hearing test procedures, two courses of action seemed possible. Discussions with the staff revealed that some audiologists were reluctant to schedule clients for series of appointments in order to complete basic testing procedures because those appointments increased costs to patients. Consequently, when children refused the earphones during the first test session, the audiologists often did not schedule supplementary appointments even though the children might well overcome their apprehension and cooperate for complete testing as they became more familiar with the situation. Furthermore, it became apparent that some staff members had limited experience in testing children of this age and had few ideas about dealing with apprehensive 3- and 4-year-olds.

Therefore, the audit committee recommended a two-part plan. The first part involved a discussion of clinic policies relative to scheduling supplementary appointments to complete diagnostic procedures. This discussion was also to involve clarification of third-party coverage for these supplementary appointments and to review institutional policies governing adjustment of fees in instances of financial hardship. The second part of the plan proposed an in-service education program led by the two staff members with the greatest interest and most experience in pediatric audiology. This program was to be reinforced both by review of a recommended reading list and by scheduled observations by the less experienced staff members of the two more proficient audiologists. These observations were to be accomplished by assigning the less experienced audiologists to serve as test assistants when young children were seen for evaluation. The audit committee referred this two-part plan to the entire staff, who enthusiastically ratified it.

A plan was next proposed to solve problems related to impedance testing. Since recording of C^1 volumes had not been routine during the period covered by the audit (it had never been discussed prior to drafting the audit criteria), the only specific action was its inclusion within the impedance testing protocol. The proposed solution to the equipment problem involved moving the complete impedance testing unit to a room where it was more accessible. Furthermore, it became apparent that the demands for use of that unit were so substantial that an additional unit was required. Therefore, it was recommended that the purchase of an additional unit be given a high priority in the next year's equipment budget. These plans were also ratified by the staff.

Deficiencies with respect to reporting observations of overall communicative behaviors seemed to relate to confusion among the audiologists about what should be reported and about the kinds of observations that should be made as a basis for these reports. The audit committee recommended another two-part plan. The first involved preparation of a checklist to serve as a guide for such observations. This checklist was to be prepared by a committee comprised of an audiologist and a speech-language pathologist. The second part of the plan called for three or four in-service education sessions for the audiologists. These would focus on the use of the checklist and would involve practice by means of videotaped examples of children's communicative behaviors. Furthermore, it became obvious in the discussion that the criterion used in the audit was probably ambiguous. The committee conceded that they were often uncertain as to whether a particular record met the criterion as it was stated. Therefore, it was recommended that the criterion be reworded for the reaudit as, "Checklist of communicative behaviors was completed." This plan was also approved by the staff.

As a part of the ratification of plans for remedial actions, completion dates were specified for each plan. All were to be carried out within the next 3 months. Consequently, the date for reaudit was set at 9 months following ratification of the plans.

When the reaudit was conducted, six of the seven actual performance levels exceeded the percentages defined as thresholds for action. On the criterion concerning impedance testing the actual performance level increased from 80% to 88%. Although the improvement was gratifying, it still fell short of the 90% threshold for action. A further study revealed that, although the increased accessibility of the impedance testing unit had been an improvement, its heavy utilization still involved substantial delays. When children were becoming tired or uncooperative, audiologists still opted for use of the portable tympanometer when the other unit was in use. This finding, then, reinforced the need for an additional complete testing unit. After reporting the results of the reaudit to the entire staff, the audit committee provided a summary to be forwarded to the center's administration.

This attempt to construct an example of a patient care audit is probably both oversimplified and overcomplex. It was oversimplified in its failure to detail many of the steps in the process. It was overcomplex in the sense that a good audit would probably focus on fewer issues than were raised in the illustration. (They were raised to exemplify some conceivable outcomes of patient care audits.) Withal, I would hope that it is apparent that patient care audit can be an extremely effective tool for accomplishing quality assurance.

Child Services Review System (CSRS)

Patient care audit is obviously a system that both derives from and is designed for implementation of particular types of human services programs, especially programs that follow health services models. Nevertheless, the fundamental concepts of patient care audit can be applied, perhaps with some adaptations, to virtually all settings in which we deliver our professional services. In response to the obvious need for quality assurance approaches applicable in school settings, ASHA developed an adaptation of patient care audit called the Child Services Review System (American Speech-Language-Hearing Association, 1982; Barnes and Pines, 1982).

CSRS can be used by single-discipline groups, such as might be represented either by all of the speech, language, and hearing specialists employed by a school district, or by some subgroup of speech, language, and hearing specialists within a district. It can also be applied by multidisciplinary groups, such as the instructional personnel and the providers of related services responsible for a particular program for handicapped children, or all of the members of a multidisciplinary assessment team.

The precepts of patient care audit also apply in CSRS: a group of professionals assesses the quality of the services they provide according to standards set by consensus and utilizes the results of that assessment as the basis for planning improved services. Finally, the success of that planning is assessed through reaudit.

The nine steps of the CSRS cycle are based on patient care audit, but some terminology has been modified for application in school settings: (1) select audit topic; (2) draft criteria statements; (3) ratify criteria statements; (4) review records; (5) identify and analyze problems; (6) develop solutions; (7) ratify solutions; (8) implement solutions; and (9) reaudit.

CSRS clearly meets the intent of several provisions of PL 94-142 which requires documentation of appropriate and effective services, review of outcomes specified for individualized education plans, team management of handicapped children, and continuing personnel development in accordance with objectively assessed needs. Even more important, CSRS offers an approach to accountability in school settings that documents the strengths and weaknesses in the services delivered to children, offers an opportunity to assess the impact of those services, and, most importantly, requires, as an inherent part of the process, planning to ameliorate whatever shortcomings are discovered. CSRS would seem to offer the potential for significant contributions to quality assurance in school-based services.

SELF-ASSESSMENT

In the final analysis, the only truly effective approaches to quality assurance depend upon individual professionals monitoring the services they provide. Most clinical services involve interaction between only two participants, a client and a clinician, and the ultimate assessment of the quality of those services must involve one or both of those participants. Although one can draw some conclusions about what has occurred throughout those interactions during supervisory sessions, during the various steps entailed in accreditation, and by auditing clinical records, none of these approaches fully reveals the real quality of speech-language pathology and audiology services. Inevitably, therefore, the responsibility for assuring the quality of all services rests with the speech-language pathologist or audiologist who is providing those services.

No matter how conscientious the clinician, it is not easy to maintain the detachment necessary for a significant appraisal of one's own services. Even self-assessment, therefore, usually requires a structured format to be truly effective.

As the quality assurance movement has progressed, there has been increasing emphasis on self-assessment. To some extent, this emphasis is a response to the antipathy of many professionals to any kind of outside interference. But, to a greater extent, it also acknowledges that self-assessment is essential for effective quality assurance. Consequently, new systems for quality assurance are likely to focus increasingly on self-assessment. At the present time, the options tend to fall within four categories: *profile comparison*, *videotape analysis*, *single-subject studies*, and *follow-up studies.*

Profile Comparison

This procedure is akin to the records audits procedures described earlier; it, too, entails the comparison of the management of individual clients with established standards. As a self-assessment procedure, however, it involves an individual clinician's comparison of his or her management of clients to profiles representing established standards for management.

Three approaches are possible. As a part of quality assurance efforts—or sometimes to assist insurance carriers seeking information about usual and customary patterns of care—groups of professionals, at state or local community levels, devise profiles defining standards of care. An excellent example of such profile development is found in the manual of the Iowa Quality Assurance Program discussed earlier. The first approach, then, consists of individual speech-language pathologists or audiologists comparing their client records against these profiles.

The second approach is essentially similar. When such a quality assurance program as patient care audit or child services review is in place, an individual clinician may compare the records of clients he or she has served against the audit criteria. Such an assessment is quite separate from the audit, since it actually violates the fundamental principal that audits aim at improvement of group performance and are not intended to identify deviant care provided by individual speech-language pathologists and audiologists. Nevertheless, after an audit has been completed clinicians should have the privilege of reviewing the records of clients they have served—usually records that were not included in the audit sample—to compare their performances to the established criteria.

The third approach involves the establishment of profiles specifically for self-assessment. Ideally, these profiles should be established through discussion among a group of clinicians, as, for example, a group comprised of all speech-language pathologists employed by the same institution or by the same school district. Lacking the opportunity for more formal efforts, clinicians serving similar client populations in the same community can meet to develop profiles. If no other option is available, individual clinicians can, based on reviews of the literature or discussions with other clinicians, devise their own profiles. Although this last option may be better than nothing, it contains the risks of continuing shortcomings in client management that result from misinformation and other knowledge deficits.

As an approach to self-assessment, profile comparison shares many of the limitations of records audits. Inevitably, the profiles must deal with the kinds of information that are entered in client records and, especially, with information that can be entered in absolute or quantitative terms (e.g., whether particular tests or other evaluation procedures were or were not administered, whether particular essential information was entered in the record, the total number of therapy sessions provided to a client, or the frequency of failed appointments). All of these factors may offer helpful clues for the assessment of quality of care, but they do not tap many of the most important features of clinical services. Therefore, although profile comparisons may be useful, this approach is best employed in conjunction with other kinds of self-assessment.

Videotape Analysis

The analysis of videotape recordings of actual clinical sessions can be one of the most valuable approaches to self-assessment. When videotape equipment is not available, audiotapes can be used, but many important features of clinical management may not be observable unless both visual and auditory information are available.

Videotape analysis is widely used in the training of student clinicians. Although experienced clinicians should find it equally useful for self-analysis, they seldom avail themselves of it. Under ideal circumstances these videotapes should be recorded automatically, without a camera operator present either in the same room or even in an adjoining observation room. Such tapes, to be of real value, should represent typical evaluation or therapy sessions. The presence of a camera operator may be sufficiently distracting to the clinician and the client to render a session atypical. Furthermore, tapes should be made as spontaneously as possible; special planning in anticipation that a recording is to be made will also make a session atypical. Tapes for self-evaluation should be made only for that purpose and available only to the clinician involved. Although we can gain many clues from tapes that have been recorded for demonstrations, for research, or for some other purpose, those sessions must be considered atypical.

No matter how discomforting, self-analysis tapes should be replayed several times to exploit their value fully. The most important information is frequently not the most impressive on initial viewing. Such factors as clinician mannerisms and previously unobserved client behaviors may be immediately striking but are not necessarily the most important factors to be observed in the recorded interaction.

The effectiveness of videotape self-analysis can be substantially enhanced by the introduction of a formal analysis procedure. Boone and Prescott (1972) described a procedure that can be used either for clinician self-analysis or for joint analysis by supervisors and supervisees. It involves a detailed analysis of the content of excerpts from therapy sessions. The clinician first records the middle 20 minutes of a half-hour session. As soon as possible following the session, the clinician or supervisor selects an appropriate 5-minute excerpt for detailed analysis. The clinician views that excerpt before beginning the analysis and then replays it, allotting each event within the excerpt to 1 of 10 categories as shown in Table 12.4.

The next step in analysis involves comparing the total number of events ascribable to the clinician (i.e., those falling in categories 1 through 5) with those ascribable to the client (i.e., those falling in categories 6 through 10). Finally, the number of events within each category is expressed as a percentage of the total number of events within the excerpt. This offers a view of the distribution of events according to type.

Boone and Prescott suggest some general guidelines for assessing the results of an analysis. They note, for example, that "successful therapy is usually characterized by a 60% to 80% client success rate" and "therapy must be designed so that our clients experience this percentage of correct responses." Furthermore, they suggest comparison of analyses with goals of the session. For example, frequent events in category 5, in which the clinician engages in behavior that is not therapy goal oriented, may be quite appropriate under certain circumstances but deleterious under other circumstances.

Self-analyses of videotape recordings of clinical sessions do not necessarily permit objective assessment of all aspects of clinician effectiveness, even when some formal

Table 12.4
Categories for Content and Sequence Analysis

Category Number	
1 Explain, Describe	Clinician describes and explains the specific goals or procedures of the session.
2 Model, Instruction	Clinician specifies client behavior by direct modeling or by specific request.
3 Good Evaluative	Clinician evaluates client response and indicates a verbal or nonverbal approval.
4 Bad Evaluative	Clinician evaluates client response as incorrect and gives a verbal or nonverbal disapproval.
5 Neutral-Social	Clinician engages in behavior which is not therapy goal oriented.
6 Correct Response	Client makes a response which is correct for clinician instruction or model.
7 Incorrect Response	Client makes incorrect response to clinician instruction or model.
8 Inappropriate-Social	Client makes response which is not appropriate for session goals.
9 Good Self-evaluative	Client indicates awareness of his own correct response.
10 Bad Self-evaluative	Client indicates awareness of his own incorrect response.

approach to assessment is applied. However, given a clinician with well defined standards for competent practice, video recordings can assist that clinician to assess his or her work according to those standards. This approach is probably more effective than any kind of self-monitoring during the actual conduct of clinical sessions.

Single-subject Studies

However much it is needed, most speech-language pathologists and audiologists find it difficult to conduct clinical research at the same time they are discharging their daily responsibilities to clients. To some extent, this derives from the popular conception that research deals with comparisons among matched samples of subjects or among manifold measures obtained from a single-subject sample. Seldom do the practical constraints of most clinical programs permit this kind of research, at least when all investigative responsibilities must be assumed by the people who are also providing the clinical services the subjects require.

In recent years, some researchers have developed increasingly sophisticated designs for research carried out on single subjects. Two excellent discussions of single-subject designs were written by Herson and Barlow (1976) and by McReynolds and Kearns (1982). These designs can be applied to achieve comparisons of the effects of alternative approaches to treatment on the same subject. They may also be used to assess management options such as frequency of therapy sessions, group or individual instruction, or continuous versus interrupted series of therapy sessions. Although such studies can increase our knowledge about therapeutic strategies, they can also be a powerful tool for clinician self-assessment.

The ethical constraints on using clients for research were previously discussed. Such constraints usually do not apply to this kind of research since it is worthwhile only when a clinician is comparing alternatives that might be reasonably applied to the client's care. In other words, the fundamental purpose is to select the alternative that yields superior results for the particular client. It may be proper to inform the client or the client's family that various options to management are being compared to select the best (so long as this does not invalidate the experimental design), but any kind of consent to serve as an experimental subject is unnecessary when the studies are conducted primarily to monitor the effectiveness of the treatment program.

We often assume that the only worthwhile research leads to the publication of results. Such single-subject studies, conducted during the course of clinical programs, might well make useful contributions to our literature. But single-subject studies, carried out only for clinician self-assessment, are also worthwhile, even when the results only serve to enlighten the clinician who conducts the research.

Follow-up Studies

Some self-assessment can be carried out through retrospective follow-up studies. To be valuable, such studies must have well defined topics and be something more than loosely structured reviews of unselected client samples. Studies may be designed to appraise the outcomes of all services provided to particular client groups, or they may focus on the outcomes among clients who were subjected to a particular regimen for evaluation or management. Follow-up studies may be conducted shortly after completion of services, or they may be conducted months or even years later.

Some follow-up studies are informal, consisting of interviews with former clients, with their families, or with other professionals who are now serving those clients. Informal follow-up studies are most easily conducted when clients are still being served in the same agency where the speech-language pathologist or audiologist is employed. School settings may be ideal for this kind of study, because the children who were previously served may still be enrolled within the same school, or at least within the same school district where the speech, language, and hearing specialist is employed. Furthermore, there may be somewhat objective data, in the form of achievement test scores or other measures, to complement informal observations by teachers or other educational specialists. Informal follow-up studies can also be accomplished when former clients are scattered throughout the community, but such studies are more difficult and time consuming.

Many clinicians have used questionnaires for follow-up studies. These questionnaires may be distributed for written responses or may serve as the basis for telephone or in-person interviews. Questionnaire studies are always precarious, however, and may yield misleading data. They are probably best when seeking fact rather than opinion. Client opinions as to the effectiveness of specific approaches, particularly when secured by questionnaires, can be attributed to all manner of extraneous factors. Questionnaires are most useful in securing straightforward data that can then be interpreted for clues to the services that were delivered. For example, questionnaires sent to clients a year after they were seen for hearing aid selection and orientation might ask questions as to whether the recommended instrument is still in use or whether another hearing aid was purchased instead, questions about the frequency of use (perhaps corroborated by data regarding battery life), and questions that elicit information about situations in which the aid is most and least helpful and about specific problems that have been encountered. Analyzing such a questionnaire might offer clues as to the relative success of whatever services were provided and identify areas in which program modifications should be considered.

Follow-up studies can sometimes be conducted as though they were prospective rather than retrospective when clinical procedures have followed consistent protocols for evaluation or therapy. For example, when a clinician has followed a consistent approach to the assessment of clients falling into a particular population (i.e., clients in the same age range, clients with the same kinds of communicative disorders, etc.) the data from those assessments can be applied in follow-up studies. The efficacy of the assessment tools applied can be surmised through determining how well they predict subsequent achievement. Since most clinicians make predictions based on the evaluation techniques they employ, it can be very revealing—and often disconcerting—to determine whether those predictions were at all accurate. Similar follow-up studies can be conducted for the reappraisal of specific aspects of intervention when that intervention followed a structured regimen.

It has been often observed that our field needs more long-term studies of the outcomes and efficacy of the services we provide. This is probably true, but longitudinal research is extremely difficult to conduct. The studies proposed here would probably never withstand the rigorous scrutiny that must be applied to research before its results can have widespread application. Nevertheless, so long as clinicians recognize the limitations inherent in informal follow-up studies, the results of such studies can be useful for self-assessment.

SUMMARY

Human services professions are increasingly committed to quality assurance procedures that aspire to implement optimal standards of client care. These procedures go well beyond the limits of consumer protection afforded by legal and ethical standards. Among the quality assurance systems that are applied are supervision, accreditation, peer review, records audits, and various self-assessment techniques.

It is no happenstance that this text ends with a discussion of quality assurance. Assuring the quality of the services we deliver is the paramount responsibility of every speech-language pathologist and audiologist. In the final analysis, the one essential criterion, by which all the accomplishments of each member of our profession and of our profession as a whole can be judged, is the influence of those accomplishments on the quality of clinical services delivered to children and adults with communicative disorders. All of our achievements in research, in the development of new clinical programs, and in preparing the students who will enter our profession, must ultimately be assessed in terms of their effect on the quality of speech-language pathology and audiology services.

References

Adair MN: Accountability in hospitals. *Semin Speech-Language Pathol* 4:159–167, 1983.

American Speech and Hearing Association: *Patient Care Audit Manual.* Washington, DC, American Speech-Language-Hearing Association, 1978.

American Speech-Language-Hearing Association: *Child Services Review Manual.* Rockville, MD, American Speech-Language-Hearing Association, 1982.

American Speech-Language-Hearing Association Professional Services Board: Standards for PSB accreditation. *ASHA* 25:51–58, 1983.

Barnes, KJ, Pines DL: Assessing and improving services to the handicapped. *ASHA.* 24:555–559, 1982.

Boone DR, Prescott TE: Content and sequence analyses of speech and hearing therapy. *ASHA.* 14:58–62, 1972.

CMA/CHA: *Educational Patient Care Audit Manual.* San Francisco, California Medical Association/California Hospital Association, 1975.

Commission on Accreditation of Rehabilitation Facilities: *Standards Manual for Facilities Serving People with Disabilities.* Tucson, AZ, Commission on Accreditation of Rehabilitation Facilities, 1982.

Culatta R, Helmick JW: Clinical supervision: the state of the art. Part I. *ASHA.* 22:985–993, 1980.

Culatta R, Helmick JW: Clinical supervision: the state of the art. Part II. *ASHA.* 23:21–31, 1981.

Dublinske S, Grimes J: Program planning evaluation. In: *Health Management Institute Syllabus.* Rockville, MD, American Speech-Language-Hearing Association, 1979.

Ellis GL, Sadin RR: Potential roles of nonphysician health care practitioners in the PSRO program. In Bussman JW, Davidson SV: *PSRO: The Promise, Perspective, and Potential.* Menlo Park, CA, Addison-Wesley, 1981.

Goran MJ, Roberts JS, Kellogg M et al: The PSRO hospital review system. *Med Care* 8 (Suppl):1–33, 1975.

Gouran DS: The role of leadership in supervisor/supervisee relationships. In Anderson JL: *Proceedings: Conference on Training in the Supervisory Process in Speech-Language Pathology and Audiology.* Bloomington, Indiana University Press, 1980.

Griffin KM: *Multidisciplinary Quality Review.* Rockville, MD, American Speech-Language-Hearing Association, 1978.

Hare R: Ambulatory review—overview of current methodology. In Bussman JW, Davidson SV: *PSRO: The Promise, Perspective, and Potential.* Menlo Park, CA, Addison-Wesley, 1981.

Herson M, Barlow DH: *Single Case Experimental Designs.* New York, Pergamon Press, 1976.

Iowa Quality Assurance Program: *Manual.* Cedar Rapids, IA, Iowa Speech and Hearing Association, 1977.

Joint Commission on Accreditation of Hospitals. *The PEP Primer.* Chicago, Joint Commission on Accreditation of Hospitals, 1974.

Joint Commission on Accreditation of Hospitals. *Accreditation Manual for Hospitals.* Chicago, Joint Commission on Accreditation of Hospitals, 1983.

Kandushin A: Games people play in supervision. *Soc Work* 13:23–32, 1968.

Kaplan KO, Hopkins JM: *The QA Guide.* Chicago, Joint Commission on Accreditation of Hospitals, 1980.

Kaplan SH, Greenfield S: Criteria mapping: using logic in evaluation of process of care. *Quality Rev Bull* 4:3–9, 1978.

McReynolds LV, Kearns KP: *Single Subject Experimental Designs in Communicative Disorders.* Baltimore, MD, University Park Press, 1982.

Mushlin AI, Appel FA, Barr DM: Quality assurance in primary care: a strategy based on outcome assessment. *J Community Health* 3:292–305, 1978.

Nelson AR: The national professional standards review council: intent, function and future. In Bussman JW, Davidson SV: *PSRO: The Promise, Perspective, and Potential.* Menlo Park, CA, Addison-Wesley, 1981.

Odiorne GS: *Management Decisions by Objectives.* Englewood Cliffs, NJ, Prentice-Hall, 1969.

Oestreicher VC, Smits HL: Professional standards review organization: utilization review and quality of care. In Eisenberg JM, Williams SV: *The Physician's Practice.* New York, John Wiley & Sons, 1980.

Schoeni PO: PSRO and the quality of medical health care. *ASHA.* 16:679–681, 1974.

Shriberg L, Filley FS, Hayes DM et al: *Wisconsin Procedure for Appraisal of Clinical Competence (W-PACC) Applications Manual.* Madison, University of Wisconsin, Department of Communicative Disorders, 1974.

Shriberg L, Filley FS, Hayes DM et al: The Wisconsin procedure for appraisal of clinical competence (W-PACC): model and data. *ASHA.* 17:158–165, 1975.

Supplementary Readings

Adair M, Griffin K: Quality assurance: a professional quest for speech-language pathologists and audiologists. *ASHA.* 21:871–874, 1979.

Anderson JL: Supervision of school speech, hearing, and language problems—an emerging role. *ASHA.* 16:7–10, 1974.

Averill RW: Implications of PSRO to independent health professions. *ASHA* 16:677–678, 1974.

Bussman JW, Davidson SV: *PSRO: The Promise, Perspective, and Potential.* Menlo Park, CA, Addison-Wesley, 1981.

Culatta RA: Clinical supervision: the state of the art. *ASHA* 22:985–993, 1980.

Culatta R, Seltzer H: Content and sequence analysis of the supervisory session. *ASHA* 18:8–12, 1976.

Culatta R, Seltzer H: Content and sequence analysis of the supervisory session: a report of clinical use.

ASHA 19:523–526, 1977.
Curlee RF: New Mexico Foundation for Medical Care—a computer-assisted professional standards review organization. *ASHA* 15:415–417, 1973.
Gerstman HL: Supervisory relationships: experiences in dynamic communication. *ASHA* 19:527–529, 1977.
Griffin K: Quality assurance through patient care audit. *ASHA* 18:800–808, 1976.
Jonas S: *Quality Control of Ambulatory Care.* New York, Springer, 1977.
Pannbacker M: Bibliography for supervision. *ASHA* 17:105–106, 1975.
Pickering M: An examination of concepts operative in the supervisory process and relationship. *ASHA* 19:607–610, 1977.
Schubert GW: Suggested minimal requirements for clinical supervisors. *ASHA* 16:305–307, 1974.

Index

Absenteeism, 214–215
Accidents, reporting, 107
Accountability, 219–221
Accounting record (*see* Service accounting record)
Accreditation (*see also* Joint Commission on Accreditation of Hospitals; Commission on Accreditation of Rehabilitation Facilities; American Speech-Language-Hearing Association, Professional Services Board)
  definition, 15
  of educational programs in speech-language pathology and audiology, 291
Acute inpatient health care institutions, 52–53
Adolescent medicine specialists, 24
Advertising, 89, 267–269
Affirmative action programs, 273–274
Aid for Retarded Citizens, 248
Aid to Families of Dependent Children (AFDC), 235
Aides (*see* Support personnel)
Alexander Graham Bell Association for the Deaf, 70
Ambulatory care centers, 54–55
American Board of Medical Specialties, 22
American Cancer Society, 248
American Hearing Society, 70
American Heart Association, 70, 248
American Speech-Language-Hearing Association
  certification, 17–19, 254–256
  child services review system (*see* Child services review system)
  Code of Ethics, 254–279
  Education and Training Board, 291
  patient care audit procedure (*see* Patient care audit)
  Professional Services Board, 105, 163, 172, 292–294
    accreditation procedures, 291–294
    clinical record standards, 163
    retention of records standards, 172
    standards for accreditation, 292–294
    therapy plan standards, 105
  Professional Standards Council, 292
  Task Force on Private Health Insurance, 232
Application data, in Unit Records, 139–140, 143
Assessment, 8–9
Assignment of payment (*see* Insurance, health, assignment of payment)
Authorizations, in Unit Records, 142, 144
Automated clinical records (*see* Clinical records, computer-assisted)
Average daily attendance (ADA) (*see* Public schools, financial support, per-pupil reimbursement)

Behavioral pediatrics, 25
Blue Cross, 227, 233
Blue Shield, 227, 233
Bureau of Indian Affairs, 247
Burnout, 215

Camp programs, 71
Cancellations and failed appointments, 212–213
Cardiovascular disease specialists, 25–26
CARF (*see* Commission on Accreditation of Rehabilitation Facilities)
CASE Classification Schema, 185–186
CASE Information System (*see* Clinical records systems, Comprehensive Assessment and Service Evaluation)
Case managers, 78–79
Certificates of Clinical Competence (see American Speech-Language-Hearing Association, certification)
Certification (*see also* American Speech-Language-Hearing Association, certification)
  definition, 15
  of medical specialists, 22–23
CHAMPUS (*see* Civilian Health and Medical Program of the Uniformed Services)
Child abuse, 260–261
Child care centers, 68–70
Child development centers, 66
Child guidance centers, 64–65
Child neurology, 26
Child psychiatry, 43
Child services review system (CSRS), 320–321
Chiropractic, 32
Civil rights
  for the handicapped, 59
  movement, 272–273
Civil Rights Act of 1964, 273
Civilian Health and Medical Program of the Uniformed Services (CHAMPUS), 238–239
Classroom teachers, as instructional services providers, 34
Client directory, 137–138
Client profiles in Practice-Oriented Record, 157–158
Clinical records
  accreditation and licensure standards, 162–164
  audits of, 309–321
  centralized vs. decentralized, 137, 168
  client, 138–162
  components, 136–138
  computer-assisted, 168–172
  confidentiality, 259–261
  economy in maintaining, 136
  filing, 165–168
  numbering, 166
  permanence and retention of, 172–173
  release of, 259–260
  storage, 165–173
  subpoena of, 280
  systems, 128–162
    Comprehensive Assessment and Service Evaluation (CASE), 159–162, 185–186, 204–205
    Practice-Oriented Record, 156–159
    Problem-Oriented Record, 145–156
    Unit Record, 139–145

Clinical reports
  characteristics, 111–123
  conclusions and recommendations in, 119–123
  forms for, 109
  language usage in, 123–127
  organization, 108–111
  types of, 102–108
CMA/CHA educational patient care audit, 310
Code(s)
  diagnostic, 174–186
  procedure
    nonstandard systems, 190–193
    standard systems, 186–190
Code of Ethics (*see* American Speech-Language-Hearing Association, Code of Ethics)
Coding systems for clinical information, 174–194
Commission on Accreditation of Rehabilitation Facilities (CARF), 296–297
Community agencies
  cost computation in, 207–208
  making referrals in, 96
  models of, 66–71
  receiving referrals in, 88–89
Community colleges, 73
Community Mental Health Centers Act, 65
Community speech and hearing centers, 67–68
Complaints, reporting, 107
Comprehensive Assessment and Service Evaluation (CASE) (*see* Clinical records systems, Comprehensive Assessment and Service Evaluation)
Computer-assisted clinical records (*see* Clinical records, computer-assisted)
Concurrent review, 304
Confidentiality, 259–261
Consent
  implied, 259
  informed, 256–261
Consultation, 11–13
Consumer advocacy, 59, 252
Continuing education
  and licensure renewal, 255
  in seeking new referrals, 90–91
Continuity of services, 13
Contracts
  as basis for payment for services, 239–241
  factors to be covered in, 240–241
  with Medicare providers, 239–240
  with school districts, 239
Coordination of services, 13
Copayment (*see* Insurance, health, copayment)
Copyrights, 278
Cost(s)
  accounting, and bad debts, 204
  direct, 196–205
  equipment, 202–203
  facilities, 199–202
  indirect, 196–205
  insurance, 203–204
  personnel, 197–199
  public relations and information, 204
  staff education expense, 204
  supplies, 203
  taxes and license fees, 204
  travel, 203
Cost-benefit ratios, 219–221
Cost computation, 195–208
Cost containment
  equipment and supplies, 217–219
  facilities costs, 216–217
  legislative and regulatory measures, 208–210
  personnel costs, 210–216
Counseling
  definition of, 10–11
  procedure codes, 190–193
Counselors, 42
CPT (*see* Physicians' Current Procedural Terminology)
Crippled Children Services (CCS), 237–238
Criteria for care, 304, 313–314
Criteria mapping, 310
Data
  base
    in Practice-Oriented Record, 157
    in Problem-Oriented Record, 145–146, 151–153
  input, in computer-assisted records, 170–171
  operational, in Practice-Oriented Record, 157–158
  output, in computer-assisted records, 171–172
Day health care centers, 55
Debts, bad, 204, 267
Deductibles (*see* Insurance, health, deductibles)
Dental expense insurance, 228
Dentistry, 27–29
Department of Defense, 247
Deposition, 280–281
Deteriorating performance, reporting, 107
Developmental disabilities, service models, 62–66
Developmental Disabilities Act, 63
Developmental pediatrics, 25
Developmentally disabled
  definition, 63
  facilities for, 62–66
    day treatment and care centers, 64
    information, referral, and coordination of care, 65
    inpatient treatment and care, 63–64
Developmentally Disabled Assistance and Bill of Rights Act, 63
Diagnosis, 8
Diagnostic and Statistical Manual of Mental Disorders (DSM), 180–183
Diagnostic centers, 48–49
Diagnostic codes (*see* Codes, diagnostic)
Diagnostic-educational teams, 48
Dictionary of Occupational Titles, 5
Directory (*see* Client directory)
Disability determination, 285–287
Disability insurance, 228, 285–286
Discharge summaries, 108
  in Problem-Oriented Records, 149
Discrimination (*see* Nondiscrimination)
Dispensing products, 241–244, 269–272
DSM III (*see* Diagnostic and Statistical Manual of Mental Disorders)
Due process (*see also* Education for All Handicapped Children Act, due process), hearings, 284–285

Early and Periodic Screening, Diagnosis, and Treatment Plan (EPSDTP), 7, 80, 235
Easter Seals Societies for Crippled Children and Adults, 248
Economic Opportunity Act of 1964, 69
Economy in services (*see also* Cost containment), 13, 14

Education for All Handicapped Children Act
assessment requirements, 86
classification of
education professions, 32
handicapped children, 34–35
definition of
learning disabilities, 35
speech-language pathology and audiology services, 6
due process, 275–276, 284–285
Individualized Educational Program (IEP), 106
legal rights under, 275–276
payment for services by nonpublic agencies, 87, 95, 239
requirement for speech, language and hearing services, 47
Education professions, 32–38
Efficacy of services, 13
Eligibility criteria (*see* Referrals, eligibility criteria)
Equipment (*see* Cost(s) equipment; Cost containment, equipment and supplies)
Ethical constraints in delivery of speech-language pathology and audiology services, 255–279
Evaluation
definition, 8–9
procedure codes, 188–193
reports of, 103–104, 140, 143, 160–161
in CASE Information System, 160–161
in Unit Records, 140, 143
Extended care facilities (*see* Long-term inpatient health care institutions)

Facilities (*see* Cost(s), facilities; Cost containment, facilities)
Fair hearings (*see* Due process hearings)
Family practice, 23
Federal Trade Commission
advertising practices and, 268
hearing aid industry regulation, 268, 270
price fixing and professional fees, 225, 266–267
regulation of professions, 277
Fee(s)
disputes, 267
ethical constraints, 267
legal constraints, 266–267
Fee schedules
approaches to development, 223–226
functional, 224
pragmatic, 225–226
relative values, 224–225
unit of service, 223–224
basic considerations, 223
Financial support for services
based on individual client services, 223–244
program-based, 244–251
Fiscal intermediaries, 233
Follow-up studies for self-assessment, 324–325
Food and Drug Administration, hearing aid regulations, 268, 270–272
Foundation for medical care, 58
Foundations, private and corporate, 250
Fraternal organizations, 249–250

Genetics, 25
Gerontological nursing, 31
Gerontology, 24
Governmental hearings, 288–289
Group health insurance (*see* Insurance, health, group plans)

Head and neck surgery (*see* Otolaryngology and head and neck surgery)
Headstart (*see* Project Headstart)
Health care programs
cost computation in, 206
making referrals in, 94
receiving referrals in, 84–86
Health Maintenance Organizations (HMO), 58, 228
Health professions, 22–32
Health services, models for, 50–59
Health Services Agency (HSA), 209–210
Hearing aid dispensing
by audiologists, 241–244, 269–272
ethical considerations, 272
income and cash flow, 242–243
inventory maintenance, 242
legal regulation of, 270–272
supplies and repair services, 243–244
Hearing impaired, specialists in education of, 36–38
Hearing impairment, definition for long-term disability, 286–287
High-risk infant programs, 65–66
Hill-Burton Act, 274
Home health agencies and services, 55–56, 233, 235
Homebound services (*see* Hospital and homebound services)
Hospital(s) (*see* Acute inpatient health care institutions)
Hospital and homebound services, 50
Hospital expense insurance, 227
Hospital Survey Profile, 295
HSA (*see* Health Services Agency)

ICD-9-CM (*see* International Classification of Diseases)
Independent living centers, 62
Individualized Educational Program (IEP) (*see* Education for All Handicapped Children Act, Individualized Educational Program)
Industrial health programs, 58–59
Industrial hygienists, 32
Infant services (*see* Child care centers, High-risk infant programs, Parent-infant instruction services)
Inservice education (*see* Continuing education)
Institutional research boards, 264–265
Instructional services providers
definition, 33–34
regular instruction, 33–34
special instruction, 34–38
Insurance
health, 227–236
assignment of payment, 230
claims procedures, 232
coinsurance, 230
copayment, 230
coverage, 228–232
deductibles, 229
group plans, 228
Health Maintenance Organizations (HMO), 228
individual plans, 228

Insurance—*continued*
method of payment, 229–230
speech-language pathology and audiology services coverage, 230–232
types of, 227–228
required by speech-language pathologists and audiologists, 203–204, 262
Integration classes (*see* Transition or integration classes)
Internal medicine, 24
International Association of Laryngectomees, 70
International Classification of Diseases (ICD), 178–180, 188
Interprofessional relationships, constraints of
ethical, 278–279
legal, 276–278
Intraprofessional relationships, constraints of
ethical, 278–279
legal, 276–278
Iowa Quality Assurance Program
client management criteria, 306–307
purposes of, 306–307
system for disorder classification, 184–185

Jargon in clinical reports, 124–125
Joint Commission on Accreditation of Hospitals (JCAH)
accreditation procedures, 294–296
clinical record standards, 162–163
definitions of long-term inpatient health care institutions, 53
PEP procedure (*see* Performance Evaluation Procedure for Auditing and Improving Patient care)
purposes of, 294–295
retention of records standards, 172
standards for speech-language pathology and audiology services, 295–296
therapy plan standards, 105
Junior League, 249
Juvenile offenders facilities, 66

Learning disabilities, definition, 35
Learning disabilities specialists, 35–36
Legal controls of speech-language pathology and audiology services, 253–279
Legislative hearings (*see* Governmental hearings)
Licensure
definition, 15
for hearing aid dispensing, 270
legal implications of, 254–255, 277
of speech-language pathologists and audiologists, 20–22, 254–255
reciprocity, 21
sunset laws, 21
Litigation
clinical records and, 106–107, 280
expert witness in, 279–284
Long-term health care facility, 53
Long-term inpatient health care institutions, 53–54
Lost Chord Clubs, 70

Major medical expense insurance, 228
Malpractice, 261–264
Management by Objectives (MBO), 298–299
Master-servant principle, 278
Maternal and infant care projects, 247
Medicaid
categories of covered services, 235
coverage of speech-language-pathology and audiology services, 235–236
description, 234–236
increased availability of health care through, 274
optional services under, 235–236
rights to health care under, 274–275
Medical Care Evaluation (MCE) Studies, 304
Medical profession, 22–27
Medicare
coverage of speech-language pathology and audiology services, 233–234
definition of speech pathologist, 18
description, 233–234
rights to health care under, 274–275
Mental health and social services professions, 42–46
Mental health facilities
centers for information, referral and coordination of care, 65
day treatment and care, 64
inpatient treatment and care, 63–64
outpatient mental health centers, 64–65
Mental health service models, 62–66
Mental Retardation Facilities and Community Mental Health Centers Construction Act of 1963, 63
Middle digit records filing, 166–167
Military hospitals, 247
Mobile health clinics, 56–57

National Association for the Deaf, 70
National Commission for the Protection of Human Subjects of Biomedical and Behavioral Research, 264
National Health Planning and Resources Act, 209
National Research Act, 264
Negligence, 261–264
Neighborhood health centers, 57
Neonatal nursing, 30
Neonatology, 25
Neurologic surgery, 26–27
Neurology, 26
Nondiscrimination, 272–276
Nondiscrimination on the Basis of Handicap (Section 504), 273
Norms for appraisal of care, 304
Nurse practitioners, 30–32
Nurse specialists, 30–32
Nursing, 29–32
Nursing home (*see* Long-term health care facility, Resident care facility)

Occupational health nursing, 31
Occupational therapy, 40–41
Oral surgery, 29
Orthodontics, 28
Osteopathy, 32
Otolaryngology and head and neck surgery, 26
Outpatient medical clinics (*see* Ambulatory care centers

Parent contacts, reporting in CASE Information System, 160
Parent-infant instruction services, 50
Part A (*see* Medicare)
Part B (*see* Medicare)
Participation in services, 13

Patents, 278
Patient care audit, 311–321
Payment for services (*see* Financial support for services)
Pediatric nursing, 30
Pediatrics, 23–24
Pedodontics, 28
Peer review, 303–309
Peer Standards Review Organizations (PSRO)
and health care practitioners other than physicians (HCPOTP), 305–306
concept of, 303–304
development of norms, criteria, and standards, 304
PEP procedure (*see* Performance Evaluation Procedure for Auditing and Improving Patient Care)
Performance Evaluation Procedure for Auditing and Improving Patient Care (PEP), 309–310
Personnel (*see also* Cost(s), personnel; Cost containment, personnel)
categories of, 197
clerical, 216
Philanthropy, private, 250
Physical medicine and rehabilitation, 38–39
Physical therapy, 39–40
Physician expense insurance, 227
Physician's Current Procedural Terminology (CPT), 188–190
Plastic surgery, 27
Point of entry, 81–82
Practice-Oriented Record (*see* Clinical records systems, Practice-Oriented Record)
Prepaid group medical practice, 58
Prescriptions
for speech-language pathology and audiology services, 85, 278–279
in clinical reports, 121–123
Pretrial conferences, 281–282
Primary care medical specialists, relationships to speech-language pathologists and audiologists, 23–24
Private practice
cost computation in, 206–207
defined, 73–75
making referrals in, 95–96
receiving referrals in, 87–88
Problem list
in Practice-Oriented Record, 157
in Problem-Oriented Record, 146–147, 153–154
Problem status index-outcome (PSI), 310
Problem-Oriented Record (*see* Clinical records systems, Problem-Oriented Record)
Procedure codes (*see* Codes, procedure)
Productivity, 211–215
Profession, characteristics of, 2–5
Professional Services Board (PSB) (*see* American Speech-Language-Hearing Association, Professional Services Board)
Profile
analysis, 305
comparisons for self-assessment, 321–322
Program management, in CASE Infomation System, 161–162
Progress notes and summaries
general description, 106–108
in Problem-Oriented Records, 149, 155–156
in Unit Records, 140–141, 143–144
Project Headstart, 69, 247
Prosthodontics, 28–29
Providers of services under Medicare, 234
Psychiatry, 42–43
Psychology, 43–45
Public health departments, 57–58
Public health nursing, 30–31
Public Law 88–164 (*see* Mental Retardation Facilities and Community Mental Health Centers Construction Act of 1963)
Public Law 91–517 (*see* Developmental Disabilities Act)
Public Law 92–603 (*see* Peer Standards Review Organizations)
Public Law 93–384 (*see* National Research Act)
Public Law 93–641 (*see* National Health Planning and Resources Act)
Public Law 94–103 (*see* Developmentally Disabled Assistance and Bill of Rights Act)
Public Law 94–142 (*see* Education for All Handicapped Children Act)
Public reporting statutes, 260–261
Public schools
cost computation in, 204–206
CASE Information System approach, 204–205
Rand Corporation approach, 205
credentials for speech, language, and hearing specialists, 19–20
financial support, 245–246
per-pupil reimbursement, 246
special reimbursement, 246
unit reimbursement, 245
making referrals in, 94–95
models for speech, language, and hearing services, 47–50
receiving referrals in, 86–87
Publicity, 89, 204, 267–269

Quality assurance, approaches to, 291–326
Quality circles, 310–311
Quantification in clinical reports, 117–119

Rand Corporation study on cost of special education, 205
Reciprocity (*see* Licensure, reciprocity)
Records (*see also* Clinical records), audits, 309–321
Referrals
acknowledgment of, 103
coordinating, 78–79
developing new sources of, 89–91
eligibility criteria, 80
making referrals, 91–96
policies, 79–81
procedural criteria, 80–81
purposes of, 78
receiving, 81–89
reporting, 107
in CASE Information Systems, 159
Registration, definition, 15
Regular classroom placement for handicapped children, 49–50
Rehabilitation Act of 1973, 273
Rehabilitation Codes, 183–184
Rehabilitation counseling, 41–42
Rehabilitation facilities
inpatient, 60–61
outpatient, 61
Rehabilitation nursing, 32

Rehabilitation professions, 38–42
Rehabilitation services
  models, 59–62
  state, 237
Rehabilitation workshops, 61–62
Related services providers, 38
Relative values scales
  and health insurance, 229–230
  in developing fee schedules, 224–225
Reports (*see* Clinical reports)
Research, use of clients in, 264–266
Resident care facility, 53
Residential schools, 50
Resource rooms, 49
Resource specialists, 34
Rights
  of clients, 253
  to services, 272–276

School nursing, 31
Screening services
  definition, 7–8
  in seeking referrals, 90
  mobile clinics, 56–57
Secondary and tertiary care medical specialists
  definition, 23
  relationships to speech-language pathologists and audiologists, 24–27
Section 504 (*see* Nondiscrimination on the Basis of Handicap)
Self-assessment approaches, 321–325
Self-help groups, 70–71
Senior centers, 70
Service accounting record, 138
Service clubs, 249
Services delivery, characteristics of, 13–14
Single subject research, 324
Social Security Act
  provisions for long-term disability, 286–287
  Title II (*see* Social Security Act, provisions for long-term disability)
  Title V (*see* Crippled Children Services)
  Title XIII (*see* Medicare)
  Title XVI (*see* Supplemental Security Income)
  Title XIX (*see* Medicaid)
Social service, 45–46
  aides, 45
  technicians, 45
Social workers (*see* Social service)
Special classes, full-time, 49
Special education teachers (*see* Instructional service providers, special instruction)
Specialty certification (*see* Certification of medical specialists)
Speech and language disorders, definition for long-term disability, 287
Speech-language pathology and audiology
  definition, 4–6
    legal, 5–6
  qualifications for practice (*see also* Licensure; American Speech-Language-Hearing Association certification; Public schools, credentials for speech, language, and hearing specialists), 15–22, 254–256
SSI (*see* Supplemental Security Income)
Standard Nomenclature of Diseases and Operations, 175–178
Standard Terminology for Curriculum and Instruction, 187–188
Standards for care, 304, 307
Subpoena, 280
Sunset laws (*see* Licensure, sunset laws)
Supervision
  approaches to, 297–299
  as interpersonal process, 299–303
  competencies for, effective clinical, 300
Supplemental Security Income (SSI), 286
  and Medicaid, 235
Suppliers of services under Medicare, 234
Supplies (*see* Cost(s), supplies; Cost containment, equipment and supplies)
Support personnel, 213–214, 255–256
Surgical expense insurance, 227

Teacher of
  deaf (*see also* Hearing impaired, specialists in education of), 34
  emotionally disturbed, 34
  learning disabled (*see also* Learning disabilities specialists), 34
  mentally retarded, 34
  physically handicapped, 34
  visually handicapped, 34
Teaching, use of clients in, 264–266
Tel-communicology, 56
Terminal digit records filing, 166–167
Tertiary care medical specialists (*see* Secondary and tertiary care medical specialists)
Testamentary capacity, 287–288
Therapy
  definition, 9–10
  plans, 105–108, 147, 154, 161
    in CASE Information System, 161
    in Problem-Oriented Records, 147, 154
  Procedure codes, 189–193
  reports in Unit Records, 141–144
Third-party payment
  definition, 226
  governmental, 232–239
  influence on fee schedules, 226
  philosophy of, 226–227
  private, 227–232
Transfer summaries, 108
Transition or integration classes, 49
Trials, 282–284

UCR (*see* Usual, customary, and reasonable charges)
Unit Record (*see* Clinical records systems, Unit Record)
United Cerebral Palsy, 248
United givers funds, 247–248
United Way of America, 207–208, 248
United Way of America Services Identification System (UWASIS), 207–208
University speech and hearing clinics, 71–73
Usual, customary, and reasonable charges (UCR), 230
Utilization review, 209–210, 304–305

V Code, 179
Veterans Administration, 246–247
Videotape analysis for self-assessment, 322–324

Visiting Nurse Associations, 55–56
Vocational rehabilitation services (*see* Rehabilitation services, state)
Voluntary health associations, 248–249

Wills (*see* Testamentary capacity)
Wisconsin Procedure for Appraisal of Clinical Competence, 298
Witness, expert
  definition, 279
  roles and responsibilities, 279–289
Workers' compensation, 236–237